Culture and Mental
Health Services

T0264575

Culture and Meaning in Health Services Research

A Practical Field Guide

Elisa J. Sobo

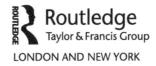

Routledge
Taylor & Francis Group

LONDON AND NEW YORK

First published 2009 by Left Coast Press, Inc.

Published 2016 by Routledge
2 Park Square, Milton Park, Abingdon, Oxon OX14 4RN
711 Third Avenue, New York, NY 10017, USA

Routledge is an imprint of the Taylor & Francis Group, an informa business

Library of Congress Cataloging-in-Publication Data

Sobo, Elisa Janine, 1963-
 Culture and meaning in health services research : a practical field guide/Elisa J. Sobo.
    p. cm.
 Includes bibliographical references and index.
 ISBN 978-1-59874-136-0 (hardback : alk. paper) -- ISBN 978-1-59874-137-7 (pbk. : alk. paper)
 1. Medical anthropology. 2. Medical care--Research. I. Title.
 GN296.S597 2009
 306.4'61--dc22
 2008052925

Cover design by: Andrew Brozyna

Hardback ISBN 978-1-59874-136-0
Paperback ISBN 978-1-59874-137-7

Contents

Foreword

This is a book about bridges. Following years of impassioned disciplinary feuds between opposing critics and proponents of the scientific paradigm, it is invigorating to read *Culture and Meaning in Health Services Research*. Rather than the all-too-common dichotomizing of interpretive (meaning-centered) and empirical (positivist) research, of quantitative and qualitative methods, of theoretical and applied orientations, and of scholarly versus popular inquiries, this book occupies a unique niche as a guide to translation that emphasizes connections rather than disjunctures.

As the subtitle suggests, this is a practical field guide: It describes the health services world as if a field site, making it much more than a "how-to" manual. Elisa Sobo has tackled a massive task as she moves between the "local knowledge" of anthropologists and health services researchers, explicating for each the practices and discourses of the other, successfully managing to normalize the "Otherness" of academic medical anthropology and health services research for practitioners in these differing yet intersecting fields. For those of us who have, throughout our careers, attempted to explain what we do as (medical) anthropologists, whether in academic or other institutional settings, this book offers answers as well as questions for contemplation.

But to say that this is just a field guide does not do justice to this volume, which ranges from concise histories of anthropological theory and the origins of health services research to the details of diverse methodological approaches. Throughout, the reader is engaged by Dr. Sobo's use of case studies and examples drawn from her own multifaceted research experiences. There is much to be gained here for medical anthropologists who intend to work in clinical settings, such as the author herself, or for nonanthropologists employed to conduct fieldwork in health care contexts. Ultimately, although the book is aimed at both these audiences, the fundamental objective is to validate "anthropologically informed qualitative health research." I also see this volume as highly pertinent to medical anthropology graduate students; it is replete with exemplary cases for premed students who will benefit from the comparative histories of anthropological and health services research and from illustrations that show how relevant anthropologically informed methods can be for clinical practice.

This endeavor leads to a rich and broad discussion that underscores the uses of ethnography for health services research. Dr. Sobo convincingly argues that qualitative methods hold much promise for health service research, an assertion that she backs with a foray into the philosophical premises underlying these methods and with illustrations from her own work. Whereas many of us assume that ethnography necessarily involves long-term immersion in the study population, thus intensive participant observation, the projects and methods described in this book raise thoughtful questions concerning the feasibility of doing ethnography in settings far different from the remote field sites of many anthropological classics.

In my own hospital-based research, I have often encountered the contention that this book counters: Social relations and meanings are not relevant to health outcomes. Stories or narratives are considered of marginal importance relative to quantitative data. Anthropologists in similar situations will be gratified to find a thorough examination of the power of qualitative data in clinical contexts and how those engaged in health services research can collect, analyze, and present ethnographic and other qualitative data in ways that will drive policy and influence decision-making.

Ultimately, the book's objective, to introduce anthropology's "holistic, systems-oriented, comparative agenda" to health services professionals, is impressively accomplished. At the same time, anthropologists will find in this volume an invaluable introduction to diverse terminology and typologies of research conducted in clinical settings such as QI (quality improvement), health services research, and IS (Implementation Science). Readers, whether experienced with anthropological methods or not, will find the review of how to use free lists, focus groups, one-time interviews, five-minute interviews, telephone interview protocols, not to mention variations on the theme of participant observation, in health services research intriguing—the making strange of the familiar—as we follow the author's explication of how particular methods were deployed strategically in health services research.

The description of focus groups—their advantages and disadvantages, formation, interview protocols, and data analysis—is especially helpful, given the contested status of this method in different disciplines. More generally, the discussion of cultural competence, which is used as a vehicle to examine the value of bringing culture into "the health care equation," is timely and provocative. Readers will be drawn into the debate on whether the cultural competence movement has the potential to reduce health inequities or even, at a much more minimal level, to generate awareness of cultural (and class) diversity that will actually produce meaningful results.

In the introduction to this book, Elisa Sobo recounts a conversation with the famous neuroscientist Francis Crick, co-discoverer of the double helix. He asks her to explain that absurd concept, the "social" sciences. As I was writing my dissertation, I had a parallel experience. While visiting friends doing doctoral research in genetics at a prominent university, I was introduced to the lab director. When told that I was an anthropologist, he inquired, "What's your organism?" I replied (without much reflection), "Humans." With furrowed brow, he asked "Don't you find them a little complex?" An understandable comment, perhaps, from a scientist whose lab specialized in one-celled organisms! Reading *Culture and Meaning in Health Services Research* might have gone far in answering the implicit questions: How do we study humans? How do we interrogate meanings and interpret social relations? Are we obliged to choose *either* the scientific method or ethnography? Quantitative *or* qualitative methods? This text shows us the possibilities of translation across disciplines, collaboration among specialties, and creative uses of anthropological methodologies in the interests of enhanced insight and effective action in the health care arena.

Carolyn Sargent
Professor of Anthropology
Washington University in St. Louis
December 2008

Preface

CRICK'S QUESTION

Years ago, at an academic party, I met neuroscientist Francis Crick. With colleagues, Crick had co-discovered DNA's double helix in the 1950s. He now lay in repose on a chaise lounge, wearing a straw hat.

Our (somewhat mischievous) host presented me to Dr. Crick as a social scientist: I was one of the few guests from that "other side" of the university. Summarily, disdainfully, and maybe even with a wave of his hand, Dr. Crick asked me to please explain the concept of *social* science, implicitly declaring the whole thing ridiculous.

Having no pithy retort, and lacking any taste for confrontation with this Nobel Prize winner, I mustered my best party laugh—and changed the subject. Even as I did, I felt regret. Crick's question represents one of the greatest challenges to responsible social scientists and health researchers who seek to improve the outcomes and experiences of patients and to help the people who provide and support patient care along the way. This book presents the methodological foundations for anthropologically informed qualitative health research, which is my main field of study. It focuses on the importance of achieving ethnographic insight in the health research context.

We can only understand and answer Crick's question if we understand the sociocultural milieu within which questions like his make sense. The implication in Crick's remark that social science is somehow substandard reflects a vision regarding data collection and analysis methods and, indeed, what research questions can be asked, that has been institutionalized in the health services arena. It is part of a cultural worldview. I intend to help readers interested in meaning-centered research to function effectively within this world. To this end, in these pages, I have combined an ethnographic-style look at U.S. health services with substantive methodological instruction that includes a sound explanation of the benefits of an anthropological perspective.

/ AN ALTERNATIVE VISION?

For a host of historical and practical reasons, the official U.S. health care or health services system favors a statistics-based or quantitative gold standard for "evidence," against which only things that can be measured and counted count. We all know that this mode of evidentiary valuation has flaws. We all know that, despite its immeasurable use to us when we or others are ill, there are problems with the quantitative standard of clinical research when it is applied in other arenas of health study. Indeed, there are great gaping holes in our health services–related knowledge base that simply cannot be filled by the quantitative approach to discovery and documentation.

Most of these holes relate to social interactions in which human beings play an active central role. They are found, for instance, in regard to diagnostic biases, patient-practitioner communication issues, care-plan "compliance" or agreement problems, and the application of preventative practices. Because willful human activity holds a central place in such situations, scholars often appeal to our need to understand the "human experience" as a justification for qualitative or meaning-based research regarding these and similar topics. They point to the uniqueness of local situations, claiming a deep inherent value for empathy-promoting description—a value forfeited, they say, in quantification.

The descriptive richness and evocative flavor of ethnographic accounts do have significant value. However, I find it far more efficient to explain my position in the language already known and appreciated by those who research, administer, or deliver nursing, medical, and allied health care today: the language of health outcomes and process improvement. That is, I get better reception when I point to the actual advances in care that work like mine has brought about and describe the advances in a way that science-minded colleagues can understand.

/ TRAINING IN METHODS

Scientific language did not come naturally to me. When I went to graduate school in anthropology (1985–90), we did not study methods at all, let alone scientific ones. This was not because the merits of systematic empirical investigation were unappreciated by my professors. Their work was soundly structured. But, as John Hast Weakland has noted, in anthropology's earlier days, when the field was in the flower of its youth and cross-disciplinary translation was neither yet expected nor necessary, anthropologists focused on presenting their conclusions rather than documenting or discussing how they reached them. Their methods were implicitly understandable to those with like experience in the field—those with whom they exchanged ideas (Weakland 1951).

By the time I was trained, this legacy had led to a somewhat dismissive and sometimes even suspect view of explicit research methods among many in anthropology. This view was bolstered by the then well-entrenched rift between positivist-minded and interpretive or hermeneutic scholars—a rift often termed the "two cultures" or science-humanities split, a la C. P. Snow (1993 [1959]). Suffice it to say that concerted methodological training was not part of our program.

My graduate experience was exemplary in many ways. Nonetheless, the methodological tradition in which I was educated did not serve me well when I ventured into the territory of clinicians and other health service professionals. Had I read in graduate school Weakland's mid-century (1951) effort to catalog how anthropologists do what they do, written to offset anthropology's appearance as "haphazard from outside the field" (p. 55), and had I taken in his concomitant observations on the hazard that "methodological vagueness" (p. 56) poses for cross-disciplinary discourse, I might have been a bit better braced for what was to come.

As things stood, I was not prepared to describe, systematically, what I had done in the field. I knew my ethnography was solid, but how many people, exactly, had I talked with? What questions, exactly, had I posed? What conceptual model drove my study? What techniques had I used to gain my data? I might begin an answer by explaining that I collected data by talking to people whenever they would indulge me—at the shop, before a church meeting, sitting on my landlady's veranda, walking through the market, waiting for the rain to stop, down at the soccer field for a holiday match, at the shore or riverside. But what was the technical term for such interviews? And how could I express the merit of my approach in a way that would seem sensible to those with a quantitative orientation?

Translation proved a significant challenge. As a result, I had trouble engaging myself productively in project planning. I had problems preparing an application for National Institutes of Health funding. I was undone discussing the anthropological approach with medical residents in a course that I was asked to teach. In short, *I lacked the cultural competence necessary to function effectively in the health services world.*

My story is far from exceptional. However, the world around us changes. Anthropological employment outside of academia has eclipsed employment within it, interdisciplinary collaboration is now common, and, to some degree, even the public seems prepared to ask, although not always for the right reasons, "How do they *know* that?" These developments all increase anthropologists' need for methodological explicitness. Because of this shift, but also because of a growing internal demand for methodological clarity as anthropologists take questions of epistemology or knowledge's basis head on, all good programs today require methods training.

I was, however, on my own in this regard. So I sought remediation, first through self-study and mentorship and then in a formal methods training course. I studied not only with anthropological texts and teachers but also read widely, expanding my grasp of science's vocabulary—and of the worldview that the quantitatively oriented sections of this language represented.

/ METHODOLOGICAL CROSSROADS

Over the years, I have grown quite comfortable at explaining my work in terms familiar to the health services audience. This has been for me a useful approach to building a program of research—but it sometimes feels intellectually impoverished and distracting, if not downright manipulative. Yes, it works like a Trojan horse to get my methods in the door. In the long run, however, the when-in-Rome strategy falls short for several reasons.

To begin with, the use of scientific jargon can hide the crucial difference between the anthropological approach, on the one hand, and qualitative methods as practiced in the normative health research framework on the other (the latter practice is highly quantified). It enables continued denial of home truths regarding the sociocultural construction of health services—even as it uses knowledge of these to gain advantage. It sidesteps the question of how one can practice science on social and cultural phenomenon, and altogether begs the questions "What is science?" and "What is biomedical science?"

What I aim to do here, therefore, is address those issues directly. I intend to share anthropology's promise by describing and illustrating select anthropologically informed qualitative methods for health services research, providing philosophical justification for their use, and supplying real-world examples of the advantages they can confer. The book's subtitle is "A Practical Field Guide" because I also mean to impart to readers a sense of what it is like to work within the sociocultural world of modern health care—a world that, like so many worlds that we moderns inhabit, can be far more exotic and foreign than any that traditional anthropological fieldworkers ever worked within. It is a world in which medical anthropologists and other outsiders must become culturally competent if they are to be effective, and if they are to address, to the health services world's and perhaps even Dr. Crick's (hypothetical) satisfaction, the call for scientific research methods.

/WHO WILL FIND THE BOOK HELPFUL?

Although the puzzle represented in Crick's question serves as the ultimate cause for this project, a proximate cause exists, too: market needs. A colossal array of books awaits the reader interested in qualitative and ethnographic methods. There is much methodological overlap between most disciplines, but for insight into how anthropologists in particular approach such work a good place to start is Bernard's *Handbook of Methods in Cultural Anthropology* (1998).

However, this text is among the first to bridge the holistic, meaning-centered anthropological sensibility with the health services research or HSR perspective (for efficiency, I use HSR broadly, to include *all* health services system–related research, including nursing). Indeed, no other full-length practical guide to applying interpretive qualitative methods to pressing health services problems exists. This book's uniqueness in this regard, and its grasp of and effort to convey the anthropological sensibility that HSR so requires, is reinforced through the substantive examples I used to build its case. The book's goals are further bolstered by its ethnographically informed exploration of the HSR enterprise.

Anthropologists and other social scientists interested in health research careers will find this book a valuable introduction to the world they seek to enter. It will also provide them with a relevant review of anthropology's history and major teachings. Readers belonging to the world of health services or students preparing to work in this area will find in the book a rich source of extra-disciplinary inspiration. The lessons of the text will build readers' methodological knowledge and anthropological wisdom. Applied, they will lead to concrete gains including better research designs, more sophisticated or meaningful analyses, and—ultimately—enhanced health services processes and improved health outcomes.

It may be worthwhile at this point to mention what the book will not provide. First, this is not a guide to traditional, academically oriented research methods; rather, it focuses on methods to be used in *applied* HSR endeavors. That these methods can also yield ample data for academic writing is manifest, for example, in my discussion of the findings from my study of surgical risk in Chapter 12—but that is not the point of this volume. Rather, my goal is to bring more cultural meaning into HSR efforts directly aimed at promoting positive change.

Second, the book does not provide a detailed guide to research design. Although I will discuss the general category of randomized controlled trials, at least in terms of their significance for HSR norms and expectations, I do not review the fine points of, say, crossover or quasi-experimental designs and such, nor do I spend much time on instrument development per se. I also do not cover the specific how-tos of research protocol development and writing or human subjects research regulations (except in passing), nor do I provide guidance regarding various HSR or clinically applied research funding streams. Grant writing does gain some attention but only incidentally, for instance, in relation to the links between promised protocols and research-in-practice. Although a lack of knowledge in these areas will not hinder the reader, he or she is advised to look elsewhere for detailed information.

The same holds true for theory. The book does review some of the theoretical paradigms important to the philosophy of science, postmodernism included, but it has little to say regarding the theoretical models that might underpin specific research questions. Readers unfamiliar with the basic theoretical paradigms of the social sciences or the conceptual models favored in HSR should at least understand that all facts are framed by one or another theoretical orientation toward them.

Examples used in the text do not cover all problems or all angles. Health care has been widely studied by insiders and outsiders alike. My tendency to favor anthropological accounts should not be taken as if a bold (and wrong) claim that no other discipline has considered the topics in question. Similarly, although I sometimes simplify the storyline to better squeeze my treatise into the space of this single book, I would never deny the true complexity of the situations detailed. Indeed, if the problems this book means to tackle were truly simple or could be solved from a single standpoint, the complementary vision I offer would not be so badly needed.

All this leads me to what the book does aim to do and who it is meant to serve. I will review its pragmatic targets first. To begin, then, because of its ethnographically inspired treatment of the sociocultural context in which HSR is so often undertaken, this book will be of great interest to anthropologists, sociologists, and other social scientists who wish to work effectively in HSR. Such readers will enter the field with a feeling of familiarity, empowering them for effectiveness from day one. Accordingly, anthropology as well as sociology, psychology, communication, and other departments seeking to capitalize on student interest in the developing qualitative HSR job market can use this text to prepare students for such work.

The book also holds value for HSR scholars seeking to add anthropologically informed methods to their toolkits—or to infuse their present use of qualitative methods or ethnography with the anthropological perspective. It will have appeal for evaluation and quality improvement specialists similarly wishing to broaden their knowledge and skills. Health care administrators and leaders interested in bringing the anthropological perspective into their organizations to underwrite quality improvement and other forms of positive organizational change can benefit also.

On a more academic level, because it reviews anthropology's history and medical anthropology's emergence, the book is valuable for introductory medical anthropology courses more generally, too; it could easily serve as a core text for such. And, because it contains substantive material on what anthropologists refer to as "the culture(s) of biomedicine" and various patient populations as well as the cultural competence movement, anyone seeking a deeper understanding of health services delivery in the United States will find the book useful. The emphasis on context even in the Specific Methods section means that the book could, in fact, be read or assigned for its ethnographic content alone.

Beyond disciplines already mentioned, the book will contribute to curricula in schools of nursing and social work and to the many disciplines that focus on child health: A majority of the examples will describe problems in pediatric care. The book may also be helpful in bioethics courses.

As the above potential readers' list suggests, this book ambitiously seeks to serve both social science and health services audiences. So, at times, small sections of the text may seem redundant for members of one group or the other. Therefore, in addition to taking pains to define technical terms as I use them, I try to alert readers from either segment to the few cases where they may find the text basic and to flag key sections that each will find extra useful.

However, the lion's share of this volume covers what will be new territory for both groups or, at the least, offers a new view on old territory: a view in which the familiar is made strange—and therefore more meaningful. It is my hope that the book will convey this new view with a minimum of jargon and plenty of heuristics to enhance conceptual clarity, making it ideal for self-study by professionals seeking to enhance their skill set and expand their understanding of the complexities of both research and health services as well as for classroom use at the upper division or graduate level.

/ ROADMAP FOR THE JOURNEY

Understanding is built in this book in a spiral manner through the deliberate layering of connected ideas and examples. Part I begins with an overview of the anthropological approach and an introduction to qualitative data in which socioculturally relevant stories are integral. Part II examines the anthropological view of ethnography in detail, explains what medical anthropology entails, and offers a critique of anthropology's superficial application in HSR as, for example, has historically been the case in "cultural competence" programs. In the process, a more complete understanding of the culture concept is forged. Part II also introduces readers to the health services landscape, which is a nuanced territory that the successful researcher must learn to navigate well.

Part III takes methodology head on. It examines theory-rich questions of epistemology as it probes the chasm that some feel exists between science proper and interpretive, humanities-influenced sociocultural research. Basic scientific concepts are explored in relation to the latter's goals. The historical reasons for science's presently narrow conception in HSR are outlined, and a way forward is justified and described. To prepare readers for the more specific methods instruction offered in the next part of the book, the last chapter in Part III reviews some of the more generic aspects of project planning and implementation.

In Part IV, I explain and explore various techniques for group and individual interviewing. More context-sensitive methods are also introduced, including participant observation and various systematic data collection techniques that can augment this traditional anthropological approach to ethnographic fieldwork. Finally, I examine the need for rapid approaches, address action research, and describe suitable methods for it.

Part V revisits the politics of research, including the ways that organizational and professional structures help shape it. I included this part to ensure that readers come away not only with an understanding of how findings can actually have an impact on practice and outcomes but also with insight into the power dynamics that research inevitably entails.

Throughout the text, I use concrete examples from my own experience in various health care settings, with the aim of adding clarity, coherence, and life to the important concepts discussed. I introduce ideas in a deliberately layered or spiraling way to scaffold the reader's slowly growing understanding as his or her journey through the book progresses. All key vocabulary terms, set in bold type, are searchable in the index.

/ ACKNOWLEDGMENTS

In drafting this no-doubt-too-ambitious volume, I relied on help from many others. Misrepresentations are, of course, my own responsibility and my own fault. For that reason, I do not single out mentors and collaborators within the main text where I otherwise might.

Among those deserving thanks are anthropologists F. G. Bailey, Jill Korbin, Mark Nichter, and Alice Schlegel, who, in the late 1980s and early 1990s, ferried me through my graduate and postdoctoral studies, first teaching position, and initial publications, encouraging me in ways they may not even realize. Nutrition scientist Cheryl Rock helped me see that leaving academia proper opened many doors and supported my early clinically applied efforts. Key HSR collaborators who helped me navigate my culture shock when working centrally within health care included first Paul Kurtin and Michael Seid, then Candice Bowman and Allen Gifford. Methods mentors include Russ Bernard and Victor de Munck. Ronnie Frankenberg and Carolyn Sargent also have each provided sage advice to me at different points in my career, and I have been honored again by their gracious contributions of the Foreword and Afterword for the present effort.

In addition to those named above who offered comments on this text or contributed to work that is referenced in it, I have been influenced as well as directly assisted by countless others, too, in this endeavor. Before space defeats me, I wish to thank several people who played key frontline roles in the research efforts described within the book: Kimberly Dennis, Erica Prussing, and Elizabeth Walker (for the Down syndrome work) as well as Glenn Billman, Wilken Murdock, and Elvia Romero (for many Children's Hospital efforts), and Leticia Reyes Gelhard, Susan Hedges, and Diana Simmes (for many of the community-focused pediatric projects). I am also grateful to Jennifer Collier, H. Russell Bernard, Matthew Lauer, Mimi Nichter, Michelle Ramirez, Shoshanah Feher Sternlieb, and a number of anonymous reviewers for invaluable comments on my initial ideas for the book and the evolving manuscript.

In drafting this text, I drew upon and adapted sections from many of my previous publications; all are referenced in the bibliography. I thank my coauthors and previous publishers for supporting with permission this repurposing. The entire Department of Anthropology at San Diego State University kindly supported me in various ways, too, throughout this project; at the least, Phil Greenfeld's generous provision of historical information must be mentioned. My students also deserve thanks for pushing me to clarify wooly ideas and to consider seriously this book's utility for them as eventual contenders in the research job market. I dedicate my work here to all readers who seek to be part of an anthropologically inspired research workforce, and whose efforts with this book will, I sincerely hope, be paid off in great dividends. Finally, in part because I have previously failed to do so (perhaps it did not seem "scientific"?), I thank my entire family, including David and Naomi Sobo and Harvey and Milo Smallman.

The author thanks the publishers who granted permission to reprint or to revise and incorporate into this book as examples materials from the following publications written or co-written by her: Bethell et al. 2006; Huby et al. 2007; Loustaunau and Sobo 1997; Prussing et al. 2004; Prussing et al. 2005; Sobo 2004; Sobo 2005; Sobo 2007; Sobo et al. 2002; Sobo et al. 2003; Sobo et al. 2008; Sobo, Bowman, and Gifford 2008; Sobo and Kurtin 2003; Sobo and de Munck 1998; Sobo and Seid 2003; Sobo, Seid, and Gelhard 2006.

PART I

The Value of Meaning

"If you were gravely ill, would you prefer a clinician with excellent technical skills or one with a great bedside manner?" This question, melodramatically posed to me many times over in the course of my health services research, suggests that social relations and the meanings they entail are irrelevant to health outcomes. But are they?

Good social interaction means next to nothing when weighed against saved lives for those with acute or emergency afflictions, such as stem from the deadly Ebola virus or warfare wounds. Indeed, the official health services system was created largely on the back of military medicine, which, in the field, had little time for bedside manner. However, the lion's share of care today is chronic (long-term) or preventive and behavioral (i.e., involving lifestyle change). Although anthropology has long been interested in the sociocultural dimensions of health and healing, the sensationalist question pitting technical skills against relationship building has not caught up to this fact. By focusing on the patient-clinician duo, the question also ignores all other types of necessary and meaningful relations that set the stage for high-quality care.

Part I examines the value of research that accounts for socioculturally relevant meanings in understanding and improving health services. Chapter 1 introduces the anthropological approach, describing ethnographic methodology as anthropologists define it, summarizing the role of both qualitative and quantitative techniques in achieving the kind of ethnographic understanding that can form the basis of robust insight. It also recounts the genesis of my own ethnographic knowledge of the field and provides some foundational definitions.

Chapter 2 establishes the utility of the anthropological approach for health services research and it does so on the basis of meaning's pervasive importance. The chapter explains why it is often the so-called anecdote and not the evidence that drives policy- and program-related decisionmaking. In doing so, the chapter imparts some basic lessons about culture and about why qualitative data, when treated interpretively, can be so powerful. This power makes it incumbent on us to learn (as we later will) how to collect, analyze, and present qualitative data using an anthropological perspective.

CHAPTER 1

The Journey Ahead: Aims and Means

/ORIENTATION

One day, I got sick, as people everywhere do. Fortunately, I was not too sick to move or think. I had insurance and there was a clinic not too far away that I was told would take it. I made an appointment and dragged myself there. When I arrived, I checked the office listings and floor plan. "Where am I?" I asked; "Where do I need to be?"

The clinic map oriented me to the physical space of the facility. However, navigating a health care system requires much more than spatial knowledge, even when one is well. Especially for complicated or chronic conditions involving care that extends over time, but even for ostensibly simple tasks such as acquiring and taking prescribed medications as recommended for acute or time-limited ailments, navigating health care requires grappling with a new language and a new set of rules. In this way, seeking care can be compared to cross-cultural travel.

The need for better orienting health care consumers—patients—has not gone unnoted by health services professionals and researchers. In the past ten years, an increasing proportion of health services research has sought to find ways to help minority group members and people with limited English proficiency to access and navigate care. Anthropologists, by definition scholars of human diversity, have sometimes participated in such efforts. But, for the most part, health services research's access and navigation endeavors have failed to take advantage of what anthropology has to offer. Anthropology's promise is foregone when studies focus, for example, on what "ethnic" foods must be put on the cafeteria menu to please "diverse" customers or what "health beliefs" form a categorically bounded group's "barriers to care."

My own disorientation on seeking care stemmed not from a so-called cultural conflict, as most in health care would define it (see Chapter 6). That is, there was no clash between my health beliefs and my medical knowledge. The cultural issues at play, and those that we must conquer if we are to improve our system of care, are many times more complex and more flexible than common wisdom suggests. Further, they are connected in crucial ways to social, political, economic, and other issues.

For instance, impoverished people living in Haiti's central plateau generally explained tuberculosis or TB as a disease sent by sorcery in the 1980s; but, in the 1990s, after an effective TB treatment program that included financial assistance, they more often explained it as a treatable airborne disease. Sorcery might still be implicated as the ultimate reason that one person got TB while another did not. But the fallacy of blaming sorcery for keeping people from seeking treatment was exposed when access was expanded (Farmer 2004).

An anthropological approach—especially the approach called critical medical anthropology, which combines an appreciation for historical and contemporary political and economic arrangements with interpretive sensibilities (Baer, Singer, and Johnson 1986; Singer 1986)—takes complexity into account. Further, the anthropological perspective extends into key backstage areas, such as clinical education and training as well as provider-provider relations, like those expressed in doctor-doctor communication. Moreover, it explores how unexamined, culturally based program assumptions can—even when shared by populations served—underwrite profound miscommunications.

For instance, in my own research on HIV/AIDS education efforts in the early 1990s, women continued to have unprotected sex even after being educated regarding its risks. Why? Condoms were promoted to the women as conferring protection from promiscuous partners. Using condoms was therefore culturally construed as evidence of being involved in a flawed conjugal relationship. From this perspective, condom use might be necessary for other women, but not those meeting (or needing to be seen as meeting) gendered cultural expectations for monogamy. The ethnographically informed study revealed the ultimate inappropriateness—and ineffectiveness—of suggesting that women's partners were disloyal, as well as its cultural basis (Sobo 1995).

Similar misunderstandings regarding whom a health education message is meant for can occur when clinicians use terms in the medical sense but patients understand them as lay terms. Take, for example, a pediatrician's recommendation to avoid introducing an infant to "solids" before six months of age. The doctor may mean the term to include soups, beverages, and anything other than breast milk or formula. But without explaining this, the new mother may interpret the term literally, to mean solid foods such as slabs of meat or whole potatoes. If asked whether her baby has eaten solids at a future appointment or in a survey question, then, the mother may answer "no" quite sincerely. Cultural semantics, or the particular meanings that words have in particular populations, are clearly meaningful. When not shared across communities, confusion and even life-threatening miscommunication can result.

/ NO BRIDGE

As cancer researcher V. R. Potter noted in 1971 when he coined the term "bioethics," the "bridge to the future" connects science and the humanities. Scholars and clinicians from many disciplines have worked to build such a bridge, and great progress has been made. But still, the bridge is not ready to bear much weight.

Increasing the amount of anthropological research attending to meaning can have profound implications for the bridge's strength and health services' success. But anthropologists often go about such research in a way that scholars trained in the scientific method may find problematic. Rather than controlled and preplanned hypothesis testing in contrived situations, anthropologists often pursue open-ended research in naturally occurring social settings. Although anthropology's disciplinary breadth does support varying methodologies, anthropologists interested in sociocultural phenomena generally prefer that research categories and the topics they examine closely reflect participants', not researchers', agendas. In other words, they often adopt an ethnographic strategy.

Scholars in health services settings often find such practices difficult to live with. But this is not the only cause of the difficulty anthropological work has had in reaching the health services. Some anthropologists expect health services professionals to find and read papers published in anthropological journals, in an anthropological genre, although the majority of such journals are not referenced by literature search engines that most health services people use, MEDLINE (see http://www.ncbi. nlm.nih.gov/sites/entrez), or are seen by this audience as "obscure."

Why don't anthropologists publish in journals read by health professionals? For one thing, anthropological papers are generally much longer than these journals (and their readers) allow. A second reason relates to the tired old division between academic and applied or theoretical and basic research. I will say more about such false dichotomies later; here, our focus is the very real tensions that they do entail. One of the most central of these has to do with researchers' willingness to communicate across the so-called divide. For example, health services research has always justified its work by pointing to its applications, as in cutting costs or improving health outcomes. Anthropologists, though, have often been over-modestly reluctant to make specific recommendations based on their work. Even those eager to demonstrate their findings' applied significance often do not know how to articulate their implications for action in a way that makes sense within health services research's purview.

The difficulty of the bridging acts is compounded further by the time frame of ethnography, a central anthropological research strategy. Because one to three years of data collection is not uncommon in anthropological ethnography, it has not been well integrated into health services decision cycle timelines: Results may come in too late to be helpful in regard to targeted processes and procedures. In sum, many in anthropology lack the basic cultural competencies necessary for smooth interactions, especially with applied health services research.

/ A SOLUTION?

In this book, I seek to counter anthropology's ignorance of health services research and to increase the quality and quantity of anthropology's contribution to it. But the book is not just for anthropologists or those in other social sciences who favor ethnography: I crafted it with health services professionals specifically in mind. Through it, I mean to introduce anthropology's holistic, systems-oriented, comparative agenda and to provide some of the tools needed to begin to implement it. Rather than presenting methods as discrete pieces of an ostensibly objective research design puzzle, I want to shed light on the entire investigational enterprise, encouraging readers to view this as a situated and negotiated process. Power dynamics, including those that affect field entry, data ownership, research deliverables, and authorship decisions are also directly addressed.

With this book, I wish to fuel excitement about the potential that anthropologically informed research has for advancing health care improvement. For example, without anthropological inspiration, researchers would not have noticed, let alone attended to, the pill sharing engaged in by some chronically ill patients whose partners or relatives also are ill but have no access to care. As a result of pill sharing (in which everyone might get some pills, but at lower-than-would-be prescribed doses), diseases may actually spread further and evolve drug resistant strains. Patients who do not seem to be improving as they should with the medication prescribed may receive counterproductive new care plans (Andrea Sankar, personal communication, May 13, 2008). Another example of how attention to ethnographic detail can be helpful comes from research revealing that women who thought they had been tested for HIV actually had not been tested at all (Sobo 1994). In both cases, the need for further patient education and the development of organizational processes that can reform the cultural logic leading to the actions or assumptions described is clear—and clearly would not have become apparent without anthropologically informed study.

Results from Carolyn Smith-Morris and others' research among the Pima Indians of southern Arizona have been used similarly. There, diabetes is so endemic that many people consider it simply part of life. Smith-Morris studied how health communication messages were received in this context. Findings regarding the local interpretation of ambiguous or conflicting test results as indicating borderline diabetes (which in biomedicine does not exist) led to a revision of clinicians' test result communication strategies. Moreover, data regarding Pima responses to health services delivered in acute care settings have led to a reorganization of the diabetes care model that acknowledges the disease's truly chronic nature. Attention also was turned toward addressing the structural causes of long-term under- and unemployment among the tribe's members and undoing the effect this has had on diet and activity by adding recreation and diabetes prevention programs to what had previously been merely a simple curative model (Smith-Morris 2006).

As noted, ethnography requires long-term participatory immersion in the cultural milieu in question. Although there are ways to do this that fit with the timeline for academic health services research, fitting it into the specifically applied mode of action can be more challenging. However, as we shall see, the anthropological perspective is transferable even when full-scale ethnography is not. After establishing the philosophical bases for their use, practical anthropologically inspired research methods that have been successfully adapted specifically for health services research are described. Some failures are recounted, too, for perspective.

In addition, I describe in an ethnographic style the world of health care in general and health services research in particular. Some of what I will say stems from an institutionally approved study of health services research itself and of its role in organizational change. I also draw freely on my extensive experience as an applied health researcher. Besides referencing relevant literature, I use critically informed observations to help situate the formal lessons of this book and support readers in accomplishing their effective application.

Before embarking on these lessons, I must define my terms a bit more precisely. After doing so, I summarize the experiential basis for my observations and describe how I learned to conduct anthropologically informed research within the health services.

My professional career includes ten years in the field doing health services–related research in addition to the more orthodox forms of medical anthropology I have also practiced in the nearly twenty years that have passed since receiving my PhD. By reflecting on that, I provide readers new to health services with my impression of the differences between working in health services and academic anthropology. Readers new to anthropology may at first be unused to the self-referential and self-reflexive way I convey this. However, doing so is essential because my experiences and my reactions to those experiences situate and thereby inform this book.

/ STARTING ON THE SAME PAGE

The Health Services System: Delivering Medical Care

Following the example of my colleagues in the field, in this book I call the system holding our interest the health care system or, more directly, the health services system. It is a system that, however well hung together it may be in some circumstances, is not always actually systematic or coordinated. In any case, for our purposes, the health services system includes all the services provided in support of health care as well as the care services themselves.

This is important because it is why in this book **health services research** (HSR) also refers to, for example, much nursing research. Having said that, the gloss includes no laboratory research nor does it pertain to the efficacy questions asked in controlled clinical trials. Those types of studies aim to establish treatment standards, whereas applied HSR (this book's focus and therefore, hereafter, simply HSR) is concerned with optimizing the delivery of such treatment. It does so through the study of staffing and financial issues but also, and increasingly, through the study of patients' experiences of care and health services workers' experiences of providing or supporting the provision of that care (e.g., when implementing new care guidelines). When patient outcomes are measured, HSR focuses more on effectiveness (whether patients show improvement in real-world settings) than efficacy (improvement under ideal [i.e., laboratory or experimental] conditions).

Our systems deliver what is sometimes termed "medicine" in the generic, although, as noted above, the health services system actually delivers services of many kinds. Clinical services gathered under the umbrella term "medicine" include: nursing, physical therapy, dietetic, and other like services as well as the technical services that support them (e.g., X-ray, laboratory, and facilities management). Administrative and other services (including keeping financial, legal, and social records) also support the edifice. So do those known by insiders as payors (insurance organizations, including the state's), because coverage plays a big part in what can and cannot be provided.

Just like the term "man," the term "medicine" is as exclusive as it is inclusive. Some health services workers have no problem with this; others (generally nurses, midwives, and some surgeons) are more outspoken about the fact that what they practice is not, actually, medicine per se. Medicine, however, does form the overarching theoretical paradigm for the entire health system's endeavors.

As an anthropologist, I would be remiss if I did not note here that the medicine delivered by the dominative U.S. system is only medicine of a certain kind. There are, in reality, many other kinds of medicine: herbal, Ayurvedic, homeopathic, and so on. There are healing traditions associated with or practiced as part of a religion, such as *curanderismo*. Therefore, what most Americans call medicine (as I will in this book) is given other names by scholars elsewhere in an effort to increase accuracy. Scholars use adjectives such as allopathic, cosmopolitan, modern, Western, or official to increase the accuracy of their descriptions, much as I did by using the term "dominative" (after Hans Baer 1989).

Along these lines, I should note that "American" is similarly problematic. In this paragraph and elsewhere in the book, "American" refers only to the U.S. populace; it is trumped by more specific designators whenever possible. Further, the U.S.-based focus of this book stems only from my concomitant professional residence in the United States. Despite their U.S. derivation, the methods described here should be applicable in all health services arenas.

In any case, because the dominative form of medicine in the United States and globally is based on the Western science of biology (and off-shoots of this, such as genetics), its most common anthropological designation is "biomedicine." When scholars paraphrased in this book say "biomedicine," I shall try to do the same, with proper attributions. In fact, I generally use the term in anthropological writing myself, but as this book is somewhat ethnographic, and aims to reach biomedicine's insiders as well as social scientists, here I follow my health services colleagues and collaborators, generally using the generic "medicine" designation.

I also have followed health services tradition in shortening the phrase "health services research" to HSR. Health services language is full of acronyms, many of which will be introduced. Some acronyms are part of the spoken vernacular. Others, like HSR, are more generally encountered in written form. HSR can be spoken, as when used in an organizational division's or journal's name. But, under most conditions at present, when speaking, HSR's full alliteration as "health services research" would be the better bet.

Science, Social Science, and Anthropology

The terms "science" and "anthropology" need a bit of deconstructing while I am at it. Used on its own, **science** refers to research that uses the scientific method of hypothesis testing, generally in controlled environments, findings from which are made and described in scientific, generally quantitative, terms. It is empirical or based on sensory observation as opposed to introspective or metaphysical perceptions. In this light, "social science" overgeneralizes: Many social scientists do interpretive work more akin to what gets classed as humanities scholarship. However, there is one aspect of science that does apply across the board, and it is a key one: systematicity. Good social science is systematic and methodical even when the scientific method (as defined above) is not directly followed. For this reason and because most HSR people use the term "social science," I will, too.

And what of the social science anthropology? Defined literally, **anthropology** is the study of humankind. In the United States, following the legacy of founding father Franz Boas, the designator traditionally refers to what are known as the "four fields." These are: archaeology, which is concerned with material culture or artifacts; biological or physical (or biophysical) anthropology, which is concerned with biological adaptation and diversity; linguistic anthropology, which is concerned with communication; and cultural anthropology, or ethnology, which is concerned with the diversity of peoples' shared, learned ideas about the world, as expressed in economics, the arts, religion, history, medicine, and so on. In addition to describing these, this subfield asks what culture really is and how it works.

When anthropology first emerged, its practitioners generally worked in all four fields and then some—formative figures included professionally trained experimental psychologists, geographers, medical doctors, and others. Today, single anthropologists rarely practice within more than one of the four initial subspecialties—although cultural anthropology or ethnology has broadened so that it is often termed "sociocultural," and linguistic anthropology has in many ways become part of the sociocultural branch. Cross-field communication is increasingly rare, even within individual anthropology departments where all fields are represented (Segal and Yanagisako 2005).

In the European anthropological tradition, archaeology has long been its own discipline, having developed and even guarded its particular methodological and institutional boundaries. Moreover, the teachings of comparative sociology and a vested interest in the varied ways that societies structure themselves (and related social categories such as class and caste) acquired great sway. Therefore, rather than cultural anthropology, Europeans practice social anthropology. Although there is much overlap with the U.S. cultural subfield, European anthropology has, historically and generally, been more interested in the links between cultural ideas and social order than in the ideas themselves.

Another major difference has been that universities in Europe often maintain separate social anthropology and biological anthropology departments. A number of U.S. anthropology departments have followed suit. Divisions arise not only from the hiving off that may naturally accompany a bourgeoning knowledge base, but also from deep disagreement over whether the anthropological endeavor should be more—or less—scientific (as we have defined that term; see also Chapters 7 and 8).

Subdisciplinary divisions notwithstanding, holism (a systems perspective) and cross-cultural comparison permeate all subfields of the discipline. Ideas about culture and society infuse archaeology as well as biological anthropology. Most social anthropologists also take culture into account, and vice versa. As a result, people often classify the social or cultural approaches together as sociocultural anthropology. For efficiency's sake, here I will use the single word anthropology to refer to the presently constituted sociocultural branch.

/ THE ETHNOGRAPHIC PROCESS

In the U.S. tradition, anthropology promotes **holism** and endorses **systems thinking** in regard to whatever may be under investigation. Why? Because, as Aristotle noted in *Metaphysics* long ago, "The whole is more than the sum of its parts." That is, the properties of a system as such can be neither explained nor determined by examining its parts alone. A system derives from the relationships between its parts—not merely their addition.

Some systems are mechanical and therefore totally predictable. For example, a thermostat-regulated heating unit will switch on and off when the temperature moves below or above a certain set-point. But the systems that interest anthropologists are human systems. These are **complex adaptive systems**—systems in which "emergent, surprising, creative behavior is a real possibility" (Plsek 2001, p. 310). This is because a complex adaptive system can alter itself, evolving in tandem with or fitted to environmental changes rather than breaking down in their wake.

One complex adaptive human system that has captured anthropology's interest is culture. During the late 19th and early 20th centuries, when academic anthropology was founded, anthropologists made long field trips to far-away places where they could study native non-European cultures. They spent a great deal of time creating descriptive written accounts of the natives' social structures and cultures—literally, **ethnographic** accounts. They practiced ethnology: They made cross-cultural comparisons to understand the situated significance of the cultural variation that they had documented as well as to test for universality.

At times, ethnology has been associated with **ethnocentric** ideas regarding cultural evolution—ideas emanating from the often unconsidered assumption that one's own culture is the best or that everything can be understood from within one's own cultural purview. However, **ethnology**, as such, is simply a comparative practice. Cultures are compared with each other and with the cultures of the anthropologists themselves. The latter comparisons can be manifest or intentional as well as latent or natural to the ethnographic process. That is, the simple act of thinking about and striving to describe other cultures inherently invites— no, requires—self-comparison. But not ethnocentrism. Ethnographic research was considered by many early anthropologists as one way to help ensure that ethnological comparisons were as free of ethnocentric bias as possible.

Although early anthropologists often stayed in temporary camps or with missionaries, and hired native interpreters to help them in the day-work of data collection, by the 1920s long-term immersion had grown common. Anthropologists lived not near those under study but *among* them, learning their language, eating their food, and participating in as much of their daily lives as was possible. **Participant observation** is the name for this approach, and it soon formed the primary method for creating ethnographic accounts.

Anthropologists are not the only participant observers. Sociologist Beatrice Webb was doing it back in the 1880s (Bernard 1998, pp. 13–14). It is not methods themselves but the questions that methods are used to illuminate that mark disparate disciplines; research concerns may divide disciplines, but methods interlace them.

Figure 1.1 depicts the ethnographic process, showing the paramount position of the ethnographer (the funnel) in the interpretive process and the centrality of his or her interaction with research participants in deriving, over time (depicted vertically), an ethnographic sense of what is going on in the circumscribed cultural milieu under study. Because the major method for this is participant observation, that is the biggest bubble in the ethnographer funnel. I have included smaller qualitative and quantitative methods bubbles there with participant observation to demonstrate that, as central as participant observation is, it is not the only ethnographic method. Ethnographers commonly supplement it with the systematic collection and analysis of other forms of qualitative data. They collect quantitative data, too. For instance, ethnographers commonly undertake village surveys in which demographic data are collected; they record the words to myths and songs; and they photograph artifacts and collect botanical specimens, which are all important features of the field

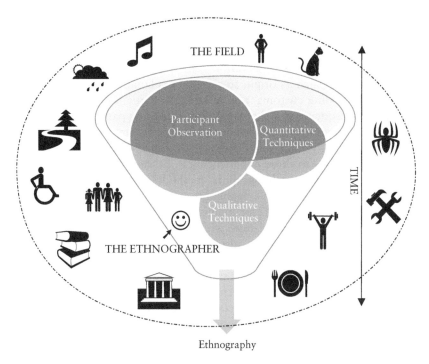

THE FIELD

Participant
Observation

Quantitative
Techniques

TIME

Qualitative
Techniques

THE ETHNOGRAPHER

Ethnography

Figure 1.1   The ethnographic process; time is depicted vertically and the funnel signifies the ethnographer him- or herself and his or her interpretive process. The shapes outside of the funnel represent (very broadly) the people, places, things, and events encountered by the ethnographer in the field.

although they are not well indicated in the figure. Ethnographers also may conduct formal interviews and administer questionnaires or other data collection instruments.

For example, in addition to spending long bouts of time in Melanesia, Margaret Mead collected children's drawings and administered and systematically scored projective ink-blot tests. As part of her investigation of the then common idea that "primitives" think like children, she asked Manus youngsters whether a canoe that slipped its moorings did so intentionally (1932, p. 185).

Such techniques can provide interesting data on their own. Overwhelmingly, the children in Mead's study told her that this idea was silly and that the canoe was just not fastened right; so much for the "primitives-equal-children" model. But—and this is crucial to the aim of this book—without the rich, multi-layered knowledge one gains from long-term participant observation, data's meaning cannot be discerned in full or explained in its entirety. *Without an intimate understanding of the sociocultural background of the data in question, their extended ramifications—and roots—cannot be seen.*

It is true that the systematic techniques with which anthropologists complement participant observation generate both meaning-related or qualitative data (such as origin stories and explanations of marriage or shamanistic healing customs) and numerical or quantitative data (such as marriage frequencies or shamans' cure rates using particular rituals or medicines). Nonetheless, the ethnographic project's key results are generally quite qualitative in nature: They are concerned with lived experience and what it means to those experiencing it. Ethnographic epistemology or, more specifically, **ethnographic methodology**—the philosophical basis for doing ethnography—highlights context and seeks to situate all findings, whether qualitative or quantitative, within the fabric of daily life and the encompassing systems within which daily lives are lived.

Ethnographic methodology also includes a focus on relationships between people of various social types. Exploring socioculturally important relationships in context and examining how these relationships generate different and often unexpected results in different circumstances allows anthropologists to understand system dynamics and their key outcomes, providing insight into complexity.

Ethnography is, thereby, not only a strategic process and a product but also a perspective. This *holistic, systems-oriented, comparative perspective* is not just ethnology's purview, it infuses anthropology's other subfields, too. Indeed, it comprises one of anthropology's characteristic approaches to studying human systems and their interrelations. If I may build on Brink and Edgecombe's observation that participant observation is ethnography's "signature" (2003, p. 1028), ethnography is certainly the signature of anthropology. Again, this is not to stake an ownership claim. Many disciplines have developed ethnographic traditions: sociology, communication studies, nursing, political science, and others. However, the ethnographic tradition in anthropology, in general, and in its subfield of ethnology, in particular, is longstanding and highly elaborated. As such, it provides an excellent starting point for fostering an appreciation of culture and meaning in HSR.

Many who already work in the ethnographic tradition are concerned not only with explicating cultural systems but also with studying the ways that such systems (and concurrently social organization) affect—and are affected by—human health. As demonstrated by this volume's focus, the ethnographic project can specifically include the study of systems developed for health maintenance or creation and improvement—medical systems, wherever in the world, however organized. In this book, the medical system of interest is the dominative, government-sanctioned, employer and insurance industry–endorsed U.S. system of health care.

/ THE FIELD

The idea that anthropologists might study health care here at home may seem new. Anthropologists have, traditionally, gone to the field (far-away, unindustrialized places) to undertake their studies. They have sailed around the world to witness native ceremonies and record ostensibly ancient myths.

Today, however, anthropology has broadened its scope. **The field** now refers to anywhere that formal anthropological studies are undertaken. The phrase connotes the fact that these studies are **naturalistic:** Ideally, human activity is studied in its natural setting and conditions are not controlled as they are in experimental research. Anthropologists undertaking ethnographic fieldwork interfere only in the sense that they ask questions and, more obliquely, in that they live with the people under study or otherwise occupy a space as participants in the social structure under consideration.

In my case, the field has included a rural Jamaican village, Cleveland's inner-city, the town of Las Cruces, New Mexico, and Durham County, England. For this book, my field sites were generally U.S. organizations: hospitals and health care systems. The methods I discuss in Part IV were all designed in the context of formal, institutionally approved research projects undertaken in health services settings.

I have come to realize, however, that the broader background against which these studies were undertaken is itself of scholarly interest. My most recent formal project, in fact, was designed specifically to examine the socioculturally situated nature of HSR. This project grew directly out of my previous health services experiences.

Clinical Settings

As a medical anthropologist focused on health care, I have worked with many community-based health services agencies as well as with community members themselves. My work within the hospital-centered care system forms the central basis for this text. That work, which I did not actually anticipate in my original career plan, began with some service on various program and planning committees at Rainbow Babies and Children's Hospital, undertaken while completing postdoctoral studies at Case Western Reserve University in Cleveland, Ohio (1991–1993). It was fortified when, after several fruitful years as a faculty member in academic anthropology (1993–1997), for family reasons and with a good deal of ambivalence, I dismounted the purely academic track and took up a clinical trials–related post within the University of California at San Diego's School of Medicine (1997–1999).

My clinical trials job entailed setting up and running the San Diego site for what was known to the public as the National Study of Nutrition and Health (NSNH). NSNH investigated adoption and patterns of use of particular foods in representative samples of the U.S. population (Kristal et al. 1998). The San Diego site occupied an office suite and included eight interview offices, a phlebotomy (blood-draw) room, lab, waiting area, and several administrative offices.

In addition to managing all site operations, which provided my first participation-based insight into non-anthropological health research, I conducted several substudies of my own (e.g., Sobo et al. 2000; Sobo and Rock 2001). These experiences led to a fascination with the backstage politics that go into designing scientific protocols, and the various "workarounds" (informal, off-the-record, and time- and energy-saving processes) that study staff devise so that they can meet enrollment and other goals. I realized that research questions *about* the trials were more interesting to me than the trials themselves—that and the action orientation of the project kept me quite motivated.

In light of my growing interest in applied pursuits, I followed my two-and-a-half years at NSNH with nearly five years as a core research staff member in the Center for Child Health Outcomes (CCHO) at what is now Rady Children's Hospital San Diego (hereafter, "Children's"). Staffed by nearly 3,000 employees (including more than 1,000 nurses), Children's is the region's only pediatric hospital. The region is large, thus, Children's is large: The hospital has 248 licensed beds and last year provided care to 142,754 sick or injured children. This entailed over 1.4 million medication doses, 125,000 X-rays, 133,000 bandages, and 21,000 popsicles. (http://www.chsd.org/body.cfm?id=969; last accessed June 6, 2008). In addition to its main facility, Children's has many satellite offices and participates in a number of community health programs.

The hospital's finances ran into dire straits in the early 2000s, leading to CCHO's effective closure. The Rady donation that led to the name change came too late for my colleagues and me. My employment was terminated as part of a programmatic reduction in forces (RIF). In other words, I was "riffed." This is not a happy memory, but I share it here because it offers an important lesson: Work in health services is subject to market whims and budget pressures (as well as to swings or changes in the immediate priorities that leadership may hold, more of which in Chapter 14).

My tenure with Children's entailed my first full-fledged participation as a worker in the health services system. Labeled a "research scientist," I was to help improve various safety, quality, and satisfaction outcomes. To help assess needs and effect change, I was involved in designing, proposing, undertaking, managing, and disseminating findings from research and quality improvement projects. In the process, contracts were executed for a number of outside health services agencies, such as California's Department of Health Services and the state's Emergency Medical Services Authority. I was also charged with helping improve the hospital's publication record. Although grants were good, they were not my salary's source. It was a dream job.

Children's did have as affiliates a number of academic researchers and my own unit was, ostensibly, a research unit. But the organization's principal deliverable (concrete, consumable aim or end product) was health care. Very few who worked directly for the organization had research preparation. Those who did have experience constructing studies generally approached them from a **quality improvement** or QI perspective, which prioritizes pragmatic over academic concerns and application over publication.

However, like me, some members of my unit also did HSR. This is different from QI although it may share the same ultimate goals. Health services research—HSR—takes the scientific method as central and has relatively long-term time-frames, whereas QI uses business improvement methods and seeks short-term gains. HSR, being **research** per se, seeks generalizable knowledge and intends to share this through publication and presentation to extramural audiences; QI is focused on local issues without an eye to sharing results or disseminating methodological advances. In the United States, as in many nations, research is regulated. HSR must be approved by an institutional review (or research) board; QI does not, as its goal is simply improvement of the business. Career advancement in QI, as opposed to HSR, depends directly on improved outcomes, not publication output.

Like the vast majority of hospitals and health care systems today, Children's was at base a business. Moreover, again as is common (see, for example, Good 1998), Children's had a long history of competition with the local school of medicine and this manifested itself in a form of identity politics that favored clinical action over the academic approach. In part because of QI's related ascendancy over HSR at Children's, I encountered—and was at first quite shocked by—widespread use of or reference to others' work without what I thought was proper acknowledgment. I have vivid memories of a visceral reaction I had to a visiting physician who, in a truly wonderful motivational speech, used ideas clearly attributable to anthropologist Claude Lévi-Strauss—without once mentioning the scholar's name. Attribution was academic: It was simply not important when compared to application.

In the same sense, publication was superfluous to Children's core mission—except as it might bolster the organization's business plan—for example, by helping the organization qualify as the kind of cutting-edge hospital where research takes place. This desire existed, despite the organization's tendency to bad-mouth academics in other contexts, because of the gains it could lead to in terms of both grant-related income and respect from the academically affiliated. Against these measures, research and publications were treated as commodities by senior leadership. This reinforced my less-educated (less-academically indoctrinated?) coworkers' ideas about intellectual ownership.

All this fostered a certain degree of culture shock on my part. For example, within the first few months of my tenure, I was caught wholly off guard when one of the MDs for whom I was writing up a case study for publication actually yelled at me for having what he saw as the audacity to put my name with his and his supervisors' on the author by-line—despite the fact that I alone gathered the case materials and wrote them up.

As with all normative behavior, prevalent views on research and publication were much more complex than they appeared on the surface. They actually did make sense in context. They followed a kind of cultural logic and fit well with the organizational norms and social or structural constraints that people labored under. This was the case both locally at Children's and at the national level, which I witnessed through participation at regional and national meetings and in various short-term consulting engagements. Eventually, I **acculturated**; that is, I internalized and adopted, or at least expressed when appropriate, local cultural norms. More bluntly, I got over it—as I would have had to do in any other hospital or health care system.

Researching Research

In my description of the research context at Children's, I indicated that HSR and QI are somewhat in opposition, but HSR has taken an interest in QI of late. A new branch of HSR, **implementation science**, or IS-HSR, focuses on the process of translating research into practice through quality improvement initiatives. IS-HSR is also sometimes termed "quality improvement research" (QIR) or "translation science"; indeed, there is a bit of an ongoing tussle regarding preferred terminology. My use of "implementation," then, is simply an ethnographic artifact: Those with whom I worked preferred it.

Because it is aligned with HSR, IS-HSR is sometimes seen as a threat by those who practice QI. Concurrently, in light of its emphasis on actual intervention and change, IS-HSR must be more flexible and naturalistic than mainstream HSR. So, in many ways, it sits on a bridge between the two other approaches to studying health services (QI and HSR proper). In many ways, IS-HSR is like applied medical anthropology, then, and it has lots in common with the anthropologically informed approach to HSR that this book endorses. Its interstitial or bridging position and the ways that IS-HSR workers negotiate this became a central concern for me in the next phase of my health services career.

From Children's, I went to work for one of the nation's largest integrated health care systems, at first as a contractor and later as a funded investigator. At this time, I also completed a number of short-term contracts and consultancies for other organizations. I mention this to give readers a sense of the patchwork way in which independent contractors often fill in their work weeks or make ends meet. But it was the investigatory work that got me out of bed in the morning.

In the integrated system, I worked in a unit concerned with the implementation of evidence-based quality improvement interventions. This unit was part of the system's overall IS-HSR program. I wrote a proposal to research their research process, including what it entailed and the way that it was articulated with QI and organizational change. The proposal was funded and I got to work, pursuing my idea that research on research could be informative.

My project sought to illuminate not only organizational change but also IS's emergence from within HSR. Because I will be describing relevant findings later, I should say something about the project's methods. First, to collect data, I used a focused ethnographic approach that included key informant interviews much like those described in Chapter 11. To increase the national scope of the sample, many of these were done by phone (for instance, with members of the system's other IS-HSR units). Population penetration as well as saturation or data redundancy was the interview sample's limiting factor. An associate (Greg Aarons) and I interviewed forty-one people: twenty clinical personnel, eight informatics or QI specialists, and thirteen implementation-oriented health services researchers. For feasibility, we requested only half-hour interviews. However, the average length of all interviews was thirty-seven minutes, and the mean duration of the interviews conducted with researchers in particular was fifty minutes. The analysis entailed a text-based search of interview transcripts and field notes for narrative themes and patterns and a concurrent effort to link these to situational factors, such as institutional timelines and reward schemes.

Crucially—especially in the context of a major methodological message of this book—I also was immersed within my host unit just as I would have been for a formal, full-scale ethnographic study. For example, I attended and conducted unstructured observations of hundreds of meetings and conference calls (scheduled and unscheduled) where the unit's business was discussed. I closely considered relevant organizational texts such as meeting agendas and minutes and program directives and had frequent informal interactions with the researchers and support staff, both individually and in naturally occurring groups (e.g., around the copying machine, by doorways, at lunch). Prior to the formalized, funded research, I had enjoyed a six-month contracting engagement within the unit.

Although not part of the research protocol, all of these experiences served a paramount contextualizing function. As I collected and analyzed my data, I reflected on time spent with NSNH and, more so, Children's, as well as at various national and local HSR meetings and in the HSR consulting jobs that I undertook while a Children's employee and afterward also. This shed light on the larger professional research and service context affecting the unit. I present many such reflections in this book. I refer to the contextual information regarding my work within HSR as ethnographic, and indeed it is, if my long-term immersion in HSR and my systematic, theoretically informed reflection on the HSR world is considered. However, with the exception of some of the field notes from the project just outlined, records regarding the context of my work in HSR were not kept as part of a formal or official research study. There were no formally identified key informants; there were no consent forms or procedural manuals. And, although I do have email and other forms of documentation such as meeting notes regarding many of the events to be described and replies that encouraged me to write them up, there were no methodically created field notes. Some events lack any form of prospective (real-time) documentation. The ethnography-like portions of this text are based not on research proper, then, but a retrospective and reflexive recollection of my daily experience in the world of health services and signal events that reflect this.

Despite these caveats and legalistic disclaimers that much of what I will describe is not research based—caveats that readers will learn are culturally appropriate and indeed required by the norms of HSR as it is practiced today in the United States—the main lessons I intend to convey are transferable. The stories I shall recount refer to cultural practices that I know, from my broad experience and through conferring with others, to be pervasive in HSR. They reflect the culture of HSR and the professional and institutional structures that researchers must negotiate—pervasive and powerful structures that encourage researchers to behave in particular, culturally patterned, and (in context) culturally understandable or acceptable ways.

I cannot overemphasize this point. Social scientists often give fake names to the locations or people about which or whom they write; this helps maintain people's privacy. There have been times in writing this book that I, too, have considered the value of suppressing information about where or for whom I have worked. And I do occasionally, and for one project in particular because of an organizational request, cloak the specifics of time, place, or person. Now and then I do use pseudonyms and draw up composite settings or events for illustration.

However, there is also value in transparency. That is why I have been candid in this introduction. Each health services organization with which I have worked has demonstrated the highest integrity in opening itself to at least some and sometimes full scrutiny in the service of hoped-for improvement. This in itself deserves recognition. It is a brave and laudable thing for them to do.

That the stories I tell in this book did take place in particular settings should not distract readers from their transferable value, however. This value, in fact, stems from their very unremarkability. In this sense, any masking that I have done is immaterial. Indeed, *the events that I recount to give this book an ethnographic flavor might happen in any hospital, health services system, or HSR unit* that is anything like those in the United States. What I will describe is all part and parcel of health services' work-a-day world.

/ ONWARD

This book provides readers with the methodological framework and the anthropological background needed to design research relevant for, and maneuver successfully within, the health services world. It also offers a basic philosophical grounding that justifies anthropologically informed or, more particularly, ethnologically inspired HSR.

In my preface, I recounted a party conversation with Nobel Laureate Francis Crick in which, as part of the banter, the value of my disciplinary approach and focus was challenged. I pompously termed this challenge "Crick's question." Many times since, colleagues and other stakeholders who use orthodox definitions of science and evidence have questioned similarly the value of the anthropological approach. Unanticipated, Crick's question may lead to distress in researchers who favor meaning-centered inquiry, but it also pushes us to sharpen our thinking and this drives forward scholarly—and social scientific—advancement.

An appeal to improved outcomes has provided me one way to defend anthropologically informed HSR. But that skirts the larger, epistemological questions that this approach entails. It ignores the deep meaning of the query: "What *do* you social scientists do, and why should we care?" This text will, I hope, not only provide some concrete instruction in the anthropological approach to health care questions but also give the reader knowledge of exactly what to say when called on to reply to the "But is it science?" challenge.

/ MEANINGFUL DATA

Some people say that there are two kinds of data: quantitative and qualitative. **Quantitative data** are numerical. **Qualitative data** are narrative data that consist of words, sentences, or visual images (pictures, moving, or still). Qualitative data include particular stories, which often are discussed in terms of the more general story they tell. To put it perhaps too simply, so that we might begin, quantitative data can be used to discover or document how many people do this or how much our behavior is influenced by that. It can illuminate dollars saved or lived cost. Qualitative data, on the other hand, can help us get to the answers for the most-asked of all questions: "Why?" Qualitative data can help us get a feel for the storyline—for the meanings that motivate people toward action or inaction, as the case may be.

Stories are integral to culture. They inspire daily deeds and drive decisions. They are one mainstay of what good ethnography collects and analyzes. And so stories provide a fine place to begin our exploration of anthropologically informed health services research's value in theory and practice.

/ THE RIGHT THING TO DO

We tend to think of medicine as a science. However, people often justify health practices and policies by telling stories. Stories have actual endings from which concrete lessons can be learned. For instance, although not research based, a "wrong site surgery" story was, at the family's request, turned into an educational video at one organization I worked for. The video sparked individual workers' participation in safety reform in a way that carefully collected and analyzed quantitative data never could have.

Take, as another example, recent discussions about medical tourism (traveling out of one's country for health care). An editorial in no less than *The New England Journal of Medicine* introduced the practice this way: "At a recent Senate hearing, two stories were recounted that illustrated the physical and financial peril driving patients to pursue care abroad" (Milstein and Smith 2006, p. 1637). Stories, not statistics, held the Senate's attention.

As F. G. (Freddy) Bailey noted one-quarter of a century ago, meeting outcomes are highly influenced by the tactical or rational use of emotion (1983). That is, rather than or in addition to rational arguments, meeting participants often make passionate appeals, each tying their position to a moral imperative that any group member must hold (or at least pretend to hold) as "a self-evident, undeniable value" (p. 134). The rhetoric deployed is "a rhetoric of belonging": "Divergent opinions are eliminated in this form of rhetoric not through discussion but by a simple elimination of the non-believers: an insistence that any belief that departs from the orthodox need not be taken into account. ... Intrinsic values ... are ends in themselves" (p. 135).

This patterned passion is probably universal. Bailey saw it in records from British parliamentary debates as well as in city council meetings and academic seminars. He saw it in formal as well as informal settings, in India (where he did his early fieldwork), Europe, and the United States. He saw it in novels as well as real life.

In my own experience working in health care, I have seen hospital executives and staff workers justify practices and policies, including movements for change, as "the right thing to do." This is because clinical care is still idealized as something people do not do for profit. Despite the fact that it is a two-plus trillion-dollar industry (Catlin et al. 2008), we like to believe that motivation must stem from inner compassion—not from corporate bankers' instructions or a personal desire for monetary profit. Health care is still, in theory, a service vocation and we all prefer to think that, if we need treatment, the best and most appropriate care will be forthcoming—not the cheapest.

Having said that, people promoting new or altered processes within health care do take pains to identify and point out the financial benefits to certain stakeholders. Recently, one set of colleagues decided to promote increased HIV screening for patients enrolled in their organization through, among other things, a computerized clinical reminder system. They argued to relevant gatekeepers that better HIV screening would have long-term cost effectiveness because of increased capacity to identify people with HIV before they are sick, thus minimizing patients' potential future needs for expensive interventions. They had the numbers to back up their statements, conveniently contained in a frequently disseminated PowerPoint presentation.

Although financial considerations opened the door for the project with hospital administrators, when the HIV screening reminder project was set to be rolled out on the floor and put into action—when project staff requested participation from front-line clinicians and clinical directors— financial incentives were not highlighted in any discussion I heard. Cost effectiveness had disappeared from the discourse. Clinicians were asked to offer the test more frequently for the simple reason that improving screening practice was the right thing to do. In fact, my research regarding the roll-out confirmed that those who embraced the project referenced its relationship to their professional identity as caregivers who "do no harm" and who serve those in need (Sobo et al. 2008b). Money remained unmentioned. And, generally, so did any scientific justification for the program change.

The case for increased screening may seem a no-brainer; of course, it is the right thing to do. My point here is that moral and not scientific reasons were used to drive the increase on the floor; even for administrative gatekeepers, science did not carry the day. And this is in an institution—health care—that is scientifically justified and supposed to be scientifically based.

Let me give one more example to show with full clarity the persuasiveness of moralizing rhetoric and the poor actual standing that science can have in health care. In the late 1990s, emergency department physicians at one hospital ordered computed tomography or CT scans for any child brought in for a minor head injury (in common clinical parlance, a "head bonk"). This was justified as the right thing to do—despite the added physical risks faced by young children who needed sedation to be scanned without difficulty, and despite the financial burden that so much scanning placed on the system. It was right because the alternative—a missed diagnosis of a life-threatening intracerebral hematoma, perhaps— was wrong and unacceptable to the individual physicians who had heard apocryphal stories of this happening previously. Failing to order imaging was linked in the minds of many with the potential for complications and perhaps even charges of malpractice, a not infrequent occurrence in the U.S. system.

Did internal data support the high rate of CT scanning? No. Did the literature? Not really, although at that time not much research had been done. In response to this information, did practice change? Meetings were called and decisions postponed so that more expert consultation could be taken. Further exploration of the internal data as well as a more thorough review of the literature was arranged. And so things went, dampening the possibility that preferred practice patterns would be made to change anytime soon.

The above example demonstrates that when health care workers or their leaders disapprove or feel threatened by an evidence-based change suggestion—one that challenges the preferred or at least habitual status quo or insults or damages self-esteem by implying poor previous decision-making—they look for loopholes by criticizing the evidence mustered. They may find their escape in methodological limitations, such as sample size, often maligned as being too small. They may express data validity and reliability concerns. In common parlance, they may "damn the data" rather than to accept findings that disconcert.

Chapter 14 explores the ramifications of hierarchical social relations for health care improvement work, and evidentiary issues are covered in Chapters 7 and 8. Here, our concern is to understand how motivational, moralizing anecdotes carry so much more policy-setting power than research findings. If we can do this, we will be one step closer to understanding how cultures work, whether they are the health services cultures that these examples entail, those of other professions that make up the health services system, or the overlapping cultures practiced by the various populations health care serves. We will be that much closer to understanding why research that takes culture into account anthropologically is so important to the future of health care.

As noted by storytelling-proponent Stephen Denning (2001), Plato ironically noted the power of narrative a few thousand years ago: In *The Republic*, he recommended the strict censorship of storytellers and poets so that they could not unduly influence children and other vulnerable groups by telling tales. But how can storytelling be so powerful? Why is one good story worth 1,000 robust research studies, even when the story contradicts scientific evidence?

/ TO DENOTE OR TO CONNOTE?

Hospitals are full of talk. Talk serves many purposes, not least of which is literal—and often directive—information conveyance: Get me a scalpel. Bring me the X-rays. Or to the patients: Take two pills. Eat this. Sit up. Stick out your tongue. Turn left at the end of the hall. Take a number and wait your turn.

But there is more to talk than **denotative** meaning; that is, there is more to conversation than realistic description or practical direction. Words also have **connotative** meanings; that is, they connote ideas beyond those that they denote. Connotations can be local and relatively context-specific. For example, "You could see his [forehead] vein" was a warning, in one hospital, to avoid a particular senior leader until he was calmer. It also could connote that the person who shared the warning had received an upbraiding. At the same time, statements can reference a grander scheme of things. In this case, a bit more extrapolation leads to ideas about the structure of power in the unit, core values, and key mission imperatives as well as (reaching further) the political economy of capitalism. Importantly, the reach made here refers to the level of abstraction itself—not the difficulty of getting to it conceptually. Connotations are always there for the making.

In hospitals as in other health services locations, lots of connotation goes on. As Byron Good has shown in his treatise on medicine as an interpretive practice, "The language of medicine is hardly a simple mirror of the empirical world. It is a rich *cultural language*, linked to a highly specialized version of reality and system of social relations, and when employed in medical care, it joins deep moral concerns with its more obvious technical functions" (Good 1994, p. 5; emphasis in the original). In other words, doctors (like nurses, and so on) often *say* more than they say.

The way that this type of communication can be used to optimize healing has come under a great deal of scrutiny recently in regard to what has been called the placebo effect or, following Daniel Moerman, the "meaning response" (2002). Either expression refers to a situation in which patients are told they are being treated but really are given pharmaceutically inactive ("fake") pills or procedures or, in contexts outside of the health services system, undergo ritual or religious healing. Even though such treatments are not medically proven, these patients can report or show improvement in their condition via medical testing. Their improvement seems to be engendered by the treatment's meaning. That is, a pill's color, name, shape, or dispensing context can somehow underwrite a degree of healing (or pain reduction or the like)—sometimes enough so that researchers who may be comparatively testing a new drug or procedure against a placebo cannot legitimately claim the drug or procedure to be in itself a significantly better source of healing.

As Moerman notes, rather than dismissing the placebo effect in a group of people as simply "all in their heads," we should find out specifically what it was about the treatment that supported self-healing. For instance, recent research has shown that knowledge about price can support healing: In a U.S.-based placebo pill pain reduction study, subjects given the placebo but told it was rather expensive ($2.50 per pill) fared better than subjects given the placebo but told it was only 10¢ (Waber et al. 2008). The adage "You get what you pay for," or the assumption that things that cost more are better, may have been at work. Similarly, studies regarding the role of the built environment in facilitating or impeding healing in hospital settings have supported the use of features such as garden views for patient rooms (Ulrich 1984, 2006). If we knew more about the connotations that have helped make placebos so effective in various cultural contexts, including those that support ritual nonbiomedical healing, we could begin to leverage the placebo effect to optimize the meaning response and improve patient outcomes. This is one reason that studying the connotative meanings or stories that items and actions index or entail is essential. But it is not what drove me to write this book.

Connotations are made not only in care settings by patients and providers but also in boardrooms where policy and program decisions, such as for changing CT scan policies, are made. In such settings, decisions are made depending on what a given set of sentences, and how they are delivered, implies about the recommender as a professional, or patients and families as deserving of change, or decision-makers as moral beings. And in addition to being inferred from ostensibly technical directives and declarations, these types of meanings and many others can be connoted by narrative tales as well. The case history, or a recollection regarding the last time a complication happened or a patient of a certain type was treated, hereby comes into play.

Stakeholders may also offer quantitative data. But numbers are abstract. Having credited psychoanalyst Heinz Kohut for the distinction, anthropologist Clifford Geertz (1983) might have called numbers "experience far" as opposed to "experience near." Or, to follow a slightly different trope, one that Geertz borrowed from philosopher Gilbert Ryle (see Geertz 1983, p. 6), he might have explained that the descriptions numbers make are "thin," not "thick." That is, they may confer a correct measurement, but they do not refer us directly, as **thick description** does, to any "stratified hierarchy of meaningful structures in terms of which [actions or ideas] are produced, perceived, and interpreted" (p. 7). This capacity to convey meaning is a quality that stories have a lock on.

/ MAKING SENSE, MAKING STORIES, MAKING SELVES

Stories can help us create a sense of coherence and continuity. They help us interpret or make sense of the world. Concurrently, our reflection on the stories that we find ourselves a part of is a crucial step in the process of identity construction and maintenance.

In medical settings, students are turned into doctors or acculturate to the world of medicine through a number of narrative traditions. Some trainees are quite conscious of this process. As a Harvard medical student who participated in Byron Good's research explained, "In a sense we are learning a whole new world. … because learning new names for things is to learn new things about them. If you know the name of every tree you look at trees differently. Otherwise they're just trees" (1994, p. 98). Regarding patients, another student said, "I've had some real perception changes of people. … More and more, I can't help but think of us as machines" (p. 96). Narrative practices have a lot to do with such changes in perception.

We learn how to *be* as well as how to *see* by paying attention to how those around us talk. Such learning is often even more direct than the learning the students referred to because examples of how to be and not to be are made concrete. In fact, the majority of speech—perhaps about 70%—is social gossip (Dunbar 1996). By social gossip, I mean not only rumors or snippets of information about famous entertainers' transgressions but, more importantly, the stories we tell each other about members of our own social networks, such as what happened to John on his vacation or why Jane's last submission to a particular journal was rejected. Such tales remind listeners—and tellers—of cultural norms and expectations by providing concrete examples of rewards and punishments for behavior good or bad.

Narrative Forms

Many of our stories follow patterned narrative forms. A **narrative** form is a recognizable way of talking to oneself or to others about a particular set of events that relates them to particular cultural ideals. In other words, narrative forms are actually used to structure or "emplot" actions so that they are part of a meaningful whole made up of past, present, and future. (MacIntyre 1985; Mattingly 1998). They can be imposed after the fact as well as driving or motivating—and thereby becoming embodied in—current or future behavioral or interpretive choices.

As philosopher Alasdair MacIntyre explains, all narratives have "some at least partly determinate conception of the final *telos*" (1985, p. 219). This telos (end, reason, or goal) relates to some conception of morality. Narrative forms give stories their structure while linking sets of actions or events to a culture's moral norms and goals, or expectations. That is, they entail models of how the moral world should, ideally, be. So, by telling stories, we educate ourselves as to our culture's moral norms and goals.

A given narrative form may be identified as such and labeled in terms of the ideals to which it refers, or by the main organizing feature that gives it its loosely patterned, identifiable form. For example, in the mid-1990s, I described two narrative forms found in stories told by single women seeking to justify the condom-free penetrative risky sex mentioned in Chapter 1. I called one the "Monogamy Narrative" and the other the "Wisdom Narrative." In brief, these stories organize actions and relate these to listeners in ways that support a woman's claim to be "safe" by virtue of her partner's sexual fidelity, or her claim to have the ability or wisdom to identify honorable, trustworthy and, by implication, disease-free men. Thus, among other things, the narrative forms are used to protect self-esteem and status in light of dominative cultural ideals (Sobo 1995).

Although our focus here is on narrative form in general and not particular contents, permit me a brief digression to ask: Why was this anthropological finding important for health services? Knowledge about the monogamy and wisdom narratives was useful in crafting recommendations for how HIV/AIDS education and prevention programs could better meet their targets. It helped illuminate how and why the message that women could not trust their partners and the request for them to take an adversarial stance with the men by demanding they use condoms backfired: Targeted women did see that some other women had cheating husbands or boyfriends, but it was too difficult for them to apply this model to their own relationships. A health campaign that made the condom a symbol of love rather than betrayal would be more productive.

STORYTELLING CONNECTS US

We tell stories now, but was it always so? Despite older theories that credited the evolution of language to its denotative uses (e.g., Me hungry, Apple tasty, Chop here), new thinking does place causality in its connotative value. In other words, language helped our evolving ancestors cross what Walter Goldschmidt has termed "the bridge to humanity" (2006), because true language entails the capacity for symbolic thought. True language enables us to inhabit a symbolic world—one where abstractions such as love, dignity, freedom, morality, family, and community are possible.

Language supports human sociality because it allows us to form groups that extend and endure beyond the here and now. But how did it come into being?

It is generally accepted that language development and tool use in ancient humans went hand in hand hundreds of thousands of years ago. Recent discoveries regarding the brain suggest that the manual dexterity necessary for making and using tools may be intimately linked not only with the development of gesture language but also with the development of the parts of the brain implicated in manipulations of lips, teeth, and tongue that are necessary for speech. These connectionist actions, and the cognitive mechanisms behind them, are in some ways "quite isomorphic" (Goldschmidt 2006, p. 23).

Thoughts and actions may be even more connected than that: There is evidence that the neurons that control specific actions can also fire when we simply think about those actions. These are called "mirror neurons," and they go off, for example, both when monkeys themselves grasp a piece of food and when they see a trainer grasping food, as was the case when they were first scientifically noted (Gallese et al. 1996; Rizzolatti et al. 1996). In humans, mirror neurons may fire when we observe someone doing something that we would imitate. Although much more research is necessary, mirror neurons seem to be a key mechanism for this nongenetic mode of information passage (Goldschmidt 2006, p. 31; see also Ridley 2003, pp. 212–214). This indicates intense connectivity in the brain—connectivity that goes beyond linear, "engineer's logic" (Goldschmidt 2006, p. 32), and connectivity that supports complexity and emergence, such as is described by chaos theory in physics.

For now, let us return to sociality—and its connection to language in general and storytelling in particular. Social connections are created and maintained through language, beginning with body language in its broadest sense during the time mother and fetus, then infant, are physically linked. However, as Goldschmidt argues, sociality is fed not so much by denotative communication as it is by connotative communication. Here, he means mainly communication that activates and relies on the emotions—communication staged in the language of ritual.

We first see tangible evidence that humans are attending to social connections about 70,000 years ago. That is when culture seems to have emerged. In what was, evolutionarily speaking, all of a sudden, humans had multi-piece tools, such as wooden-shaft arrows and antler-tipped harpoons. They also had string, thread, and sewn clothing as well as shell and tooth beads for adornment. Many small statuettes, often depicting female figures, have been found. Less portable but no less impressive polychromatic cave paintings, for example of horses and bison, also began to appear, as did artifacts apparently meant to "support, defend, and amuse the deceased" in burials or otherwise (Ehrlich 2006, p. 170).

It is widely agreed that human beings by then had developed the capacity for spirituality and religious beliefs. Some say that without cultural belief systems to justify or at least make sense of the tragedies and trials that inevitably accompany human life cycles, the anxiety that must have accompanied humanity's increasing intelligence and self-awareness would have been too much to bear. In addition to providing a means to mitigate existential angst, culture provided a mechanism for achieving social cohesion: ritual, which Goldschmidt terms the "language of sentiment" (2006, p. 40). Rather than simply instructing, ritual motivates. It entices our cultural commitment. Ritual coerces through its ability to mobilize emotions (see also Durkheim 1915).

When human groups grew larger and cultural adaptations more complex, we began to need devices "to create the emotional cohesion that makes for effective and continued collaboration and to reduce tensions between potentially hostile persons and groups" (Goldschmidt 2006, p. 40). With the capacity to make music and partake of other sensory stimuli, humans now had the ability to convene "multimedia events that could make everybody involved feel the same way about whatever the group [needed] to feel about" (p. 40). How? According to Goldschmidt, ritual transfers feelings between people the way that mirror neurons aid motor imitation—it transfers "not information about feeling, but the feeling itself" (p. 41).

In sum, ritual is the "cultural invention that made culture work" (Goldschmidt 2006, p. 41). What it ultimately expresses is not factual, like information on where the best fruit can be found and what time of day it should be gathered (although that might be expressed too), but emotional, for instance regarding the family, kindred, or tribal solidarity created when we pick this fruit and eat it together. It is not the explicit messages that, for example, "Turtles are our clan's totem" or "This is the American flag" that are of the most import but rather the viscerally felt confirmation that "Our clan [or society] is a wonderful group to which we should be loyal." Feelings are paramount. Paradoxically, as Goldschmidt notes, imagination and sentiment are essential social catalysts for us humans, although we so often focus on our rational intelligence as the thing that makes us special (p. 42).

/ LEVERAGING EMOTION

The implication for anthropologically informed HSR goes something like this. Humans are story-telling animals: They need to tell stories to stay connected to social network members and cultural goals (among other things). Stories, like rituals, activate emotions or passions that can stay these connections. In effect, we can think of stories as mini-ritual acts, or as a subcomponent of the ritual that is the policy-making meeting (see also Bailey 1983 regarding the anthropology of meetings). Stories also, of course, can help investigators understand and explain—and devise plans to remedy or even to spread—patterns of thought and action that lead to better or worse health outcomes. That is why I am taking pains here to ensure that we understand how and why stories work. When we understand this, we can see how important it is to so carefully study them.

Stories make us feel things. Good stories resonate with listeners, generating emotional responses. Which of us has not shed tears while listening to a human-interest story on the radio or reading newspaper reports about families harmed in the latest acts of senseless global violence?

Indeed, the power of narrative is so great that even the most obvious fiction actually can, when well-crafted, evoke *real* feelings. We really do feel grief, anguish, joy, exhilaration, and the like when watching movies like *Terms of Endearment* and *Brief Encounter*—or, for that matter, *Star Wars* and *Gladiator* (Worhol 1992).

Because they make us feel things, in health care arenas stories can function like rituals do for cultural groups. But wait, someone may say, having read the works of British social anthropology's founding figures Bronislaw Malinowski and Alfred Reginald Radcliffe-Brown: Ritually told myths and legends function to remind people why the status quo is good and to reinforce the existing social structure or order. They form part of higher order collections of stories, practices, and rationalizations termed **discourses**, which are institutionalized and thereby dominative ways of thinking and acting. For instance, the monogamy and wisdom narratives mentioned previously tapped into gender discourses, particularly those regarding heterosexual relationship expectations.

Discourses can serve the same function as ritually told stories, evoking emotion-laced commitments to one's culture or community. But they do so much more pervasively and implicitly when they become internalized and habitual or assumed. For example, health discourses that favor the use of purgatives to unplug blockages in the body and thereby effect healing reinforce social norms that favor an uninhibited flow of goods and services between kin rather than supporting individual accumulations of wealth (e.g., Sobo 1993a; Taylor 1992). Similarly, the use of dye to cover graying hair in some societies reinforces normative assumptions about the value of youth, the future, and things brand new as well as the worthlessness of age and of the past—assumptions so powerful in some communities that the question is not whether someone might be dyeing his or her hair to affect a youthful visage, but why, despite the various costs entailed, anyone would fail to do so. Where the discourse on aging is positive and elders garner respect, younger people strive to affect the signs of age instead.

In any case, the viewpoint regarding the socially reinforcing nature of storytelling (and cultural discourses) is termed "functionalism" or, more specifically, "structural functionalism." And stories do do this. But not always and not completely.

Stories also may be told to gain individual goals or to help a faction meet strategic (and generally power-related) aims. In this, they can bring about change rather than maintain stasis. For instance, in one village in India members of the Pano Untouchable caste instigated a "nearer-to-chaos imbroglio" by introducing a new story (or, actually, suggesting a new discourse) regarding their right to full citizenship; this eventually came to pass when the hierarchy of caste was replaced by democracy in

India (Bailey 2001). In other communities, people have reinterpreted or altered origin stories to justify the legitimacy of their claims, for example, that certain behaviors are necessary (or the opposite), or that certain parties should (or may never) rule the group. Some have justified racism by pointing to passages in their religious community's holy texts or scriptures. Others have justified claims to power and authority by tracing their lineages to the ancestral creator's and, in the process, erasing others' claims to such a birthright. The penchant for rewriting the historical story so that it suits present political needs seems to be universal.

Stories can vitalize group commitment—whether to what is known or to a new way of thinking or acting. Moreover, when concretely nonfictional and when repeated in a situation in which action is expected, such as at a meeting of health-care decision-makers, the feelings stories conjure can be attached to goals and made motivational. In other words, the emotions they generate can drive action, concurrently leading listeners to organize their knowledge in a different way than they did before hearing the story. Storytelling can thus be a "powerful and formal discipline for organizational change and knowledge management" (Denning 2001, back cover). They are repositories of meaning with directive force.

In sum, stories are integral to culture. Stories and the meanings they index or serve as placeholders for are, to rephrase this chapter's key assertions, crucial components of what anthropologically informed HSR collects and analyzes. They must be both carefully investigated and treated so as to maintain their integrity if the study of stories, enacted or retold, is to yield actionable findings. They must not be converted unthinkingly into numbers alone or inadvertently lost in the translation process that accompanies the dissemination of research findings. But before turning to these challenges, a firmer historical and epistemological foundation is needed.

PART II

The Lay of the Land

Part I examined the value of meaning as well as exploring, in preliminary form, the anthropological approach and the culture concept. Here, we begin to take direct stock of the landscape that anthropologically informed health services research (HSR, including nursing research, etc.) both functions within and hopes to reveal in meaningful ways. We do this by taking an inventory of medical anthropology and the health services, and of various ways that, for better and for worse, they have heretofore interacted. Anthropologists and health services professionals may be tempted to skip ahead. However, one of my aims in this text is to bridge these two worlds, and I have tried to present this material in a way that focuses on nuances crucial to the project at hand. In other words, even professionals will benefit from the perspective taken in Chapters 3 and 5. All should read Chapters 4 and 6 quite closely. They warn of certain conceptually based pitfalls that truly anthropologically informed HSR protects against.

Although Chapters 1 and 2 introduced the anthropological approach and established a precedent for reliance on stories for meaning-centered data, Chapter 3 explains what medical anthropology in particular entails and offers; it also reviews some of the relevant history of this and the larger anthropological field so that readers seeking to apply an anthropological approach in their research and practice can lay fair claim to really knowing what such an approach is all about.

Chapter 4 specifically explores practice of anthropologically informed HSR. It establishes the difference between doing medical anthropology in HSR and doing studies of the health services using an anthropological perspective. In the first case, HSR's categories are taken for granted; in the second, they are not. Allowing researchers the space to pull back or widen the angle of inquiry beyond HSR's categories allows for the generation of unique and helpful anthropologically informed insights.

The chapter also explores various definitions of ethnography, arguing against its reduction to time-limited and otherwise circumscribed qualitative protocols but also demonstrating that the purist take on what counts as ethnography is, in our case, an irrelevant and distracting question. Of more importance is that investigators who allow themselves to reflect on a project in context, as it unfolds—and who attend to types of data that are frequently classified as "noise" or "merely situational and superfluous"—can arrive at valid ethnographic-like insights.

Further, if a linked series of projects is undertaken in a given research setting or with a given population, investigators can capitalize on a long-term build-up of experiences that, although officially outside of each given data collection plan, can be used to comprise an ethnographic understanding of the host organization or community. Bringing past experience to bear on data collected in each subsequent project and adopting a holistic, systems-oriented, comparative approach makes such undertakings anthropologically informed, whether or not they are considered "truly" ethnographic.

Having established, in Chapter 4, our foundational knowledge regarding the anthropological approach, we do the same for health services, with the quick tour offered in Chapter 5. In addition to describing the basic components of health services, this chapter provides insight into their sociocultural construction.

In Chapter 6, we critically examine the cultural competence movement in health services. We do this to gain an understanding of how the health services have generally handled culture, a core anthropological construct. Chapter 6 deconstructs the concept after outlining the problems that the cultural competence movement arose to ostensibly address—health inequities. It establishes the need for sophistication in deploying the culture concept as well as the sister terms "race" and "ethnicity" in addressing health inequities. It helps substantiate the claim made previously that there is much more to medical anthropology than advising organizations about non-Western traditions.

CHAPTER 3

Medical Anthropology: An Agenda

BACKGROUND KNOWLEDGE

In this chapter, we trace the history of medical anthropology and explore its present dominion, providing just enough background to fully prepare medical anthropology novices for the methodological work to come. Thus, the following pages include a concise examination of some of the subdiscipline's rudimentary concepts as well as of the links between medical anthropology and health care improvement. For further reading, I refer readers to any of the good, recently published medical anthropology textbooks (e.g., Pool and Geissler 2005; Singer and Baer 2007), or the textbook I coauthored with medical sociologist Martha Loustanau (Loustaunau and Sobo 1997; Sobo and Loustaunau Forthcoming). Carolyn Sargent and Tom Johnson's edited collection (1996) will provide a good overview for more advanced readers.

History of Anthropological Health Research

Although anthropologists have long been interested in issues pertaining to health, it was not until the end of World War II that a specialization in what is now called "medical anthropology" began to emerge. This was largely through the impetus and support built from foundation- and government-funded applied work in the arena of international public health. The data collected by anthropologists in earlier times for non-medical purposes were invaluable; anthropologists helped ensure that social and cultural aspects of health and healing were taken into account in ways that promoted health program success (Foster and Anderson 1978, pp. 7–8).

The incorporation of anthropology in international public health efforts called for a distinctly applied orientation, and medical anthropology was greatly influenced by this. Byron Good (1994) refers to medical anthropology in the 1960s as a "practice discipline," dedicated to the service of improving public health of societies in economically poor nations. Indeed, initial efforts at organizing a medical anthropology interest group occurred in the late 1960s under the auspices of the Society for Applied Anthropology (Todd and Ruffini 1979).

In 1971, the medical anthropology interest group decided instead on an affiliation with the dominant anthropological association in the United States, the American Anthropological Association (AAA), and is now known as the Society for Medical Anthropology (SMA). Although this move firmly anchored the group within academic anthropology, the influence of applied perspectives remained strong. From the viewpoint of those seeking practical solutions to specific health problems, theory seemed abstract, obstructive, and sometimes even irrelevant. The authority of medical culture, where curative work and saving lives takes precedence, was manifest (Singer 1992).

Medical anthropology has grown dramatically since the early days, partly because of increased opportunities for applied medical anthropologists. But perhaps more importantly, nonapplied anthropologists interested in health saw that they, too, had something to gain by identifying themselves as "medical" anthropologists. For some, a key benefit was access to a community of scholars with a common interest in health issues—as well as health-related data from diverse cultures that might be shared. For others, the benefits included increased credibility in medicine and easier access to medical workers and organizations. (For more on the debates about the medical anthropology appellation, see Sobo 2004b and Good 1994, p. 4.)

What Is Health?

Anthropologists generally consider health as a broad construct, consisting of physical, psychological, and social well-being, including role functionality. Such a definition works much better cross-culturally than one that links health only to **disease**, a term that refers specifically to medically measurable lesions or anatomical or physiological irregularities. Disease is something that is either cured or not. But in part because it can be present without being realized, disease itself does not spur people to seek medical treatment; illness does. **Illness** is the culturally structured, personal experience of being unwell and it entails suffering of some kind. The main goal of most people seeking medical treatment is to have their suffering removed. Illness thus underwrites the entire medical enterprise (Hahn 1984, p. 17; see also Mechanic 1962).

Illness can refer to a variety of conditions cross-culturally. In some cultures, it is limited to somatic (bodily) experiences; in others, it includes mental dysfunction; and in others, it also includes suffering because of misfortune. That is, some medical systems deal with human struggles related to love, work, finances, etc. Social, somatic, emotional, and cognitive troubles often are not separated at all but quite intertwined and even fused together.

This underscores a major criticism of the disease-illness dichotomy: that it recapitulates the mind-body dichotomy that medicine has been criticized for trafficking in. Disease, as the dichotomy defines it, is anchored in the body; conversely, illness may be seen as anchored in the mind. Disease is thus attributed a real, concrete, scientific factuality or objectivity that illness, as a subjective category, may be denied (Hahn 1984).

A second criticism of the dichotomy is that both disease and illness are located in the individual or experienced at an individual level. The term "illness" does refer to an individual's social relations, but generally it does so only insofar as these were the cause of the illness, as when an offended party places a hex, or as the illness leaves the individual unable to fulfill social or role obligations. Some scholars would link suffering more palpably to the social order by examining how macro-social forces, processes, and events (such as capitalist trade arrangements) can culminate in public health problems (such as HIV/AIDS, tuberculosis, alcoholism, or pesticide-induced anomalous pregnancy outcomes) and poorly functioning health systems (see Baer, Singer, and Johnson 1986; Waitzkin 2000).

Taking their cue from this movement, most anthropologists have heeded the call to link individual illness experience with social context, at least to some degree. Further, although illness may be defined mentalistically in opposition to physical disease, in more recent anthropological work this simplification has met rejection; illness is conceived as affecting the whole person, body included (e.g., Mol 2002). The disease-illness distinction thereby retains contemporary currency, although the term "sickness" may be used when the distinction is not important (e.g., Young 1983) or when larger social processes are being highlighted (e.g., Frankenberg and Leeson 1976).

Seeking Health

Much medical anthropology focuses on what people do when they fall ill. In all cultures, the household is the key unit in therapy seeking; members influence one another's care either directly, through resource allocation and care provision, or indirectly, through examples set and care plans recommended. In various ways in various cultures, individual problems are linked to the well-being of the group, and the group may therefore actually organize individual care. The less individualistic a culture is and the more it promotes a socially linked self, the more whole groups themselves may be seen as being in need of therapy. In some cultures, an entire group (the extended family, for example) may be seen as the patient and healing intra-group conflicts may be part of the treatment regime (Janzen 1978).

Although for some conditions, only one form of treatment will be necessary, this is not always the case. There exists a stepped "hierarchy of resort" (Romanucci-Ross 1977 [1969]) in which people first try one thing and then try another until their condition is fixed to their satisfaction. When it was first introduced, the hierarchy concept related **patterns of resort** (the patterned treatment choices people make) to acculturation issues. However, the phrase is often used today to mean that people try the most familiar, simplest, and cheapest treatment first and resort to more expensive, complex, or unfamiliar treatments later, if necessary.

Treatment choice can follow a hierarchical or stepwise sequence, but patterns of resort often involve many types of treatment in parallel or pluralistically, at once. Further, people do not necessarily adhere to all the official rules related to each type of treatment. They often combine recommendations creatively, creating personalized regimens that they feel are right for them. Health seeking is a dynamic process; people constantly reevaluate their symptoms and revise their health care plans (Chrisman 1977).

Of course, before people can begin to seek care they must recognize the need for it. Symptom recognition is generally the first step in what Noel Chrisman (1977) long ago termed "the health seeking process."

Technically speaking, a **symptom** is anything that indicates to the individual that something is not right in his or her body or being. Perceived chills, nausea, pain, or shortness of breath might count. In Jamaica, and in Britain, people who felt ill often told me that they felt "low." As opposed to a symptom, an indication of unwellness that has official recognition through some form of medical measurement, such as a documented fever, is, in medical terms, a **sign**. Medical information tracts regarding various diseases generally include a section called "signs and symptoms." Signs may matter if an individual seeks care from the health services system; but for now, symptoms are our main concern.

Symptom recognition depends on cultural definitions of normal wellbeing and cultural understandings about the causes and contexts of sickness. Because of cross-cultural differences, symptoms are not always grouped together in the same way in all cultures. However grouped, some of the important factors that people in all cultures consider when evaluating symptoms include how dangerous to life they might be and the degree to which they interfere with lifestyle or function. Also considered are the visibility and frequency of the symptoms in others and the way this compares to their visibility and frequency in the ill individual.

Another important aspect of health seeking is preventive behavior. Again, symptom recognition is important, as is recognition that a given condition's long-term health costs outweigh the immediate social, cultural, economic, and other benefits of nonpreventive behavior. This depends on the meaning of those benefits in cultural context and any effort at health education and prevention intervention must take this into account (e.g., Sobo 1995). Research also has shown the importance of keeping in mind popular interpretations of how new medical technology or pharmacology works, and indigenous methods for knowledge transfer, which may take place through plays or songs (see Nichter and Nichter 1996). That is, our way of patient education may not be effective out of context.

Medical Systems Cross-Culturally

What people do for health depends to a large degree on how they understand illness's causes or **etiology**. Early ethnology, which focused on cross-cultural contrasts and comparisons, was accordingly interested in etiological or causal schemes, and a great deal of effort went into categorizing these.

One simple model cast illness as either internalizing or externalizing. **Internalizing systems** focus on **proximate** or immediate physiological mechanisms, such as the actual germs, poisons, or spirits infesting, say, the bowels. They give primacy to biological or physical signs that can mark a disease's progression (Young 1986 [1976]). In internalizing schemes, an ailment is an individual problem, not a social problem. In contrast, **externalizing systems** ascribe importance to events outside of the ill individual's body. Such systems view pathogens (germs) as purposive; they are often human or anthropomorphized (rendered in humanlike terms). Diagnostic activity focuses on discovering what brought the now ill individual to the pathogenic agent's attention, provoking the attack to begin with. Externalizing systems focus on **ultimate** causes, not proximate ones. That is, they focus on the far end of the chain of causality rather than whatever is most immediate. The jealous ancestral spirit that causes a person to trip over a protruding root while walking down a path is to blame—not the root itself or that person's weak ankles or careless manner.

Using the externalizing-internalizing model, Allan Young offers some interesting suggestions regarding the evolution of health systems. He holds that internalizing systems evolve from externalizing systems when societies grow complex (1986 [1976]).

Externalizing systems focus on social and cosmological relations. They are interlinked with other cultural domains, such as religion, and have little conceptual autonomy (Young 1986 [1976]). Many scholars have noted that, in small-scale societies, beliefs about illness etiology generally connect with beliefs about all kinds of misfortune, including interpersonal conflicts and geological disasters. But internalizing systems are highly autonomous. So, for example, health is treated as separate from legal or religious issues. Young explains this in relation to the division of labor seen in complex societies.

In small-scale societies, specialization is uncommon and the division of labor is low. Young (1986 [1976]) argues that this explains the overlap between healing and other cultural domains in small-scale groups. Large-scale societies have complex labor division patterns that include specialization and engender distinctions between cultural domains. The conceptual autonomy of internalizing systems is linked to this. The fragmentation of cultural realms in large-scale societies supports internalizing systems, which focus on the body, paying little heed to legal, religious, and other dimensions of life.

Today, many people in complex social systems do draw lines of connection, acknowledging global or even just national or local capitalism as the ultimate cause of illness (for instance in coal miners' lung disease). Even so, because biomedicine dominates, the cures they most often practice are proximately focused. There is generally no sense that an external force targeted them particularly or personally for attack. Their aliment may make them ill, but it is treated individualistically as a disease.

The contrast between naturalistic and personalistic medicine introduced by George Foster (1976), which focuses directly on social relations, is helpful here. **Naturalistic** models explain sickness as due to impersonal forces or conditions, including cold, heat, and other forces that upset the body's balance. **Personalistic** approaches, however, ascribe illness to active external agents. The agent involved in a given case may be human (such as a sorcerer), or nonhuman (such as an evil force or ancestral ghost). Accident or chance has no role in illness here as it does in naturalistic explanations: In personalistic systems, illness is the direct result of an agent's purposive act. Therefore, people need to be certain that their social relations, with the living and the dead and with deities and other agentic forces, are well maintained. If not, others may be provoked to take actions leading to one's ill health.

Although etiological questions do have importance, categorization can also rest on the organizational characteristics of the systems in question. For example, medical systems can be categorized as either accumulating or diffusing systems according to whether they entail accumulated, formalized teachings or, rather, encourage the fragmentation of medical knowledge (Young 1983). Practitioners in **diffusing systems** generally do not communicate with one another; their knowledge is often secretly held. **Accumulating systems**, on the other hand, amass knowledge, generally in written form. Knowledge is shared at conferences and through professional associations and formal training institutions. U.S. health services medicine, Chinese medicine, and Ayurveda (practiced in India and elsewhere) are examples of accumulating systems.

Oversimplification and Other Dangers

Some controversy surrounds the fact that all of the categorization schemes discussed previously are **etic**; meant to be universally applicable, they are imposed from the outside onto the cultures in question. Yet from the **emic** or insider perspective, the distinctions they index are unimportant. Moreover, they support enforced categorization with central contrasts or binary oppositions.

Many would argue that it is a mistake if not outright intellectual laziness to cast medical systems as simply one or the other of a given contrasting pair. In Chapter 6, I discuss the danger that doing this has for diverting attention from the complex causes and consequences of health inequities (see also Farmer 2005). But here, my focus is on the fact that the contrasts just described should be thought of as occupying a *continuum*, with each system containing some of each emphasis. When determining a classification, the researcher must ask not which ideal type a given system represents but which of a given contrasting emphasis is most salient or primary in that system. So, for example, although care in the dominative U.S. medical system may entail some personalistic touches (for instance, a physician may refer to an outcome as being "in the hands of God"), the overarching emphasis is naturalistic and for that reason it is classified as such.

On the other hand, not all systems will be easily classifiable, because some systems explicitly accept both aspects of a contrast and focus on either one depending on the illness or condition in question. Take, for example, the intrusion versus extrusion contrast offered by Forrest Clements in 1932. This model contrasts the bodily **intrusion** of substances or essences to the **extrusion** of such as the cause of illness. Extrusion would include, for example, soul loss, or the loss of blood, or even the nonabsorption or leaching of nutrients, as with diarrhea. In intrusion-caused illnesses, on the other hand, noxious substances (such as poisons, germs, or evil spirits) pierce or infiltrate the body's barriers. Illness from bleeding and from soul loss are classified together in this model as extrusive; germs and evil spirits are both categorized as intrusive—although treatment for germ- or spirit-caused illness can differ. In any case, one medical system can allow for both intrusion and extrusion illnesses. So the question is not always which of a given contrast dominates but how the two are linked together and under which *circumstances* one or the other predominates.

Further, medical systems typically entail subsystems, both professional and organizational. The National Health System in England, for instance, comprises several administrative bodies and separate trusts or groups for primary care and public health, hospitals, mental health, and ambulance services. As in the U.S. system, professional groups include not only medicine but also nursing, social work, occupational therapy, dentistry, human resources, food services, and so on. Achieving care coordination as well as continuity of care over time can be problematic when the relationships between subsystems are complex.

Dominative medicine is not alone in its complexity. Most medical systems entail a diverse array of practitioners. These can include herbalists, chemists, surgeons, bone setters or body workers, midwives, sorcerers, priests, and shamans (Loustaunau and Sobo 1997). Their work—and their understandings of how health is produced, maintained, compromised, and best regained—may or may not overlap. All things being equal, in the U.S. system a surgeon's approach to cancer favors removal; a medical doctor's or internist's approach will favor chemotherapy. For more regarding the differences between medical and surgical doctors, see Chapter 5.

Here, it is worth noting that not all medical systems are actually all that systematized. Sometimes, what is referred to as a "system" is only weakly aggregated. Care must be taken to avoid using labels (e.g., "externalizing system," "the indigenous system") in a way that fosters the impression that a culture's loosely assembled set of health-related beliefs and practices is actually highly systematized.

If a continuum runs between tightly and loosely coupled systems, when does a loosely coupled medical system fall off the far end? When can we stop counting such an aggregate as one loosely coupled system and start counting it as several distinct systems? This question has not been sufficiently considered as yet, but the answer may lie in the degree to which the various components compete with each other for clients.

Generally speaking, in a tightly coupled system with specialized practitioners, an agreed-on division of labor exists, such as between a given patient's surgeon, internist, nurses, and physical therapist—all of whom consider themselves part of the patient's care team. The looser the system, the less practitioners interact and the less they share information regarding patient histories. Although at least in theory different parts of the system serve different needs, a looser system's left hand knows very little of what the right hand does. The looser the system, the less consensus there may be regarding which types of practitioners can best serve the patient at hand. And, generally speaking, when things reach the point at which various types of practitioners see each other as competitors who would fix the same problem quite differently, two or more distinct systems probably exist. When separate systems coexist under the same government, we have a **plural system**.

Within-System Distinctions

One common typology describing complex medical systems is the tripartite scheme of popular, folk, and professional medicine (Kleinman 1978). The key variables are: Who provides care and in what context. In the **popular** sector, nonspecialists like oneself or one's mother, friends, or other kin and relations provide treatment. Treatment is based on shared cultural understandings and generally occurs in a family or household context—and never for a fee. **Folk** sector healers are specialists; their practice is based on cultural traditions and philosophies. Legally sanctioned official systems make up the **professional** sector.

This three-part scheme is an advance on simple public-private dichotomizing, in which private or household care is separated from care provided within the formal health care system, and often discounted. But the three-part typology—which is known in some health services circles and so worth discussing here—does have an unanticipated shortcoming in relation to its potential for cross-cultural application: Although it specifically allows that some nonbiomedical practices, such as Ayurvedic or traditional Chinese medicine, should be classed as professional medicine because of their routinized, formalized, professionalized nature, this is easily forgotten by those who view these therapeutic modalities as so-called folk practices.

Bonnie O'Connor's model (1995) has only two parts: conventional medicine and vernacular medicine. **Vernacular** medicine subsumes Kleinman's (1978) folk and popular sectors; **conventional** medicine consists only of the official, authorized, authoritative, dominative health care industry or system—whatever that may be in a given cultural context. The contrast is simple but important, because it explicitly highlights the dominative position held by conventional medicine (seen in the fact that we just call it "medicine" in this book). The power dynamics and medical status hierarchy that O'Connor's model reflects are, to at least some extent, universal (all systems have conventional medicine of some kind).

Of course, classifying systems is not the ultimate goal of medical anthropology. Classifications are helpful only as they propel theoretical contributions to the field or make helpful action possible.

/ MEDICAL ANTHROPOLOGY AT HOME

Areas of Inquiry

Medical anthropology frequently is associated only with work done "over there" or with international health (meaning public health efforts aimed at alleviating diseases of the poor). Thus, and although many of the classification schemes and concepts already described were generated by comparisons between other ways of medicine and our own, the local application of medical anthropology often slips from notice. Notwithstanding, the interests of medical anthropologists today are varied and wide and many carry out research in their home countries.

Medical and popular social representations of the body and of disease have received a good deal of attention from medical anthropologists. For example, many have studied the differing ways in which medical and scientific rhetorics has, across time, anchored popular theories of gender in the body. Emily Martin's 1987 analysis of just this, and of the ways that women actually experience their embodied selves, spurred my own move into the subfield.

Anthropology's keen interest in embodiment also has included a focus on body size and shape. For instance, Mimi Nichter examined whether, how, and why adolescents from various backgrounds talked about weight and dieting. White girls, especially, tended to engage in what Nichter termed "fat talk"—ritualistic chat about bodies that, in demonstrating ample concern with weight and diet, both promoted solidarity and diminished girls' immediate needs, if any, for weight-related behavior change (2000).

More recently, chronic care has received much scrutiny. This is because of the increases recently seen in many chronic illness categories as part of the world's epidemiological transition away from infectious disease. The present health services system's historically derived acute care orientation leaves medicine ill prepared in some ways to cope with the needs of those who require chronic care (e.g., Manderson and Smith-Morris Forthcoming).

The ways in which people come to experience their bodies according to how they are brought up to believe that their bodies work and should feel or function has been another very productive topic for exploration. For example, Margaret Lock's research (2002) demonstrates that, despite being technologically advanced and subscribing to the same dominative medical system that we do (biomedicine), Japan has been very slow to take up the practice of organ transplantation in comparison to the speed with which the field grew in Canada and the United States. Although on the whole North Americans tend to view the brain or mind as the seat of the person and so can tolerate the idea of keeping a brain-dead cadaver's heart beating and lungs breathing so that organs might be kept healthy enough to be transferred to another body, Japanese people tend to view the person as diffused throughout the body and therefore find it difficult to cast the brain-dead person as truly dead. For these and other reasons (see also Chapter 8), organ transplantation or—to use Leslie Sharp's more socially accurate expression—"organ transfer" (2006) is not a common practice in Japan.

Issues related to the therapeutic patient-practitioner alliance have been perennially popular topics of inquiry for ethnographers, who have long been interested in psychological aspects of health and in the social and cultural context of medical knowledge and practice. Numerous studies have investigated the healing role of storytelling and the impact of illness on identity as well as the ways that professionally dominated knowledge and practice patterns are socially established, maintained, and expressed or negotiated—or subverted—during patient-practitioner interaction. For instance, Athena McLean's work with nursing home staff and residents shows how resident elders' refusal to tolerate demeaning or dehumanizing treatment, often demonstrated by withdrawal or noncooperative and sometimes disruptive behavior, is cast by providers as medically rooted rather than socioculturally generated and therefore treated by pharmaceutical means. In addition to identifying this practice, McLean describes the performance pressures on staff members and cultural features that help underwrite them (2007).

As McLean's work suggests, **medicalization**—the extension of medicine's authority into what were once nonmedical realms and the conversion of what were once normal human ailments or social problems into medical diseases, and the resulting (medical) regulation of everyday life—has continued appeal as a framework for anthropological health studies. Studies of women's health issues, perhaps especially investigations into the medicalization of pregnancy and birth, were central to the growth of this area of research (Inhorn [2006] provides an interpretive meta-analysis of this literature). For instance, Carolyn Sargent and Nancy Stark have investigated how the information imparted in childbirth classes, as well as the ways that it is imparted, can help reinforce particular orientations toward childbirth, including socioculturally supported preferences for intervention. As a result, for example, many women have positive responses to Cesarean deliveries or interpret the "elimination of feeling by means of epidural anesthesia" as "the ultimate definition of control in delivery" (Sargent and Stark 1989).

With childbirth now such a well-established arena of inquiry, recent investigations of technological intervention and medicalization have broadened. Diagnostic categories such as attention deficit hyperactivity disorder (ADHD) and male sexual or erectile dysfunction (ED) have recently commanded much attention. A 2006 satire regarding disease mongering, in which scholars introduced the spoof disease "motivational deficiency disorder"—otherwise known as extreme laziness—also is illuminating (Moynihan 2006). The increased role that medical consumers and pharmaceutical corporations can play today in the process of medicalization is concurrent with recent attenuations of medicine's power, for example, through the imposition of oversight by health maintenance organizations (HMOs) and the rise of practice guidelines (see Chapter 8).

Corporations remain, however, much more powerful than consumers in the health care game. Medical anthropology today is astutely aware of how profit motives and global capitalist arrangements shape health outcomes, drawing our attention to the political economy's role in this, especially (but not only) for the poor. For example, although many have chronicled the ways in which national and regional as well as global fiscal and military policies—particularly (but not only) those of the United States—underwrote the rise of HIV/AIDS and associated conditions in particular populations (e.g., Farmer 2005; Singer 1998), others have examined the reach that pharmaceutical representatives have into U.S. physicians' prescribing practices (Oldani 2004).

In this context, the pluralistic approach that many patients take to their own health and the impact of the latter on medicine is an increasingly important area of inquiry. Thus, self-care—either as an adjunct or supplement to medical care, as an alternative when medicine fails to meet people's needs, or for cases of un- and under-insurance and when people feel as if they have "no time to be sick" (Vuckovic 1999)—has received increasing scrutiny. Explorations of medical tourism, in which people travel out of their home countries for medical and surgical services, also fit in this area. The organizational aspects of the failure of systems to meet people's needs, already of concern within international health circles, promises to become a more popular area for inquiry as medical anthropology's alliance with HSR at home begins to burgeon. It is to this alliance that we now turn.

CHAPTER 4

/ Anthropology in and of
Health Services

CLOSING IN

A number of disciplines share many of anthropology's goals and methods
for research on culture and meaning, at least to some degree. However,
none push the centrality of holism and cross-cultural comparison quite
so far as anthropology. Having defined medical anthropology's purview
in the last chapter, here we examine more directly how anthropological
ideas can be applied productively to and in health services.

First, we look at various definitions of ethnography, comparing traditional or orthodox with contemporary field contexts and demonstrating
that the purist take on what counts as ethnographic distracts attention
from what counts as anthropologic and, moreover, from the value added
by an anthropologically informed approach. In the course of this discussion, medical anthropology's need to push the health services to examine
its own indigenous categories and assumptions is established, as is the
value of reflecting on one's program of research itself, and the research
process, for contextualizing data. The chapter ends with several examples
of studies that successfully and productively apply the anthropologically
informed approach to solve particular problems in health services.

DOING ETHNOGRAPHY

The Need for a Common Vocabulary

In 1999, while being interviewed for my job at Children's, someone
suggested—indeed, guaranteed me the option—that as part of my duties
I could undertake an ethnographic study of the organization. This
sounded wonderful. However, as I later learned, this interviewer had no
idea what ethnography entailed—at least not as I had learned to define
it. But within the health services research (HSR) context, the promise
made sense precisely because the definition it referenced was different
from mine.

My four year old is fond of telling his grammatically correct father, "You say it your way, I'll say it mine." This holds not only for pronunciation and syntax but semantic questions as well. However sweet this approach may be in a preschooler, it does not work so well for researchers.

Agreeing to disagree or allowing others to define terms as they have come to be defined in their disciplines only works when disciplines never comingle. However, disciplinary borders are porous. Moreover, inter-disciplinarity is a prerequisite for most HSR (see Chapter 9 regarding teamwork) and it is definitely required if findings from anthropologically informed HSR are to be broadcast beyond anthropological quarters. Successful interdisciplinarity demands a common vocabulary.

After Humpty Dumpty said rather scornfully to Alice in Chapter 6 of Lewis Carroll's *Through the Looking Glass*, "When I use a word it means just what I choose it to mean—neither more nor less," she asked him whether he actually could "make words mean so many different things." His reply was to state that she was asking the wrong question; rather, he said, "The question is: which is to be master—that's all." To answer the question of which definition should be authoritative, we must first ask: Which definition of ethnography adds the most value to our work within HSR? As a prerequisite, we must explore the various definitions already in play.

A Brief History of Loss

Ethnography emerged in anthropology and comparative sociology as part of the toolkit by which we would study other cultures. As H. Russell (Russ) Bernard has written, "Any method [or approach] that seems useful will get picked up and tried out, sooner or later, across the disciplines" (1998, p. 13). However, it may not be picked up whole and, even if it is, it may undergo change in its new incarnation. This is what happened to ethnography.

As generally happens when practices migrate, the ethnographic approach (defined in Chapter 1, along with its main method, participant observation) changed in new surroundings. It was adapted, mostly through a narrowing of scope, to the new tasks it was put to. Long-term, immersion-based participant observation dropped out of the ethnographic equation in some investigational arenas, HSR included.

One reason for this is that in the health services, as in other fields, research must receive institutional review board (IRB) approval to ensure that ethical standards are upheld (see Chapter 5). Health services IRBs are set up to expect and are used to receiving firm, circumscribed, highly detailed protocols regarding data collection, including number of subjects, time frames, and prepared data collection forms such as prewritten surveys or interview question lists. Participant observation, which requires flexibility as well as a refusal of a priori etic categories, fits very poorly in this context; it was not often proposed in HSR and even when it was, it commonly did not receive IRB approval. For this and related reasons, it was simply not imported with the ethnographic package. Yet, just as my grandma called the refrigerator the "ice box" until the day she died, some in HSR continue to call the narrower form of naturalistic study that did survive "ethnography." Indeed, in some cases, only the word "ethnography" survived; that is, some call qualitative data collection and analysis ethnography because of the family resemblance. Much ethnography is indeed qualitative. And yet, without immersion of any kind, a key process for doing ethnography does appear to be missing.

Pamela Brink and Nancy Edgecombe lament the redefinition of ethnography in this way as a "bastardization of research design" (2003, p. 1028). They complain quite rightly that, for example, asking nurses questions in focus groups or individual interviews does not, in itself, constitute ethnographic research—although it is sometimes represented as such.

Brink and Edgecombe also point up another offending practice: Some label a study "ethnographic" simply because a "culturally distinct population" is involved (2003, p. 1028). Paul Farmer has denounced the undue focus on culture as the cause of ill health as "anthro lite" (Farmer 2005; see also Chapter 6). In like fashion, what we are talking about here might be referred to as "ethnography lite." Not only is this form of ethnography less fulfilling than what traditionalists would term "the real thing," it also may mislead health services professionals to disregard ethnography and so anthropology's full potential as well as, again, to blame culture for problems caused by processes ongoing in other sectors of human existence.

But without certain key features, research—even qualitative research, naturalistic research, and research with distinct populations—is not actually ethnographic. What are these key features? In Chapter 1, I said that ethnography (or, ethnographic methodology) "highlights context and seeks to situate all findings, whether qualitative or quantitative, within the fabric of daily life and the encompassing systems within which daily lives are lived." That is, it is holistic and applies systems thinking. Further, it honors emic or insider views, while at the same time acknowledging their constructed nature. In this, it is aided by a comparative perspective and participative immersion.

Keeping a Critical Distance

Anthropologists coming to HSR may know well the above stipulations. However, honoring them can be quite difficult when doing research in, for, and under the auspices of the health services. In Chapter 3, I noted medical anthropology's interest in medicalization: the extension of medicine's authority into what were once nonmedical realms, such as childbirth. As Carole Browner has noted, medical anthropology, too, can become medicalized; this happens when its practitioners lose touch with the principles of the mother discipline (1999).

The medicalization of medical anthropology is, Browner says, "one of the risks of 'going native'" when working within the health services (1999, p. 135). Browner respects the anthropologist's need to find a common language with which to communicate with colleagues in the health services and to adopt some of medicine's cultural practices, if only to gain credibility in that world. She understands the likelihood that many anthropologists will already to some extent have internalized medicine's categories because of their own reliance, at times, on the system. She wisely notes that our medical studies are inherently different to traditional cross-cultural ones. For one thing, the definition of community is different: We often study aspects of culture or partial cultures rather than whole ones (such as the Trobriand Islanders); concurrently, it is very difficult to achieve full immersion or to participate fully in some aspects of the world under study. But, Browner warns, one of the grave dangers of being medicalized—of being absorbed into HSR and of accepting medical categories as given—is the sacrifice of our "critical distance" (p. 137). **Critical distance** entails the ability to question categories from an outside or detached perspective; this promotes our recognition of their socioculturally constructed dimensions as well as of ways in which categories do and do not overlap across cultures.

Take, for instance, a study regarding abortion rates and practices. In Jamaica, women have abortions but they also practice menstrual regulation when a period is late—as any woman reading this knows it occasionally will be—even if fertilization and the implantation of a healthy embryo in the womb's wall has not occurred. Menstrual regulation removes the cause of the menstrual blockage by washing it out with herbal medicines (much as constipation is flushed through when treated with a dose of fiber and lots of drinking water). The "washout" purges the body of the potentially toxic menstrual blood build-up. An abortion study, framed from a medical perspective, might try to count menstrual regulation (if researchers even were told about it) with abortion. But to Jamaican men and women, this practice is of a different order entirely and, as such, they might not even mention it in the context of discussions with investigators regarding abortion (Sobo 1996a).

Another turn on medicalized medical anthropology would be framing malignant, aberrant pregnancies—seen locally in Jamaica as caused by witchcraft—as if they were stillbirths or miscarriages, or explaining that what a woman thought was a monster baby was really a molar pregnancy (an unviable embryo that grows without the genetic information necessary to take a human form) or was otherwise misconceived in the natural course of things. To do so forfeits an ocean of cultural meaning and culturally informed experience (Sobo 1996b).

In Melissa Parker and Ian Harper's opinion, the main problem with anthropology in health services (including public health, which is their focus) is that "research that sets out to generate data that fits within pre-existing categories embraced by the 'factorial' model frequently compromises what anthropology has to offer as a discipline" (2005, p. 2). In other words, it pulls experience to bits, focusing attention on parts rather than the whole. The factorial model separates health-related situations or experiences into discrete, static units or factors to be counted. It fails to acknowledge its own socioculturally situated and historically contingent nature and is further faulted because "it embraces conceptual splits that may be more misleading than they are helpful" (p. 1).

Building on Geertz's notion of convergent data (referred to in a 1983 Huxley Memorial Lecture) and invoking Marcel Mauss's idea of "totality" from *The Gift*, Michael Oldani also has commented on this (2004). He sees factorial scholarship such as can be found in medicalized medical anthropology as a "divergent" force that "limits our ability to conceptualize the 'totality' of everyday activities" (p. 332). Such activities are, Oldani argues in reference to his work on pharmaceutical sales, socially embedded, evolve over time, and refer to multiple goals.

Along the same lines, Parker and Harper argue that—and this is crucial—*culture should not be seen as just another factor or variable in a researcher-imposed equation*. Rather, "complex interpretive strategies" (2005, p. 4) should be applied. Further, although fidelity to a preapproved research protocol is sacrosanct in HSR, anthropological researchers should be free to redefine their questions and methods as the research moves along, if more interesting and important questions come to the fore.

Anthropology of—as opposed to in—health services is anthropology that takes such a path. It maintains that research should be an open-ended, iteratively interpretive process. Moreover, it keeps its critical distance (Browner 1999); it questions the health services frame of reference rather than simply accepting it as given. It is medical anthropology, not medicalized. But there still are differences between it and old-time ethnologic inquiry.

Farewell Malinowski?

I stand firm with others in demanding critical distance, primacy of the emic perspective, and holism or systems thinking in ethnography.

Justifiably making the claim to doing ethnography hinges on "observing what is going on while it is going on" (Brink and Edgecombe 2003, p. 1029). "Asking about what is being observed, while it is being observed" (p. 1028) also is important.

Having said that, ethnography so defined is not always possible. For example, sexual practices are not generally observed by ethnographers. Living at the study site also may not be desirable and, in fact, institutional powers may not permit it. For instance, researchers who work in crime-infested areas (where health problems commonly also are rampant) generally have home addresses elsewhere. Further, some places are institutionally difficult to enter, such as the trauma resuscitation room at Children's hospital (no visitors—not even parents—could be there while a resuscitation effort was ongoing, nor could video tapes be made because of a policy decision already in place).

Others also have noted the increasing frequency with which anthropological fieldwork in general has become partial and fragmented. For instance, Els van Dongen considers it in an essay entitled "Farewell to Fieldwork?" (2007). For his fieldwork with elders in South Africa's Western Cape Province, key limiting factors were violence and the need to travel between the sites where elders were rather than settling down in one single location. In this, his work differed essentially from that of, say, Bronislaw Malinowski, or any old-time anthropologist-ethnographer who might speak fondly of "my village."

However, in addition to differing dynamics, and the "day job" rhythm of his data collection efforts, van Dongen's fieldwork (and the fieldwork of countless others, myself included) differs, too, from the old-time ideal because our specific questions are not the same. Although Malinowski, Boas, and other anthropological ancestors were generally interested first and foremost in just getting things down—in recording other life ways—thanks to them and others, anthropologists today have a vast ethnographic record on hand to consult. That is, we are not starting from scratch and can often begin the immersion process through the literature before even getting to the field (this is absolutely essential for rapid assessments, as noted repeatedly in Part IV; and see Pelto and Pelto 1997).

Partly because such a grand ethnographic record exists, but also because of postmodernism's contribution to our conceptualization of culture (see Chapter 6), we now ask about culture not as a thing but as a process—a process that everyone everywhere partakes in. *Anthropology's disciplinary essence is maintained in our interest in culture and our methodological heritage.* But, rather than simply describing culture's actualization in practice, we are more interested now in how practice creates, maintains, and modifies culture to begin with; we are more interested than previously in how groups cope with the cultural milieus that humankind has created. We also now know that cultural discourses can be contradictory or even indeterminate and that cultures themselves are partial, porous, and articulated in complex webs of power and authority.

Indeed, in some ways our increasingly partial and itinerant anthropological work practices much better reflect our core construct culture's true complexity and flexibility. Do these practices constitute "real" ethnography? Perhaps not. But I think there is a better question to ask: Do they promote anthropological understanding? Are they, at the least, ethnographically informed? If they do not include the full-time, long-term immersion that really "being there" entails, do they at least include critical distance, prioritizing the emic perspective, and holism or systems thinking?

Is the Aim True?

In the early 1990s, I conducted a mixed-methods HIV/AIDS education and prevention study among inner-city women in Cleveland, Ohio (1995). The study included surveys as well as both interviews and focus groups (or, as I termed it originally, "focused discussion groups"), but no direct participant observation. I slept in my own home at night, in another part of town. I never ran into respondents on my home turf, although I often thought about them.

The interviews were fairly standard stuff: one-time meetings centering on the participant's responses to a number of open-ended questions pertaining to the topic at hand (see Chapter 11). The focus groups were different. Although focus groups, technically defined, meet once to discuss a focal topic (and see Chapter 10 for a fuller discussion of this method), each of the three groups in this study met once a week for four weeks. This allowed my main research assistant Margaret Ruble, her assistants, and me to establish some rapport with participants.

Moreover, the groups were not convened specifically for study purposes, as focus groups are meant to be; rather, they were parenting support groups that met anyhow, every week. Each group's members graciously agreed to participate in the research by considering my questions, instead of their usual agenda, over the course of four weeks. In other words, participants were known to each other and would have gathered anyway. However, as is typical with standard focus group research, I never went home with any of the participants.

Brink and Edgecombe do not mind "a little tinkering around the edges of a design" but they say that the "signature" must remain true if a project is to be described as ethnography per se (2003, p. 1030). I agree. Total immersion was impossible, and immersion beyond the clinic was not even attempted. So the work was not, technically speaking, ethnographic.

Most HSR cannot qualify as ethnography per se, simply because of the nature of what the communities under study are engaged in and the necessity for researchers to respect their workplace, health and rehabilitative, and sickroom and deathbed needs (see Chapter 9). Nonetheless, in the HIV/AIDS project my perspective was holistic; I was interested primarily in the sociocultural system that supported HIV/AIDS risk denial. I prioritized participants' perspectives and let them determine the direction the work did take. My point is: It may not have been traditionally ethnographic, but the work was anthropologically informed (as defined in Part I); anthropology's "signature" was valid.

Another example, but a different kind, would be my work at Children's, from which I will draw many of the methods stories I use in Part IV for illustrative purposes. While at Children's I undertook dozens of research and QI studies, each separately reviewed and approved by the relevant authorities. Each was, therefore, an island, technically speaking. But my experience of them was far from modular. And, as is par for the course, each protocol was not really as circumscribed as their official reification in document format would imply. Let me explain.

First, in translating each separate protocol from the ideational world of its paper format to real life, many extra-curricular lessons were learned, including lessons about the sociocultural context in which the participants' experiences were created, enacted, and perceived. Second, from my holistic, systems-oriented (anthropological) perspective, the studies were serial and part of a larger program of work. They spiraled into one another, with the next building on lessons learned during the first.

Taken together, all of my work at Children's includes not only each particular study I organized or helped with, but also the experiences I had in setting projects up and disseminating the findings from them to foster in-house improvement. All this provides me with ample data for the ethnographic-like account I deliver in certain parts of this text. More important in the context of this inquiry into the definition of ethnography is that as time went on—after a year or so of my immersion in the system had passed—I could truly say that my analyses were ethnographic when I brought my broader, participant observation–based understandings to bear.

Taking an Anthropological Stand

Definitional Clarity

We have established that neither qualitative studies nor naturalistic ones nor studies undertaken with delimited populations are, as such, ethnographic. Further, we established in Chapter 1 that ethnography and anthropology are distinct terms and we have been using them that way so far. Yet, they overlap because anthropology inherently subsumes an ethnographic epistemology—even when it does not entail the full-fledged ethnographic research process.

This is complicated stuff, so let me add a clarifying declaration to keep us on track: *The anthropological approach is, by definition, ethnographic in aim, even when contingencies mean that it cannot be truly ethnographic in scope (i.e., when immersion cannot happen). In either case, priority is placed on holism and a systems perspective that favors emic points of view, achieves critical distance, and takes a reflexive stance toward the research context.* It effectively evades, inasmuch as is possible in light of any given research question, the unnecessary imposition of researcher-driven categories on the data.

Spreading the Word

With that, the following comments from Brink and Edgecombe must be considered:

> Research studies, mislabeled as ethnography, are appearing everywhere in the health care literature. Why? Is it that the teachers of research misunderstand the design and teach from their own ignorance? Is it that anthropologists don't really care what other people are doing with their design? Are anthropologists so protective and secretive about their design they hesitate to share it even when it is becoming widely misused? Or is it that editors of research journals do not know the design and publish these flawed articles, which are then quoted and used as the basis for other flawed research? (Brink and Edgecombe 2003, p. 1030)

I have mentioned the role that the expectations of institutional review board (IRB) committee members have played in narrowing ethnography's scope in health services. Brink and Edgecombe (2003) add editors, reviewers, and anthropologists to the list. It is true that editors and reviewers are often ignorant regarding how to evaluate qualitative let alone ethnographic submissions. A number of recent editorials, essays, and white papers attempt to help correct for this (see, for example, Huby et al. 2007; Mays and Pope 2000; Office of Behavioral and Social Sciences Research 2001; Patton 1999; Sofaer 1999).

But what about anthropologists? In addition to the overall lack of attention paid to methodological details in anthropology (but see Bernard [1998] and my Preface), anthropologists are notorious for preaching to the choir, complaining to each other about ethnography's misuse. Only recently have those who actually practice anthropological ethnography made the effort to speak out to health services audiences regarding the approach in a language that such audiences can easily understand.

In addition to Brink and Edgecombe (2003), anthropologists such as Helen Lambert and Christopher McKevitt (2002) and Jan Savage (also a nurse) (2000) have attempted to educate their peers. They have cunningly done so via the *British Medical Journal* or *BMJ*'s "Education and Debate" section, thus getting the message into the medical mainstream. Each essay takes a slightly different angle on ethnography, and I will report here positions that add to or reinforce, from a new perspective, the foundational understanding of the ethnographic process that we just built. Lambert and McKevitt (2002) enter the debate by questioning the present need to pin down ethnographic methods to the extent that they become separated from theory. Reducing the ethnographic approach to a delimited set of techniques that interchangeable research assistants can carry out virtually guarantees the superficiality of the findings. This is partly because one key to doing ethnography is interpreting data as you go. Factory models in which interchangeable research assistants take on different parts of a project generate substandard data and, moreover, substandard analyses because investigator continuity—and investigator familiarity with all parts of the data collection and analysis process and with the cultural context in question—is a crucial aspect of the ethnographic enterprise (Sobo, Seid, and Gelherd 2006).

Further, deciding prior to an investigation exactly what will be done and how limits anthropologically oriented researchers, cutting them off from potentially important insights that can come about when inspecting unanticipated turns of event. Similar to Brink and Edgecombe who deride the tendency to label mere interview research as if ethnographic, Lambert and McKevitt note that, "Words cannot be taken at face value"; they add that "naturally arising informal situations involving talk and action are more useful than formal interviews in highlighting this" (Lambert and McKevitt 2002, p. 211). That is, the hidden meanings of words sometimes only emerge when we observe speakers' actions, in context.

Lambert and McKevitt also call for health services ethnographers to push back from initial research assumptions so that the very categories under investigation can be probed. We should "question the familiar" when embarking on ethnographic research and we should do so with the express goal of "reconfiguring the boundaries of the problem" (2002, p. 212). I would add that the categories to be questioned often are multiply defined; in other words, such reconfiguration is aided immensely when we compare and contrast *all* of the varied perspectives at play in the complex social arenas that are so often our field sites in HSR (Huby et al. 2007).

It follows that the category of human subjects for which research protocols are framed also needs reconfiguring. In the health services, it is often assumed that the only eligible human subjects are the patients (or, in the case of pediatrics, their parents or guardians). This should not be so (Lambert 2006; Savage 2000). Making good on anthropology's promise depends on following all threads in the social fabric of the health services arena. *All* stakeholder groups—nurses, systems analysts, respiratory technicians, administrators, etc., including even researchers—merit anthropologically informed examination and illumination. So does the way that each stakeholder group is organized into the complex system that we call health care. I will soon provide some examples of why this is so, but first we must understand why, in most cases, outsiders rather than insiders should do this illuminating.

Nonnative Points of View

Outsiders Inside?

Although I have been a worker in some of the organizations I have examined anthropologically, I also have always been an anthropologist with academic affiliations. I have always maintained dual citizenship, so to speak. This is important for anyone who wishes to evaluate the validity of my ethnographic insights or those of other scholars who, like me, are positioned along the borders of a number of professional worlds.

In her recent review of the literature regarding structured observational research, which is described specifically as a version of ethnography adapted by and for health services, Jane Carthey of the National Patient Safety Agency in London asks "Who is the most appropriate observer?" (2003, p. 15). The choice was between health services insiders and researchers from the outside.

The answer? According to Carthey the literature reviewed shows not much difference overall, although "medical experts are better at assessing content specific attributes, while non-medical observers are better at assessing interpersonal factors. Research in other industries has shown that researchers who develop good domain knowledge can make consistent and meaningful observations." Carthey goes on, noting, "Medical professionals sometimes do not recognize an event as an error or problem and may also be reluctant to report errors if it makes the team being observed look bad" (p. ii15). If I may generalize from the two quotes—leaving aside the implications of drawing an equation between health care and other industries—insiders lack awareness regarding certain social system issues and they have vested interests (see Chapter 14).

It is true that a number of insightful autoethnographies and ethnographic-like texts exist in which insiders have penned self-reflective and theoretically informed accounts of native worlds (e.g., Murphy 2001).

However, good autoethnography is nearly always informed by the fact that the author has inhabited a different life-world at one time or another. Such ethnographers often have gone abroad for college or have been the first members of their family to go to college. They may alternately (or concurrently) have experienced marginalization by virtue of membership in some kind of minority group, as was common among many pioneering anthropologists. Adults who moved frequently as children, for example, as dependents of diplomats or military personnel, also can have gained the anthropological benefit of having experienced the outsider-insider tension necessary to productively reconfigure the boundaries of what is being explored.

Although many people forced to confront other cultures simply reject them, those who take advantage of the border-crossing experience to gain a relativistic point of view and an appreciation of the holistic perspective on meaning are well equipped to do ethnography. Those who have not studied anthropology intensively or truly immersed themselves in another cultural world simply do not have the prerequisite perspective needed to attempt such work.

So, health services insiders can be trained to collect and analyze data using an anthropologically informed protocol, but there are certain limitations to this. It works best when the project in question is squarely situated in, rather than being a study of, health services. Otherwise, when the researcher is a member of the community of practice under study from the start, and thereby already "medicalized," the critical distance that informs really good ethnography can go missing (see Browner 1999). This is one reason to bring in a trained ethnographer rather than to try to do ethnography or anthropologically informed HSR from the inside out. Alternately, with proper training (and see Chapters 11 and 12), students or those new to health services can be a boon to a project because, not having habituated to what are seen from the inside as standard attitudes and practices, they still can be surprised and alert to things that insiders cannot see.

Here, it is worthwhile to explore the processes that underlie the achievement of critical distance. Key to this attitude is not accepting all categories at face value. I say "all" rather than "any" because the research process would be paralyzed if everything had to be questioned. Moreover, some point of overlap must exist with the health services system for findings to be useful. This is why, in many of the projects I describe in Part IV, I use health care acronyms. But accepting some assumptions to facilitate translation does not mean buying into everything wholesale.

The simultaneous use by the nonnative ethnographer of immersion through participant observation and structured data collection highlights the tension between the emic view of social life that ethnographers strive to gain and the etic view of the systematic data collector. This forces the researcher to consider, as well as compare, different perspectives on a practice or topic, both from within and without the setting under study. The everyday can be seen in new light, allowing us to "reconfigure the boundary of [the] problem" as per Lambert and McKevitt (2002) and suggest new ways to address old woes.

Outsider ethnographers or anthropologists also can help bridge the research-practice gap because of the relationships that they build with key stakeholders. Seen as outsiders, their recommendations can be less threatening than those of insiders whose interests may compete with those in the area targeted for change.

Examples

To illustrate, here are some examples (see also Huby et al. 2007). An anthropologically informed ethnographic approach was used to study the liaison between hospital care and community care for people with HIV/AIDS in Lothian, Scotland (Huby 1999). The program's assumption was that liaison was poor, that general practice (GP) or primary care physicians were not involved in discharge arrangements, and that postdischarge care was therefore inadequate. A survey of postdischarge service contacts among a sample of patients was conducted in parallel to participant observation. This was followed by a longitudinal study of service use by a group of eleven people that entailed immersion in and observation of the system in question.

Although the survey showed that GPs did not liaise to a great extent with hospital-based services, observation revealed that patients valued their GPs' input precisely because of GPs' position outside pervasive and controlling service-provider networks centered on hospital services. The key gap in services, from patients' point of view, was actually the complex system of welfare benefits. On the basis of these findings, welfare rights provision was strengthened.

Another example of anthropologically informed research that benefited from the fact that the researcher was an outsider able to maintain critical distance was an evaluation of a community stroke service that involved ethnographic immersion in and observation of the organization, delivery and use of care with patient, service provider and manager interviews, and review of documentary data such as care plans. A number of patients had experienced setbacks, which service providers deemed an inevitable consequence of stroke and patients saw as the result of their individual circumstances (Hart 2001).

However, a significant number of these setbacks could be explained as a consequence of patients' interactions with the care system. This was seen when emic and etic accounts were compared and contrasted from a range of patient and professional perspectives. This process made visible individuals' relationships to a wider system of care and highlighted patterns in these relationships that had implications for care improvement in the way preventable sources of setbacks became identifiable, such as poor liaison at care transfer points and inappropriate placement in passivity-inducing care settings (Hart 2001).

The anthropological approach has a crucial role to play in the actual implementation of recommendations also. For example, one very large integrated health care system has included an HIV-screening test reminder in its computerized clinical reminder system. If patients have risk factors, this reminder appears on the coversheet of their electronic medical record, prompting an HIV-screening test offer. My own investigation of the screening program's roll-out revealed several discrepancies between different stakeholders' perceptions of the intervention. These discrepancies, which slowed progress in implementation, were reinforced by the organizational structure and by the norms and goals of each professional group involved. As a result, procedures meant to foster better communication and collaboration between groups were put into practice as the project expanded (Sobo, Bowman, and Gifford 2008; Sobo et al. 2008a, 2008b).

Optimizing the potential that anthropologically informed HSR has to affect health services is not without challenges. For one thing, anthropologists have had to adapt to the short time scales of some HSR: With care, we can accelerate the pace while not compromising quality. Still, we must do more to demonstrate to colleagues and funding bodies exactly what the anthropologically informed approach offers. A better understanding of the health services perspective will facilitate this.

CHAPTER 5

Health Services: An Insider's Guide

THE "DECEPTIVELY FAMILIAR"

As Sjaak van der Geest and Kaja Finkler argue in their introduction to a special journal issue focusing on hospital ethnography, we lack studies of hospitals and related facilities because "on first glance they appear to be deceptively familiar" (2004, p. 1995). However, as anyone who has ever used hospital or other health services knows, that sense of familiarity is fleeting. On the surface we see simply a hospital (or another form of health care facility), undifferentiated except maybe for the coarse-grained social categories of patients, doctors, and nurses. But a given facility is actually an intricate, living web of various types of relations. Further, this web—this system—is not isolated; it is interpenetrated with various other webs as well as being part of an even larger one.

Assuming that the reader has or will have the social and professional connections necessary to gain entry for study in a health services site—whether a hospital, assisted living facility, community clinic, hospice, or elsewhere—here we will examine some of the basic structures and processes of health services systems.

Although the U.S. system forms the basis for my examples, most national systems have similar pieces in play and, in any case, much of the difference between health services in the United States and other nations relates to financial arrangements. For instance, in many nations, health care is an entitlement paid for by the government, not the patient or his or her private insurance company or family. This is not to say that economics is beyond our ken; however, the focus here is on the other sorts of moving parts of health services: the units that make up any health care system, however paid for. Our examples will commence after a brief review of the origins of HSR as a delineated pursuit (see also Chapter 8).

This chapter's foray into the land of health services is not exhaustive but it will familiarize readers who are new to health services with some of the language and organizational structures that might be encountered when entering the field. It will demonstrate that individual workers' decision and action options are actually highly structured by the systems that they work within, professional cultures included.

HEALTH SERVICES RESEARCH: INCEPTION OF THE FIELD AND BASIC CONCEPTS

Research in the area of health care provision and health seeking is nothing new and it goes on worldwide. However, as Thomas McCarthy and Kerr White note (2000), the codification of theories and methodological discussions under the rubric of health services research (HSR) is a relatively recent development. My brief recap focuses on the large role that the federal government has played in fostering HSR's emergence in the United States, reflecting its power to shape scholarly inquiry; however, private foundations also have contributed a good deal to the development of HSR by funding particular programs or initiatives fitting with their particular missions. (I focus on the United States because the phrase "health services research" was coined there and, more importantly, because many of my own studies have taken place there; parallels do exist in other countries. In light of my focus, I draw heavily on McCarthy and White's review in this section; see also the National Library of Medicine's historical information page at http://www.nlm. nih.gov/hsrph.html.)

Historically, HSR emerged in the context of increasing concern about accountability in U. S. health care. It crystallized as a named field in 1960 as the result of a merger of the Public Health Research and Hospital Facilities Research study sections of the National Institutes of Health. A series of fourteen papers was commissioned and these papers, published in book form in the mid-sixties (Mainland 1966), defined HSR as it stood at that time.

About the same time (1965), the Hospital Research and Educational Trust, a charitable trust set up by the American Hospital Association, wanted to organize a journal. They eventually agreed to sponsor *Health Services Research*. The journal's inception contributed greatly to the development of the HSR field, providing a medium for disseminating information to colleagues and serving as a symbol of the field's scholarly legitimacy.

HSR got a big boost from the expansion of government health care coverage programs such as Medicare and Medicaid, which reimburse certain health-related expenditures for the elderly, certain low-income people, and people with disabilities. Interest in health care utilization, cost, and variations in services grew very quickly in light of taxpayers' and governmental interest in accountability. The Office of Research and Statistics in the Social Security Administration, which originally administered Medicare and Medicaid, developed an extensive body of research that was continued by the Health Care Financing Administration (HCFA) when it took over responsibility for the Medicare and Medicaid programs. HCFA, recently renamed the Centers for Medicare and Medicaid Services, continues to play many roles in health care delivery, including as a payor for services, in determining benefits packages, and in research.

In 1966, Avedis Donabedian developed a conceptual framework for health services that viewed care as a production system. This simple framework defined the components of structure, process, and the resultant outcomes, and it continues to provide the core paradigm for assessing and improving the quality of care (see also Donabedian 1988). Indeed, structures, processes, and outcomes are referenced by habit in most HSR-related conversations today. **Structures** include who is delivering services, where services are delivered, with what equipment, and who is receiving services. **Processes** are what is done and how. **Outcomes** are the health results of the interaction between providers and patients (Vivier, Bernier, and Starfield 1994), or a change, either positive or negative, in health status of the individual, group, or population as a result of previous or concurrent care (Donabedian, 1966).

In 1967, prior to creation of Department of Health and Human Services, the Secretary of Department of Health, Education and Welfare (DHEW) authorized the National Center for Health Services Research (NCHSR). NCHSR consolidated the health research activities in various DHEW departments. Additionally, NCHSR established HSR centers at sites such as Harvard University, the University of North Carolina in Chapel Hill, the University of California in Los Angeles, and Kaiser Permanente in North California.

Also at this time (for details see Chapter 8), randomized controlled clinical trials research was experiencing a growth spurt. Key epistemological assumptions that accompanied such trials' ascendance in clinical research were eventually generalized to HSR. That is, although quite different from clinical research, HSR does idealize and in many ways models itself on the epistemology of clinical science. This is defined in detail later in the book; at this point, suffice it to say that NCHSR was absorbed in 1989 into the Agency for Health Care Policy and Research (AHCPR), a Public Health Service agency in HHS with the mandate to support research, data development, and activities that will enhance the quality, appropriateness, and effectiveness of health services (P.L. 101-2399). AHCPR was reauthorized in 1999 as the Agency for Healthcare Research and Quality (AHRQ), which is where things now stand (see http://www.ahrq.gov).

/ ORGANIZATIONAL ELEMENTS

System Parts

However funded and however focused—whether patient-provider interaction, employee experiences, information flow, use of space, or other
issues are under study—anthropologically informed HSR generally
takes place within health services organizations. These organizations are
staffed by various kinds of workers.

Executive leaders manage facilities and operations, finances, and
administration. Large departments are committed to maintaining patient
records, billing, vendor payments, and human resources. There are also
legal departments as well as related divisions focused on regulatory compliance and risk management (often including safety issues) and departments
to manage volunteer services, shipping and receiving, public relations,
continuing medical education, information systems, and the like.

Some include individual users as part of the system. Each user may
make any number of visits in a given time frame. Use tends to be skewed
toward those with chronic conditions. Therefore, a small number of users
make a large number of visits (some refer to them as "frequent flyers").

Organizational Subcultures

Organizations articulate multiple, sometimes somewhat redundant units;
they are supported or enacted by a myriad of professionals filling varied
organizational niches. Workers in each niche have their own subculture,
entailing an at-least-slightly and sometimes radically different view of
the whole and of one's place within it.

These subcultures can be fragmenting. They may reflect differing reward
structures and professional priorities as well as structurally imposed differences in power and authority. They may exist in direct tension to unifying
global organizational understandings, which are limited to mission statements and basic or core values. Nonetheless, in any organization, at least
some functional horizontal linkages already exist between departments, as
do vertical ties that bind (e.g., ties extending from vice-president to director
to supervisor to staff nurse). These links can be capitalized on in research
and for application. However, before we ask how, let us make sure we are
familiar with central aspects of the typical health services organization.

/ INFORMATION

Health services organizations generate and maintain a huge amount of
information regarding users and visits as well as provider practices, costs

(which often do not include physician fees; see below), and so on. In 1999, when I first joined Children's, I found it quite difficult to keep up with the acronyms my new colleagues were constantly throwing at me and each other to describe various information classes. These ranged from CX (complication) through DX (diagnosis) to HX (the patient's history or the story behind the complaint that the patient "presents" with) and included other letter combinations such as LOS, or length of stay. A patient's LOS is equal to however many days he or she has been in the hospital. The latter is often used in HSR that relies on data pulled from health services information systems.

A similarly popular data point is the ICD code; the ICD is the International Statistical Classification of Diseases and Related Health Problems. All diagnoses have an ICD code. For example, K35.0 refers to acute appendicitis with generalized peritonitis; K35.1 refers to acute appendicitis with peritoneal abscess. There are 12,420 basic ICD codes in the latest version of the system. The system is updated from time to time as new disease categories are invented and old ones fall out of use. Medicine's disease classification scheme or nosology is dynamic and serves as the site for various contests regarding validity claims. For instance, using the ICD-10, one would code fibromyalgia, a disputed disease class, as M79 (other soft tissue disorders, not elsewhere classified) and M79.0 (rheumatism, unspecified). That is, it is not itself a defined disease entity, according to the ICD system.

In addition to having to conform to existing nosological notions, another problem that occurs when data registries are queried using ICD codes is that these represent diagnoses, not presenting or initial complaints. Therefore, it is hard to track how populations of patients who present with particular complaints are treated, for example for quality improvement purposes; ICDs are applied after the fact. This is one reason why an analyst who preceded me at Children's found that CT scans for children diagnosed with minor head injuries of a certain type were never associated with significant findings: Those who presented with apparently minor injuries and whose scans revealed more serious head trauma would not have been left with an ICD for *minor* head injury. There was surprisingly widespread confusion about this point.

ICD codes eventually turn into DRGs, or diagnostic related groups. These are, essentially, grouped ICD codes used for billing purposes; there are about 500 of them. A related scheme, E-codes, represent the external cause of an injury. For example, E-880 designates a fall on or from stairs or steps. E-codes 870–876 cover various "misadventures to patients during surgical and medical care."

E-codes are notoriously problematic; they are often missing from patient files and, in any case, they, like ICD codes, are sometimes put into registries by data entry clerks who are under their own time and other pressures. Even in computerized patient record systems that offer clinicians the option of real-time bedside data entry, or even (for those who are qualified) procedural and pharmaceutical order entry, errors can be made. Further, data collected during patient care are not actually research data per se, so many of the double-checks used in research protocols to ensure data quality are not in place. This is a problem in many other kinds of health services record-keeping, too, and must be taken into account when organizational information systems built for business or internal purposes are used for research studies.

When Is Research Research?

A project described as **research** is undertaken to add to the literature regarding the issue at hand; generalizable knowledge is expected. Research is, in health services and according to the U.S. federal government (see Title 45 CFR 36 §46.102), a technical term not to be confused with quality improvement activities. It also is generally viewed as peripheral to clinical or organizational concerns and therefore it is sometimes resented and often deprioritized by non-researchers in health services (see Chapter 14 and below regarding the clinic-academic split).

In the eyes of most health services workers, the prototypical research project is the clinical trial comparing outcomes in patients who serve as "subjects" and receive different medication regimens. When patients or even patient records provide study data, the project must have human subjects research approval from an institutional review board or IRB— or any given nation's equivalent (assuming that nation subscribes to or has built on the World Medical Association's Declaration of Helsinki, the Nuremberg Code, or any other convention declaring human research subjects' rights). To follow the U.S. example, it is assumed that, in research, formal written consent processes entailing forms, signatures, and so on will be used if contact with patients (now "subjects") is entailed. Even nonpatients participating in studies need to sign consent forms, although many in the health services do not realize this; it has sometimes taken me a while to convince health services workers who would participate in my own studies that the informed consent process was indeed necessary.

It is crucial that research work be labeled as such. Calling it something else (a study, for example) does not convey essential information about its intent: to generate broadly applicable knowledge that will be disseminated or shared extra-organizationally. Research means to contribute to the literature; quality improvement (QI) work does not. QI studies are developed for the immediate benefit of the organization, with no intent to publish. There is only the intent to learn and to apply that knowledge in improvement efforts.

The distinction between research and QI is, in some ways, semantic—but it is no less important for that. For one thing, all nations have regulations and good researchers must abide by them. For another, these regulations (whatever form they take) will have ramifications for the types of investigations that can and cannot be done, and for the dissemination of findings.

The U.S. government's Office for Human Research Protections (OHRP) recently barred a number of Michigan hospitals from using a five-item checklist to reduce nosocomial or care-induced infection rates—all because results were studied and published without IRB clearance. Findings demonstrated that after eighteen months of use, the checklist had saved 1,500 lives and $200 million. However, because the checklist's application was a deviation from standard practice, equivalent in OHRP's eyes to the administration of an experimental drug, and because they did not procure the written, informed consent of patients and providers whose health and actions were scrutinized as part of this deviation, those in charge of the project violated ethics regulations (Gawande 2007; see also Dingwall 2008).

This is not to say that the study organizers intended to do wrong (but regarding the pressures to publish, see Chapter 14). Nonetheless, rules were broken and an anonymous tip to OHRP led to the shutdown (Atul Gawande, personal communication, January 11, 2008). Had they simply applied a guideline-based checklist, evaluated its impact, and instigated changes in the name of a local QI effort—without purposive publicity—all would have been well. However, although local lives would have been saved, others would not have benefited from knowledge about the project because dissemination is not part of QI as it is of research.

The QI-research distinction is paramount. To an anthropologist, meaning may be negotiated and situational but, like research regulators, heath services workers generally view it as immutable. For example, at an injury prevention conference in 1999, I asked someone working for the county about her research, using the term broadly to mean any inquiry meant to further our understanding about what is going on. "It's not research!" she snapped. I found her uptight, but thought no more of it until I'd better acculturated and realized the significance of my mistake within her professional worldview.

Misunderstandings can escalate, however. In another incident, I asked an employee at a particular health care organization to grant me an interview for a research project. I asked in an email and specified concretely that the project was research. This point is important because, as noted, it does have legal and ethical ramifications. Weeks passed before this person got back to me. Such delay is not uncommon; health services workers are generally very busy. In any case, the employee did respond eventually and asked for more information about the project. This was rather unusual; most participants in the research I am referring to were satisfied with my initial explanation and justification. I answered, not remembering to reiterate that what I was doing was research per se, in part because I also sent the research proposal's official abstract (its label said as much). Further, my email is set up to include all information previously exchanged.

To make a long story short, after this worker agreed to participate and initiated the informed consent process with me, a crisis occurred. The individual became irate, contacted a director of the program hosting the research study, and argued that I had misrepresented the study as if not research. The irate individual also happened to be a key gatekeeper for the program in question; the director could not afford to ignore the complaint, however unfounded.

It turned out that the offended individual had great disdain for research in general, holding it to be (among other things) too time-intensive to be useful. In short, this was the type of nonresponder whom I would have loved to have interviewed. As part of the project in question, I actually had wanted to learn more about the distaste for research in a formalized, research-based way, and from the native point of view, so that I might draw what HSR would define as evidence-based rather than "anecdotal" conclusions regarding the significance of this negative position on research. But the individual's reaction had to be treated as a refusal and, after some crow-eating in the service of my research project, the crisis abated. In the research articles that eventually came out of the study, I could not and would not refer to this individual's opinion.

There was one other nonresponder for this study. That person faxed a very long explanation of why participation was not possible. However, without a signed informed consent statement, I could not and would not use as data what this individual told me about the research-care provision chasm in the fax. And it is certainly not offered as such in this context. Rather, this story and the story above are meant only as evocative illustrations of the potential for resistance that readers may encounter behind the scenes of the HSR landscape. (Regarding the academic-care provision chasm, see below; regarding what counts as evidence, see Chapter 8.)

/ CARE PROVISION UNITS

Aside from a glossary, I longed for an organizational chart. Figure 5.1 provides an example of what I might have seen had one existed. In a real

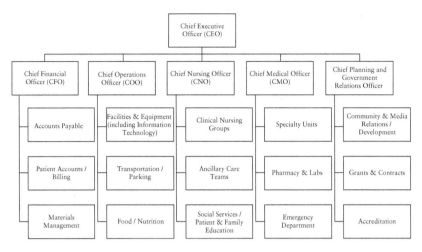

Figure 5.1 Mock hospital organization chart created using a standardized Microsoft SmartArt hierarchy graphic. Each facility's actual organization will vary and most charts will be quite asymmetric, especially when subdivision details are provided.

"org chart" maintained by a technologically well-equipped institution, one might find names and even people's pictures in the blocks representing major offices; drill-downs are also sometimes possible. Because of turnover, even well-maintained org charts are often out of date; still, they can provide a helpful orienting tool for researchers and new staff members.

Within hospitals, for instance, typically there are units or services such as intensive or critical care, cardiology, orthopedics, pharmacy, radiology, neurology, oncology, and emergency departments. There is also often a pain service, social work, psychiatry or behavioral and mental health, and some type of religious representation. Some organizations house age- and gender-specific services, such as adolescent health, geriatrics, pediatrics, neonatology, and labor and delivery and reproductive health. Rehabilitative consults may be offered, but rehabilitative services are more likely found in facilities that specialize in rehabilitative care.

The children's hospital in which I worked was a **tertiary care** center— a facility set up to coordinate and offer highly specialized care, often using sophisticated technology. **Primary care** is doctor's office or general practitioner (GP) care, whereas **secondary care** is offered by a specialist on referral by a GP (or, depending on the insurance or reimbursement scheme, through self-referral). Most HSR concentrates on tertiary care, but more and more is being done in primary care settings. Because those are generally more simply configured than tertiary care organizations, and because some tertiary care centers subsume both secondary and primary care anyway, my discussion here focuses mostly on tertiary care. Hospitals serve as the example, but nursing homes and other care facilities have at least some of the elements we consider.

Whatever the facility or organization, coordination along the **continuum of care** or the various kinds of units that, together, can contribute to patient services is not always as it should be. Primary, secondary, and tertiary care centers often do not share information as well as they might, which leaves the door open for duplication, error, and harm as well as inconvenience for the patient, who may be sent from office to office or across town to get an X-ray only to find that the X-ray center is shut. **Case management,** in which one individual provides oversight for every patient, or "case," is one answer to this problem, although not the norm.

Beside levels of care, other important distinctions are those between **acute** and **chronic** care, which are for short-term and longstanding conditions respectively, and urgent and emergency care. Although the latter distinction may seem subtle and both departments are generally under the Emergency Department's or ED's direction, urgent care is for acute conditions or flare-ups of chronic conditions that are not life-threatening or where the patient can afford to wait a bit longer than for a real emergency or emergent condition, such as a gunshot wound. **Triage,** the process by which ED intake staff sort those who enter, is meant to ensure that that those whose complaints are most serious are taken care of first.

Gunshots and many car-crash injuries are classed as "traumas": especially life-threatening injuries in which whole-body systems are threatened. EDs that are well set-up to deal with traumas (for example, with appropriate staff on call all day every day) are classed as trauma centers. Emergency vehicles carrying trauma patients will head to trauma centers, if possible, bypassing EDs that are not so equipped. Here, it is worth pointing out that, despite links to state and local agencies, for example via 911 arrangements, emergency services are generally provided by private businesses with contractual agreements to serve certain hospitals or regions.

The entire health services system was originally built to meet acute care needs. This legacy has led to much distress for chronic-care patients, so it is no surprise that a great deal of medical anthropology effort has gone into understanding the chronic care situation (e.g., Manderson and Smith-Morris Forthcoming).

EXTRAMURAL CONNECTIONS

Health services also are linked to private and governmental insurers or **payors.** Payors have a variety of modes of reimbursement, ranging from capitation, which means that they pay an organization a set price per head, no matter what amount or type of care is given, to individual indemnity plans that reimburse approved per-procedure payments after the fact. Although some nations have single-payor systems such as England's National Health Service, the United States has a myriad of insurance schemes—and a myriad of uninsured people. Legally, uninsured people have access to emergency care but this access is sometimes compromised. For a bit more on financing, such as regarding managed care, see Chapter 8.

Even among the insured, getting care ("realized access") can be challenging because of reimbursement arrangements. I refer here not to the sometimes-complicated task of getting a referral or getting coverage approved but to simply getting primary, preventive medical attention. The following example is drawn from my own work on a State Child Health Insurance Program (S-CHIP) evaluation (Sobo et al. 2003), and it involves parents who seek to immunize their three children. The parents—this family—are not afforded insurance coverage by any employer. The parents make little enough to apply for S-CHIP coverage for the children (for themselves, coverage might be secured through Medicare or Medicaid). However, this family's three children have different legal fathers, and the fathers have differing incomes. Therefore, two children are eligible for two different types of coverage (available in two different locations, for differing fees) and one is not eligible for any coverage at all. This example and the access challenges it entails is unfortunate—but not unique.

Although there is some standardization across various reimbursement plans, there is also much that varies. HSR conducted with administrative data often includes a data field for insurance information because of the potential that insurance status has to affect a person's health-related processes and outcomes. Such information can be important in understanding why particular choices are made or actions are or are not taken. In other words, it can be useful in establishing a context for findings.

Beyond Payors, health services organizations also are linked to national and local accreditation organizations, such as the U.K.'s Commission for Health Care Audit and Inspection (CHAI) and the U.S.'s Joint Commission on Accreditation of Health Care Organizations (JCAHO, often pronounced Jay-co), whose inspection timelines and shifting priorities can have a huge impact on an organization's activities. Some health services organizations also have links to academic institutions, and may house or share IRBs or other research oversight committees to ensure that in-house research is carried out according to local and national ethical and scientific standards.

/PROVIDERS OF CARE

Within and cutting across the various units are various occupational strata. Some I mentioned previously: dietary and respiratory care specialists, lab technicians, pharmacists, physical and occupational therapists, and so on. There also are physician assistants or PAs and nurses (in some nations, "sisters"). A wide variety of nurses exist; for example, from least- to most-trained and privileged there are, in the United States at least: aides, licensed vocational nurses or LVNs, registered nurses or RNs, and nurse practitioners or NPs. The main job of nurses is, of course, nursing: Nurses provide care in support of medical and surgical plans for a patient. PAs and NPs have some medical decision-making ability, but the lion's share of that is limited to "the docs."

What Is a Doctor?

In the United States, doctors who hold either an MD or a DO can be licensed to practice medicine. A DO is a doctor of osteopathy; an MD, a doctor of medicine. Osteopathic physicians are doctors whose training includes an additional 300–500 hours of hands-on instruction focused on the musculo-skeletal system. They are trained to be more holistically oriented than MDs, too. According to the American Osteopathic Association, today in the United States, 6% of doctors are osteopathic; 65% of DOs practice primary care (see American Osteopathic Assocation, n.d.) (http:// www.osteopathic.org/pdf/about_the_aoa.pdf; accessed August 28, 2008).

The majority of doctors practice **allopathic** medicine, which treats disease through medicines and behavior changes intended to oppose or counteract the signs and symptoms at hand. Allopathic medicine is therefore another term sometimes used to differentiate the type of medicine offered by the U.S. health services system from other forms (sometimes called complementary and alternative medicines or CAM by health services professionals). Medicine that uses multiple approaches is sometimes termed "integrative medicine." For the history behind allopathy's dominance, see Chapter 8.

The main distinction among doctors within U.S. health services is generally between medical and surgical doctors. The difference between surgeons and medical doctors is summed up in the following rude joke, which I first heard from an MD and will paraphrase here: A surgeon and a medical specialist are trying to get on an elevator when the doors start closing. The medical doctor instinctively stops it with his hands; the surgeon uses his head.

Although the joke suggests complementarity, it has other connotations as well: Some adversarial tension does exist between the two divisions. I had a hard lesson in this when designing my first in-house survey at Children's. I used the term "medicine" generically, as I have been doing so far in this book. This turned out to be taken as biased against surgeons.

Medicine and surgery were originally two separate healing cultures, and surgeons were definitely the lesser of the two in terms of public esteem. Surgeons were lumped in with, and often also were, barbers. Unlike medical doctors, they were not university trained and held no degrees. Indeed, it was not until the invention of modern anesthesia that their status began to rise (P. Katz 1999). In some nations, perhaps especially those colonized by the British Empire, surgeons are still addressed as "Mister" or "Miss" rather than as "Doctor" (Whelan and Woo 2004). Regarding surgeons' self-identification as a paranoid lot and the possible reasons for their fearfulness, see Cassell (1991, pp. 49–58).

Medicine entails adjusting a body's balance or alleviating symptoms through behavioral or pharmaceutical means, which is very different than cutting someone open and removing the source of the problem. Partly because of the nature of their work, Pearl Katz writes in her ethnographic account, surgeons are bold and prone to decisive, speedy action. To them, medical doctors are "hesitant, contemplative, introspective, and ... indecisive" (1999, p. 34). And to medical doctors, as suggested in the joke above, surgeons are headstrong and favor action over thought. At least these are the recognized stereotypes doctors have related to anthropologists like me, Katz (1999), and Joan Cassell (1991).

Clinical Versus Academic Practice

When I joined Children's I was, in some ways, relieved to be leaving my academic affiliations behind. For one thing, working in a hospital promised more action and application in my work. For another, although I had not been working in an anthropology department for several years by that time, my clinical trials work was done through a school of medicine where I was on a research, not academic faculty, track. New to this status, which basically entails no departmental voting rights (or committee work), I was rudely awakened to how poorly some tenured and tenure-track faculty members treat their nontenure-track colleagues. I was looking forward to joining a more unified and service-oriented organization.

Although I had little experience of my own in community hospitals and other health services organizations unaffiliated with academic centers or schools of medicine, I had been told that the academic hierarchy is not of concern in such settings. My chance to find out first-hand was stymied when, ironically, Children's and the university where I had worked decided to amalgamate—meaning that, after forty-five years on its own, Children's would become academically affiliated.

The amalgamation had, apparently, been years in the making. Some of my new colleagues were not certain it would happen this time at all; in their words, Children's and "the U" had been to the wedding altar many times before, but marriage had never been consummated.

The discourses surrounding the amalgamation were illuminating. Comparable discourses seem to occur whenever academic or scientific and clinical or community clinic-type cultures come up against one another. Similar scenarios are reported by Pearl Katz, for example, in her work with surgeons (1999), and Mary-Jo DelVecchio Good in her work regarding medical education (Good 1998; see also Good and Good 1993 and Good 1994). They have a keen family resemblance to the infamous "town-gown" or community-university split seen in college towns worldwide.

Basically, those who were threatened by the amalgamation (generally, those with few or no publications and little or no academic status) pointed to Children's strength as a clinical care center where providers focused on service to patients, not publications. They worried that the quality of care would decrease if too many academically inclined providers came on board. They worried that the average LOS and costs would rise as patients became research fodder. LOS and costs also would be affected because "docs from the uni" were just slower than ours were, being less experienced with clinical care.

Another discourse was favored by those who were more academically inclined and those already university affiliated. In their eyes, many of our providers were parochial throwbacks to the time before science. It was in the organization's and the patients' best interests to adopt a more evidence-based stance toward care (I myself was brought in specifically to help shore up Children's publication output and academic reputation). Plus, as the only dedicated pediatric hospital in the region, we offered a wonderful training and research site. Those who were on this side of the argument often referred to the hospital as the "campus": They said things like, "I'm going to be off-campus for the afternoon," as if they were leaving a traditional university setting.

The clinical-academic divide has a sibling: the MD-PhD chasm. In medical settings, including not just schools of medicine but places where medicine and etcetera is practiced, PhDs ride second-class. For instance, at Children's, MD badges read "Dr. So-and-so" and PhD badges read "Jane Doe, PhD," as if to do otherwise would be improper. Compared to doctors in general, PhDs are considered bookworms who carry huge amounts of completely impractical knowledge in their heads. In Chapter 14, I will describe a related divide between practice and science within HSR.

Like any dichotomy or binary opposition, including that between medical and surgical clinicians, these generalizations fail to accommodate reality very well. However, anyone seeking to conduct effective HSR must be aware of these cultural discourses, their structural underpinnings (e.g., in regard to historic and political forces as well as the reward systems at various institutions), and the grain of truth that they carry.

The Right to Write Orders

Various types of doctors manage patients' medical care. Primary care and secondary care were covered above. When a patient checks in for tertiary care, however, things can get a bit slippery. The doctor specifically in charge of a patient's care is his or her attending doctor. But the attending doctor is not the only one to provide care. Much care is given by interns or residents, new graduates just completing their qualifications through rigorous on-the-job training. Sometimes, patients or families do not know who is in charge of their care because there are so many people going in and out of their rooms and introductions may be misunderstood even when made. Gender stereotypes also can come into play in fueling confusion.

Both attending doctors and other doctors can be hospitalists (staff employees, as they often are for large organizations like Kaiser Permanente or the Veterans Health Administration) or outsiders with "privileges" to visit and write orders for the care of their patients when they are hospitalized. Many doctors have these privileges because they belong to a medical group that has set up a formal relationship with a health care organization; the medical group also takes care of billing.

So, with the exception of hospitalists and doctors-in-training, many doctors are not hospital employees. The impact this has on organizational culture can be immense. For instance, at Children's, some nurses saw doctors as "just passing through" and resented their assumptions about how things should be run when, in fact, they were not employees. But where doctors are employees too, the situation is a bit different.

Workplace Culture

Although health services centers are places where life and death events occur, for workers they also are workplaces. Some health services workers find it helpful to distance themselves emotionally from the personal crises that daily surround them. Techniques for doing so are embedded in their training. Simon Sinclair (2000), for example, has shown how medical students distance themselves from patients' life stories by creating neatly structured, unreflexive histories that delete or elide the context of health-related events—and how by so doing they also constitute themselves as full-fledged doctors.

And, as in any workplace, a number of tasks must be done daily, routinely, if order is to be maintained. However, much health care work is done not in offices but in patient bedrooms, some with walls, others without. These spaces are adapted by staff for the work at hand. For instance, Mary Ellen Macdonald, Franco Carnevale, and colleagues (2005; see also Macdonald et al. 2007) report that chairs can be seen by staff as for staff primarily, not friends and relatives (who often have, anyhow, been reduced to "visitor" status). Staff members lean on beds and equipment, use bedrails to support their clipboards as they write notes, and sit on dirty laundry bins. Beds often are used to store excess medical supplies: One bed Macdonald observed was piled with a bag of intravenous liquid, a nursing chart sheet, a binder, syringes, a latex glove box, and a pile of diapers while also containing a tiny pediatric patient.

The routine nature of much work in health care supports engagement in what Macdonald and colleagues refer to as a "water cooler culture," not only behind the scenes in the clinic but also on the floor. Because of its status as a workplace, in addition to attending to their relationships with patients and families, which are often very short term, staff members attend to and maintain their day-to-day relationships with coworkers. I will not rely on only my own experience for examples (although one involving ice cream–eating nurses and a baby languishing in an ED consultation room with a differential or rule-out diagnosis of intestinal intussusception, in which the intestines collapse like a telescope and the part that is cut off from one's blood supply necrotizes or dies, is hard to shake). Instead, I quote Macdonald and colleagues writing about a particular intensive care unit:

> Jokes are told, snacks are shared, laughter is common, radios play pop songs. I watched an attending sitting at the central station eating a bag of chips; moments ago the life support had been removed from a baby who was shaken to death by a caregiver. I watched a nurse come out of a dying child's room, exhausted and wondering: "Where is my coffee?" Staff swap recipes, talk about the weather, the hockey statistics. Cleaning staff come and go with their brooms and cleaning products, pinching a baby's cheek (without washing their hands) as they pass by the bedside. The phone may ring loudly eight times before it is answered; when answered, everyone nearby can hear the conversation. The secretary delivers the pay cheques and staff joke about spending their wages. Staff birthday parties and wedding showers occur in empty isolation rooms. An administrator shows off her new belly button ring. (2005, p. 6)

All the while, business as usual must continue. Macdonald reports directly from field notes: "A rounding group carried out their conversation at the foot of the patient's bed as the bedside nurse carried out her routine tasks at the bedside. She routinely removed the diaper and inserted the rectal thermometer and removed it to take the reading. The curtains were opened the whole time" (Macdonald et al. 2005, p. 8). There was no question that the staff members observed were devoted to the care of their patients. However, bedrooms are workrooms in the hospital setting.

Sometimes, staff social activities do inappropriately take precedence over patient care. But most times, although angry patients and families may not know it, staff members who seem to be just having fun may actually be filling time with relationship work while they are waiting for a pharmacy delivery, for instance, or a physician to arrive.

ADMINISTERING IMPROVEMENT

In case of problems, or to ease the stress of accessing health services, many large organizations have patient care liaisons. In addition, even those health services organizations that do minimal research generally do QI (sometimes under the rubric of quality management). This was discussed briefly in Chapter 1, along with implementation science, when HSR was introduced. In brief, all health services organizations are interested in quality improvement, although they use various means to achieve it and have various standards for it. One area that has been a central priority in recent years is cultural competence, to which we now turn.

CHAPTER 6

The Culture Concept, Cultural Competence, and the Dangers of "Anthro Lite"

FIRST INCURSIONS

The interest of quality improvement (QI) and implementation scholars notwithstanding, and despite the variety of projects mentioned in Chapter 4 and elsewhere, anthropology's increasing presence in domestic health care is, to a large degree, related to the particular and disparate health care experiences and outcomes of U.S. subcultural or minority groups. That is, the main pull from within health services for anthropological insight has generally been narrowly linked to problems related to serving particular populations. This chapter outlines the evidence for health disparities or inequities in the United States and describes the evolution of the cultural competence movement. I deconstruct the key constructs of culture, ethnicity, and race in the service of explicating their sociocultural basis.

The cultural competence movement is then defined and critiqued to help readers get a more sophisticated and more productive grasp of key issues involved, especially regarding the nature of culture. In doing so, I further build the case for a vision of culture as something more than just ethnicity. I call for a vision of culture, long promoted in anthropology and cognate social sciences, that includes, for example, professional and organizational cultures, too. I also push further Chapter 4's assertion that culture is better understood as a process than a thing. I argue that careful fieldwork that accounts for process and meaning, for example in exploring how preexisting ideas can accommodate new ones and what this means for the negotiation of a care plan or clinic politics or any other aspect of health service provision, is paramount. The chapter also helps prepare the reader to anticipate how those in health services research (HSR) may at present conceive of anthropology's role.

HEALTH INEQUITIES

One magnet drawing anthropologists and others to HSR is increasing concern with the way that health services are distributed, or not. In the

United States, the results of this maldistribution have been and in some cases still are referred to as "health disparities." Elsewhere, for instance, in England, "inequities" is the more common term. Having been called on the carpet for the way that disparities may conceal the link between health and an unegalitarian social hierarchy, many in the United States who originally preferred that term are beginning to follow suit.

Some health differences are related to genetic differences between particular circumscribed groups. Although these may be lumped in with inequities and are to some degree environmentally triggered, for our purposes, those will not be considered as they are not directly in our bailiwick. But cultural and social as well as system-supported provider biases are. If better understood, through anthropological study for example, the negative effects of these might in practice be minimized if not alleviated and positive effects could be optimized.

Take, for instance, heart disease, the leading cause of death among women in the United States. In an extensive literature review of the role of social structure in clinical decision-making, Clark, Potter, and McKinlay (1991) noted that providers' preconceived ideas resulted in the underdetection of heart disease in women. Because women who had not yet reached menopause were considered to have one-third the risk of heart disease as men, and because U.S. women often got (as they still get) much primary care from a gynecologist whose focus is not on the cardiovascular system, heart disease was much less likely to be suspected if a patient was female rather than male.

Race and Ethnicity

Gender is not the only organizing principle implicated in health services maldistribution. Race and ethnicity figure highly. As the Institutes of Medicine reports in *Unequal Treatment*—a book-length report that begins with a patient story (see Chapter 2)—in the United States non-Whites are, in certain circumstances, less likely than Whites to receive appropriate care, including cardiac medication and surgery, dialysis and kidney transplantation, pain medication, and the like. Further, when explicit care process criteria are applied, non-Whites receive poorer quality care. Certain minority groups also are less likely to have a primary care provider or health insurance (Smedley et al. 2003, pp. 29–30).

Most of the studies of health inequities use race and ethnicity categories in their research designs. Recall my warning (Chapter 5) about the quality of data from administrative information systems. Not only is validity a concern; so, too, is reliability. As in regard to all health services constructs, race and ethnicity should not be taken for granted as if self-evident, natural categories.

Technically, a **race** would be a biological subspecies differentiated by anatomical or physiological characteristics. Historically, however, among humans, racial categories have been forged from traits that are easily seen, such as skin color and facial features; this visual, racializing focus has helped those in power use racial categorizations oppressively. Research regarding existing racial categories has shown that within-race differences are by far greater than those demonstrated to exist between the so-called racial groups. In other words, race is a construct, not a biological fact (see, for example, Fluehr-Lobban 2006).

Research that lumps all members of a given racial group together leads to spurious conclusions because members can be from completely different backgrounds. For example, the category "Asian" can include people from Korea, Cambodia, and Japan as well as Americans of Asian descent. "Black" can include Somalians, Haitians, Australian Aboriginals, and African Americans. Other racial categories can include equally diverse mixes. Important between-group differences (both biological and cultural) may be masked. Likewise, between-group differences can be erroneously imputed when samples are nonrepresentative for a given racial category, as they normally will be because research is generally geographically limited.

Many health researchers have erroneously deployed the terms "ethnicity" and "race" as if equivalents. However, the ethnicity construct differs from that of race because ethnicity assumes that cultural knowledge and practices—not physical traits—distinguish groups of people.

Technically, **ethnicity** is a facet of the self that is tied to notions of shared origins that contrast with those of people with whom one shares borders (be they household, neighborhood, or national borders). In the United States, ethnicity is reflected in the classifications of African American, Mexican American, Navajo, and the like. Even without explicit continental, national, or tribal qualifiers, all of us have an ethnic heritage or a mix of ethnic heritages that we may choose to honor.

The same caveat introduced for coarse-grained racial groupings in HSR—that they conceal important differences—holds true for ethnic groupings also if too broadly defined. To further complicate matters, people often have multiple ethnicities and may participate only partially or not at all in their ethnic traditions. Research groupings based only on racialization or ethnicity can lead researchers to overlook other salient differentiating variables, such as gender, nationality and migration status, and that complex variable called "class" (often derived from a consideration of education, occupation, and income). The anthropological approach questions the overreliance on overly broad, system-defined ethnic and racialized constructs so that a fuller understanding of the situated processes at hand is attainable.

Structural Violence

Local organizational systems and individual biases certainly play a role in supporting health inequity. But higher order social structures are implicated, too—and these are perhaps even more important because they both sustain and construct individual and local system actions. When they do so in a way that robs individuals of agency or the right to self-determination and damages their well-being, something called **structural violence** is implicated.

The structural violence concept is generally attributed to Johan Galtung and dated to the late 1960s (e.g., 1969) (but see also the works of Rudolph Virchow [e.g., 1985 [1848]). It describes a socially structured situation in which particular groups of people are systematically barred from achieving their full potential. Class and caste systems are examples of structurally violent systems. Health inequities can result from the structural violence systematically inflicted on those in the lower classes or castes.

Although structural violence can be described or demonstrated with statistics, anthropologist-physician Paul Farmer starts a 2004 explication of the concept with a story. This is the type of move that will come as no surprise after the lessons of Chapter 2 regarding the power of storytelling to connect us. Farmer's story tells of the crowd of patients and families that he encounters every morning when entering the courtyard of the hospital where he works in Haiti. It is punctuated and overshadowed by another tale, this one told by an insistent patient who refuses to present her suffering to him in divergent bits of disembodied data: "She is going to tell the story properly, and I will have to listen." Not only does she talk, she takes his arm, and guides his hand to a huge lesion where once was her breast, saying, "Touch it and see" (2004, p. 306). This is the type of immediacy that good ethnography thrives on. But the larger point that Farmer wants to make with his tale within a tale goes beyond our earlier insights into the power of meaning.

After the tale is told, Farmer reflexively explains that anthropologists are generally trained to explore cultures in the here-and-now, focusing on the "ethnographically visible." That is, the master ethnographic narrative structuring the work of many anthropologists exists in the present tense and so, in our writing, we strive to evoke for the reader what it feels like to "be there," in the thick of the ongoing action (2004, p. 305). But to do this we often recount events within a timeless "ethnographic present"—as if history does not happen. Farmer's point is to draw our attention to the substantial challenge that such immediacy poses for ethnographic inquiry because of the way that it elides the reality of structural violence. Less visible than the present and local instance, and therefore often ignored, are the global ties that bind (but see, e.g., Baer,

Singer, and Susser 1997). As Farmer points out in regard to his Haitian field site: "The transnational tale of slavery and debt and turmoil is lost in the vivid poverty" (2004, p. 305).

And vivid this poverty is. Yet, "because ethnographic work relies on conversations with the living" Farmer says, "we are still not getting the entire picture." What about the dead? What about those left for dead? Why do the health problems of some groups never matter? What benefits for others is their ill health supporting? The best anthropology, Farmer advises, "seeks to understand how suffering is muted or elided altogether. It explores the complicity necessary to erase history and cover up the clear links. ... Bringing those links into view... is a key task" for anthropology in the new millennium (2004, p. 307). And, I would add, it should be a key component of anthropologically informed HSR.

Health inequities are, in good part, the literal embodiment of structural violence. However, as important as it has been for raising our consciousness regarding the impact that global and other macro-level systems have on local well-being and individual health outcomes, the structural violence concept is not without some "analytic perils" (Wacquant 2004). It is crucial for us to understand these if we are to design and conduct relevant and robust research projects relating to health inequity.

First, one thing that gives the structural violence concept its emotive power—that is, its sweep—also makes it imprecise or wooly. It therefore lacks power as a conceptual tool. There are various degrees of violence as well as various forms of it (e.g., mental, physical, political, economic, symbolic, social); further, these various forms are wielded by various entities (e.g., the state, individuals, institutions). Each of these aspects of violence's variation must be examined (Wacquant 2004; see also Bourgois and Scheper-Hughes 2004). In addition, collusion in and accommodation to structural violence must be accounted for (Green 2004). Finally, H. K. (Kris) Heggenhougen reminds us: "In the most inequitable societies not only the disadvantaged but the elite have poorer health than in societies that are less so" (2004, p. 321). Of course, this is squarely tied to the excess of luxuries that the elite in such societies take advantage of.

There are many ways to address the inequities problem. Those that can be most effective will acknowledge that it is not one problem but many, tied together in a myriad of socially intricate ways. However, most solutions suggested so far aim merely to *manage* inequity rather than to fix the system that generates it. Such fixes are hard for us to imagine from within the U.S. culture because of its individualistic ethos and related tendency to focus on individual change (Kirmayer 2004). We must be specific regarding what conditions, exactly, need to be fixed as well as in identifying how that might be done (Heggenhougen 2004).

/ CULTURAL COMPETENCE

More than global systems, local systems, and provider biases, many health services organizations have focused on patient biases that contribute to health inequities. That is, they have targeted culture as a key cause of inequities. For example, when patients do not access care or take medicines as directed, cultural reasons are sought. Culture in this light is a key barrier to care, and the cultural competence movement emerged in part to correct for this.

Cultural competence has been officially defined as "a set of congruent behaviors, attitudes, and policies that come together in a system, agency, or among professionals that enables effective work in cross-cultural situations" (Health Resources and Services Administration 2001, p. 1). In their federally funded review of MEDLINE- and HealthSTAR-indexed literature on the topic (all of which is now in PubMed), Cindy Brach and Irene Fraser observe: "Cultural competency is an explicit statement that one-size-fits-all health care cannot meet the needs of an increasingly diverse American population" (2000, p. 183).

Here, I should note that there are many ways of talking about culture in relation to health care, and a number of approaches to incorporating culture into health care exist. Not surprisingly in light of the care work they do, nurses have played a big role in this area. In the 1950s, the Transcultural Nursing Society's founder Madeline Leininger first put forth the "culture care diversity and universality" (or: "culture care") theory (2002). There is also the "cultural safety" model, which grew out of Irihapeti Ramsden's early 1990s nursing-based attempt to see Maori health care needs met in New Zealand and has subsequently been modified for extended application (De and Richardson 2008).

These and other related approaches are unique in their own ways, each with its own diverse strengths and weaknesses. My goal in this chapter is not to enter the important debates ongoing between or within disciplines regarding which model or theory should prevail but rather to do something entirely different: Expose and then constructively challenge existing assumptions regarding the value of bringing culture into the health care equation to begin with. I do this with reference to "cultural competence" only (and precisely) because of its dominative position.

In essence, the definitions of cultural competence included above suggest the value of creating, through policies and programs, a health services environment that accommodates people from various cultural backgrounds. Why? Because federal funders and program and policymakers whose goal is a reduction in health inequities have backed this approach in the hopes that it will help them in that quest. As a result, there has been a huge upsurge in cultural competency projects and programs. By the time I was formally involved with the topic in the early 2000s, 87% ($n = 118$) of medical schools offered lectures relating to cultural issues (Flores, Gee, and Kastner 2000). Residency programs are now required by the Accreditation Council for Graduate Medical Education to teach, as part of the competency called "professionalism," skills in cultural sensitivity ("sensitivity to a diverse patient population").

Reducing health inequity is certainly a worthy goal. But has the cultural competence movement led to any measurable improvements in patient and family outcomes? If not, why not, and what changes or additions might bring about such results?

/ THE CULTURE CONUNDRUM

The Culture Concept

Part of the problem with cultural competence is the concept of culture itself, or, rather, the way that people have come to define it outside of anthropology. In Chapter 2, I described culture in relation to storytelling. I did this as a way of demonstrating the salience as well as value of meaning-centered data. Here, I will expand on that description by historically tracing the culture concept's development. Although it takes more than a few pages to do so, reviewing this history (and the history of sister concepts such as society and civilization) provides us firm ground for understanding exactly what is wrong with the way that culture is conceptualized in most cultural competence programming—as well as ideas on how to make it right.

Commonly, when we characterize **culture** in introductory anthropology courses, Edward B. Tylor's 1871 definition is invoked: "Culture, or civilization, taken in its wide ethnographic sense, is that complex whole which includes knowledge, belief, art, morals, law, custom, and any other capabilities and habits acquired by man as a member of society" (e.g., cited by Langness 2005, p. 25). This definition is offered up in part because it is thought to be the first English-language definition of culture; further, most agree that it has basically withstood the test of time and is as good as any other definition around—at least for a starting point.

However, as students' anthropological expertise grows, they come to realize that things aren't so simple. Many other definitions are at play. They are often quite similar to Tylor's declaration, but never exactly so. For example, some focus on behavior only, or its results; others define culture as ideas alone. And even individual theorists can be inconsistent. For instance, Geertz finds Clyde Kluckhohn guilty of using at least eleven different meanings for the term in his introductory textbook

(Geertz 1973, pp. 4–5). Kluckhohn was aware of the problem: A few years later, in 1952, working with Alfred Kroeber and others, Kluckhohn coauthored a study of the term that cataloged 164 definitions (Kroeber et al. 1952). This lack of exactness is one reason for the truth behind Geertz's assertion that the term "culture" "obscures a good deal more than it reveals" (1973, p. 4).

Who Has Culture?

Tylor developed his ideas in the late 19th century. As L. L. (Lewis) Langness notes, after George Stocking, Tylor wrote his definition in the context of an evolutionary argument focusing on "primitives" and their "development." Note that "culture" and "civilization" are exchangeable in his gloss. "This was quite a contribution in its day, however," Langness explains, "because Tylor was implying that 'savages' could at least potentially progress to attain the civilized state like Europeans, an idea that had certainly not occurred to many western Europeans previously" (2005, p. 25).

The Determinism Debates

That "savages" could progress to become "civilized" also was an idea that many found too threatening to allow on the table for too long. It would mean, for example, allowing others access to a system of privilege that was at that time reserved for particular white populations.

Determinism is a philosophical stance holding that one thing or event has caused another and that this causal link is immutable. Racial and ethnic prejudices fueled recourse to a position termed "biological determinism," according to which people could justify institutionalized inequalities on the basis of a people's innate biologically given capacities. They could postulate, for example, that African Americans could never be educated because of their inherently inferior brains, or that Irish or Jewish people were fit only for particular marginalized occupations (the Irish and Jews were among those who were not, in early formulations, accepted as "White"; see Fluehr-Lobban 2006, pp. 180–183). Similar arguments have been used to justify gender bias.

In any case, from biological determinism it followed that not everyone could attain the pinnacle of development then termed "civilization." Although (white male) European scholars living at the time might allow that others had culture, civilization was theirs alone to partake.

A tendency emerging in early 20th-century U.S. anthropological circles to pluralize the term "culture" fueled, without intention, the primitive culture versus modern civilization demarcation that was coming to be drawn. U.S. anthropologists had, in the late 1900s, begun to see that different societies had different histories and that their cultures were therefore unique and particular. The technical term for this viewpoint is **historical particularism** and it is most associated with Franz Boas, one of America's key anthropological pioneers.

Boas was appalled by the misuse of science to support biological determinism in the name of racist injustice. He counterattacked by promoting, along with historical particularism, a strong form of cultural determinism. Aided by numerous students, Margaret Mead and Ruth Benedict among them, he mustered evidence to support the stance that culture, not biology, endowed a given population with a particular set of skills and aptitudes.

In its extreme form, cultural determinism is as bogus as biological determinism. But Boas's position did serve a purpose. His papers and speeches arguing that environment influenced bodily form, that there was no such thing as a "pure" race, and that "racial mixing" was not harmful undercut racist contentions regarding humanity's divisions. His cultural research directed attention away from unilineal evolutionary thinking. Overall, Boas's work highlighted the need for a relativistic stance—one by which cultural ideas and practices are understood not as they rank on a spurious developmental scale but rather in their own context. Culture was something that everybody had a different version of, and to understand part of a culture one had to understand the larger context in which that part made sense. Holism was essential.

Culture versus Society

On the other side of the Atlantic, changes also were taking place. As anthropology matured, those scholars interested in European pre-history ("us") migrated into classics and history departments. This left the study of non-Europeans ("them") to the anthropologists who were left. Concurrently, another discipline, sociology, had laid claim to the study of "us" in contemporary form. That is, sociology took as its main focus the study of society.

"Society" had, by mid-century, come to delineate the interactional system of relationships between people. But it also had come to cover that old term "civilization." This meant that the term, and study of, society was generally only applied to scholars' own social groupings, again leaving culture to what some still called "the primitives." That is, culture was left squarely in anthropology's bailiwick. Table 6.1 illustrates this historical shift.

The society-culture distinction was codified in 1958 when sociologist Talcott Parsons and anthropologist Alfred Kroeber—both grand men in their respective traditions—published an article saying the distinction just outlined existed. They did this, some claim, as a way of diffusing the potential for scholars in either field to become jealous of each other's

Table 6.1   Culture and society in U.S. anthropological and sociological tradition: who has what?

When?	*What?*	*Who?*
Phase I: emerging anthropological theory (1800s)	*Culture* = *civilization* = "That complex whole... capabilities and habits acquired by man as a member of society" (Tylor 1871).	Primitives (non-Europeans) have neither.
Phase II: relativism emerges (early 1900s)	*Culture* = "That complex whole ... capabilities and habits acquired by man as a member of society" (Tylor 1871); there are many cultures.	We *all* have culture but only Europeans have civilization now, although primitives can become civilized (and thus will no longer be primitive).
Phase III: sociology and anthropology stake disparate territorial claims (midcentury)	*Culture* = Shared, learned, holistically related capabilities and habits of primitive peoples *Society* = *civilization* = large-scale, complexly systematized social relationships.	Europeans no longer have culture, only civilization: Primitives still have cultures.
Phase IV: contemporary positions (the last several decades)	*Culture* = "That complex whole... capabilities and habits acquired by man as a member of society" (Tylor 1871). *Society* = systematized social relationships. *Civilization* = large-scale, complex societies.	Everybody has everything except civilization, which is differentially distributed (and there are no primitives).

territory and means (Kroeber and Parsons 1958). Of course, the distinction never really worked: The link between the two is too tight; both inform one another. Sociologists and anthropologists have long intertwined their knowledge bases and, despite conceptual distinctions, society or social structure and culture form two sides of the same coin of human group experience.

But it did not take long, in Europe or the United States, for synonymy between culture and "them" to solidify once it had begun to take shape. Culture was now an attribute of what some have come to call "the other."

So, Who Has Culture?

Today we know that us-them and culture-civilization distinctions are nonsense. Civilization, where the word is retained, means only a particular form of social organization (generally including a large population, civic or public architecture, a judicial system, centralized decision-making, and class- or residence-based rather than kin-based relationships). Culture is something that both anthropologists and sociologists today will say that everyone has, as Boas and his followers argued so revolutionarily 100 years ago.

Health services workers have, in addition to various ethnic and other cultures that they each may lay claim to as individuals, professional or occupational cultures. And those affiliated with a particular organization may have a few shared values and habits related to that organization, too; this is what is meant by "organizational culture." Having said that, often an organization's managerial culture provides all officially accepta-ble organizational cultural fodder, for example, through vision statements, dress codes, and the like. Cultural practices in the lower ranks, such as workarounds developed by data entry clerks or the use of derogatory nicknames for certain types of patients, generally are undertaken behind closed doors. Certainly managerial values can be dominative, at least in organizationally public contexts and in front of superiors (see Sobo and Sadler 2002).

The belief that only other people have culture continues to thrive in the popular imagination as well as in health services. This is partly because of the invisible, tacit, taken-for-granted nature of culture. Because of this, we rarely think about it in reference to ourselves. Unless, that is, it is challenged, for example when entering another culture or when someone from another culture enters ours. Even then, it is their way that is described as "cultural," not our own.

Sharon Traweek has labeled the culture of objectivity held by high-energy physicists a "culture of no culture" (1988, p. 162). In the physicists' cultural viewpoint, there is an objective reality out there that we can measure and fully describe, given enough observational time. Although Traweek is talking about scientific culture, I would like to push the idea further. If what I have said above about culture's taken-for-granted nature is true, most of us live in a "culture of no culture" a lot of the time. It is not just that the cultural nature of our lives is kept out of awareness but that our cultural notions are internalized to the extent that they them-selves seem objectively real. We believe that the world is a certain way and those who do not see its (acultural, true, real) reality are deluded. They are deluded or blinded to "reality," we believe, by their cultures.

It is easy to see, then, why Janelle Taylor equated the health services culture that has husbanded the cultural competence movement with the "culture of no culture" inhabited by Traweek's physicists. But there is a problem with this that goes beyond the fact that most in health services see culture as something belonging to others (minority group members, people with limited English proficiency, and foreigners) in the way that

I have just insinuated. They also define it in a way that is, as Taylor notes, at odds with current anthropological thinking about what culture is (2003, p. 161).

Relativism Revisited

Cultural competence programs have generally taken culture to be a set of beliefs that can be cataloged and recounted. In some cases, culture also has been taken as inherently problematic beliefs that can be exchanged, given good patient education programs, for accurate knowledge. Paul Farmer has faulted this approach (which he derides as "anthro lite" (2005, p. 15) for diverting attention from other causes of poor health outcomes. Building on his observation that labeling the Chiapas rebellion an "ethnic uprising" rather than a class-based social and economic rights movement distracted observers' focus from the latter, Farmer warns against the cultural "alibi" that the present-day focus on cultural competence can provide (p. 49). He warns that pointing to culture to explain health inequities provides the real culprits with a cover, diverting attention from what is really going on.

Ironically, and despite the concern it causes for today's anthropologists, the simplistic definition of culture used in many cultural competence programs is quite similar to the definition used in late 19th-century anthropology. Recall my mention above of progressive cultural evolutionism, in which savages could become civilized. This position became untenable in the face of mounting evidence for multilineal change and that is when relativism came into vogue in anthropological circles.

Originally, **relativism** (as, for example, Franz Boas practiced it) meant only that one should not try to interpret cultural practices or ideas out of context. This is what is known now as descriptive relativism. So far, so good. But remember how culture was divorced from civilization around this time, demarcated as something that others had. It was also at the time being studied with checklists containing partitioned sets of disparate traits that could be counted and mapped to determine the so-called laws of cultural diffusion. Bits of culture were individually catalogable.

Sociocultural anthropology today teaches the importance of comprehensively and holistically understanding the subject culture. This is no change from what Boas recommended when the subfield was more commonly termed "ethnology" in the United States. Be this as it may, in the old days, culture was conceptualized and measured by many as if a thing comprised of bits and pieces.

Recall how, as they matured, the disciplines of anthropology and sociology focused in on the twin topics of (primitive) culture and (contemporary) society, respectively. This kind of apportionment or hiving has long been common in academia. To claim a place at the university table, emerging disciplines must stake out a particular territory for study. Further, as knowledge accumulates, disciplines can no longer do it all.

But the fragmentation trend began much earlier, in the 18th century, when the discipline of **political economy** was subverted. Eric Wolf (who is largely responsible for political economy's resurgence in the social sciences) defines that discipline—now more of a perspective—as concerned with "the production and distribution of wealth within and between political entities and the classes composing them." As capitalism grew, a "rising tide of discontent pitting 'society' against the political and ideological order ['the state'] erupted in disorder, rebellion, and revolution" (1982, p. 8). The French Revolution is but one example.

Early social theorists such as Herbert Spencer and Émile Durkheim focused their inquiries on the ties that hold society together. It is true that Durkheim's sociology was comparative, including for example, Australian aboriginal religion, but his main interest was his own society. Although his work (and Spencer's) may be studied in anthropology courses, it is generally under the rubric of classical social theory or comparative sociology, not anthropology per se.

The grave importance of the emerging political economy for global well-being was discounted: The new social theory disarticulated large systems (transglobal national trade networks), hiding the structural violence of the new order in the process (e.g., Farmer 2004, p. 308). Each society was taken to stand on its own, divorced from even the human bodies that made it up. Society was now thought of as superorganic. It was **reified**: It was considered as a concrete, bounded thing, existing in and of itself.

The boundedness of concepts such as culture or society has social as well as scholarly implications. As Wolf explains, "By endowing nations, societies, or cultures with the qualities of internally homogeneous and externally distinctive and bounded objects, we create a model of the world as a global pool hall in which the entities spin off each other like so many hard and round billiard balls" (1982, p. 6).

This image of cultures, societies, and nations as bounded, coherent, things-unto-themselves—which Janelle Taylor has noted is the image propounded by most cultural competence programs (2003)—may be expedient, but it is wrong. It misrepresents humanity's past and present intergroup interchanges and cultural flows.

In fact, cultural boundaries are porous and flexible. Cultures have always evolved. People and practices have always moved in and out of more-or-less cohesive social groups, through trade networks, in- and out-marriage, labor migration, tourism or neighboring village visits, and so on. Today, with air travel, cars, cellular phones, and the Internet, the pace of movement is even faster. International media now permeate all corners of the world. As Wolf declares, "The world of humankind constitutes a manifold, a totality of interconnected processes" (1982, p. 3).

He goes on to say:

> Inquiries that disassemble this totality into bits and then fail to reassemble it falsify reality. Concepts, like "nation," "society," and "culture" name bits and threaten to turn names into things. Only by understanding these names as bundles of relationships, and by placing them back into the field from which they were abstracted, can we hope to avoid misleading inferences and increase our share of understanding. (1982, p. 3)

That is, only by rejecting "anthro lite" (Farmer 2005) and readopting a holistic, global systems perspective can we really get a grip on what is going on.

Should We Throw Culture Out?

We have seen in our brief historical foray how and why culture has come to be routinely applied to others and not ourselves. We have seen, too, how and why, through the process of disciplinary emergence in academia, it came to be disarticulated and reified, or misconstrued and studied as a bounded entity or thing.

Some anthropologists argue that we should jettison the term "culture" altogether, because of its connotations and the temptations it provides. These scholars have additional complaints to the ones already aired. Attending to them here will help us refine even further our understanding of the culture concept. This will support us in our efforts to conduct the highest quality of anthropologically informed HSR.

Following from and building on Wolf's argument that the term "culture" as we use it now always highlights difference and conceals variation, anti-culture advocates point out that the term also always entails relationships of power and dominance. This viewpoint reflects the present postcolonial global reality, in which populations once under the thumb of colonial rule have been left to self-rule but without the infrastructure and, in some cases, the experience necessary to successfully do so.

Importantly, self-rule is not only a political endeavor; it also is a cultural one. In addition to freedom from colonial governance, postcolonial societies are free from the hegemonic dominance of colonial cultures. Hegemony occurs when a nonindigenous or elite ideal or expectation (e.g., for light-colored foods or a certain style of comportment or medical practice) is internalized by indigenous or nonelite populations largely because of its association with power. Colonial prejudices are internalized by colonized populations to the degree that they seem to be common sense; colonized people thereby become, in many ways, self-regulating, abandoning any desire to subvert the oppressor's power.

Unlike the original "informants" of anthropology, who generally lacked access to the texts written about them and had little input into decisions made "on their behalf," postcolonial subjects talk back and even those who cannot, because of the dangers this would pose given the current global maldistribution of power, often have advocates. The health, welfare, power, and other inequities that exist in the world—the histories behind them as well as all that they presently entail—can no longer be hidden behind a falsely disconnected ethnographic representation. The timeless "ethnographic present" in which unique, bounded, homogeneous cultural groups practice their long-standing, unadulterated ways (or "authentic traditions") fails to hold up in the harsh light of the postcolonial day.

But what to do? Some anthropologists refuse to use the word "culture." Rather than falsely pretend to describe bounded cultural entities that do not really exist, many prefer to refer instead to cultural processes, such as "practice" and "discourse" (Abu-Lughod 2005). When writing an editorial on the uses of ethnography in HSR for a wholly health services audience, some of my U.K. colleagues and I decided to avoid the term completely because of the connotations it carries with that audience. Our word count was limited, so, without space to explore the term, we were not willing to risk a miscommunication (Huby et al. 2007).

Banning the term from our vocabularies is not really a tenable solution in the long run. The term "culture," like "race" before it, has broken free of anthropology's boundaries: It has escaped into the world outside of anthropology's control. It is in use now and will be in use for the foreseeable future. Furthermore, anthropology textbooks still always contain a definition of culture, and culture is still taken as central for the mainstream of the discipline.

Widespread usage of the term is not in itself a sufficient reason for retention. But there are other holes in the argument for culture's excommunication.

One cannot deny that some nongenetically acquired or learned values and habits of body or mind *do* co-occur in particular groups (at least for some periods of time) and "culture" provides an efficient and effective shorthand for referencing these. Christoph Brumann, using the (so-called?) Japanese as an example, notes: "There are many situations in which 'Japanese culture' is a convenient shorthand for designating something like 'that which' many or most Japanese irrespective of gender, class, and other differences regularly think, feel, and do by virtue of having been in continuous social contact with other Japanese" (2005, p. 62). The "that which" is held in common would fill a bigger basket if a subgroup was referenced (e.g., the Japanese middle class). But even for the large group, some "that which" will always be there.

A certain amount of consensus does exist among people who spend time together, whether physically or virtually. Even if ideas differ, as those less central to group membership can do, those who share culture generally agree on how such differences should be expressed; witness for instance the patterned divergence between how anthropologists, clinicians, and football or soccer fans resolve their differences. This does not discount the facts that people may belong to many cultures and most cultures are partial; that is, taken alone, most cultures (e.g., organizational cultures, professional cultures) do not cover all life's questions. It does not discount cultural change or internal dynamism or idiosyncratic uses or interpretations of culture. It does not deny that there are aspects of human nature that we all share. However, used with care, the term "culture" does allow us to convey to others a point of reference regarding human groupings, and that is a useful thing.

Further, it is that point of reference that processes such as "practice" and "discourse" often revolve around, negotiate, or strive to create and maintain—or tear down. So culture may well exist both as a thing (or a reified point of reference) *and* a process, much like light exists as both particle and wave, according to many physicists.

Therefore, bearing in mind culture's complexity as well as the need to move quickly to process-related matters once the cultural group in question has been identified or outlined and the dangers of such delimitation have been at least acknowledged, I will continue to use the term "culture" to refer in the first instance to a group's or groups' shared values and habits (e.g., Japanese culture/s, student culture/s, nursing culture/s, health services research culture/s). The reference will, of course, be coarse-grained. Fine-grained references to practices and discourses will necessarily follow.

Such mindfulness frees us from holding ourselves aloof from the term "culture." And it allows us to engage in the ongoing conversation that health services programs do want to have regarding their cultural competence needs. It enables us to provide the cultural competence endeavor with some anthropological moorings.

/ REDEFINING CULTURAL COMPETENCE

Language Barriers Are Key

Culture is supposed to be anthropology's bread and butter. Still, there is much more to successful cultural competence than that, and knowledge of its other various dimensions strengthens our grasp of the context in which much anthropologically informed HSR takes place. A number of disciplines, not least health psychology and health communication, have been making inroads into understanding them. On a more programmatic level, the National Standards on Culturally and Linguistically Appropriate Services (CLAS) mandate several practices and recommend others in support of cultural competence and these include not only Culturally Competent Care (Standards 1–3), but also Language Access Services (Standards 4–7), and Organizational Supports for Cultural Competence (Standards 8–14) (http://www.omhrc.gov/templates/browse.aspx?lvl=2& lvlID=15, last accessed August 28, 2008).

Given organizational support, a necessary (but not sufficient) condition for cultural competence is people's ability to communicate using one shared verbal language. Therefore, strong translation service policies and programs are essential. Better translation leads to better communication. This helps both decrease the probability of misdiagnosis and increase patient comprehension of the care plan. Better communication also leads to improved patient satisfaction. Satisfaction correlates with adherence to recommended care plans, which, in turn, correlates with better health outcomes (Betancourt, Carrillo, and Green 1999).

Adequate translation services rely on trained, professional translators rather than bystanders, family members, or untrained staff members who happen to speak the language in question. For one thing, nonprofessionals may not actually speak the language as well as is necessary for adequate communication. For another, they may for some reason edit or elaborate on speakers' messages. And any social closeness with the translator may lead to self-censorship in the patient or family. This is perhaps especially true when household members are asked to translate; health information may be considered private by the patient or the person translating because of the implications it can have for social standing. Finally, nonprofessionals may lack background in medical terminology and mistranslate, however unintentionally, leading to miscommunication (Loustaunau and Sobo 1997).

Communicative Competence

Although adequate translation is necessary, linguistic concordance is not sufficient for culturally competent communication. Medical miscommunications occur even when translation is not an issue (Clark et al. 2002). As many have noted, the content of what is communicated may be poorly understood if it is not explained in terms that are familiar to the listener. This is critical in clinician-patient communication because, as Hahn (1995) and Good and Good (1993) have demonstrated, the intensive training that the clinician receives creates a gulf between patient and healer. To quote Hahn, patients and healers "inevitably conceive of the world, communicate, and behave in ways that cannot be reasonably or safely assumed to be similar or readily compatible"; in other words, "*All medicine is cross-cultural*" (1995, p. 265; emphasis in the original).

As I have argued elsewhere (Sobo and Seid 2003), the type of competence that clinicians need to master if they are to better serve people from all cultures—including cultures that are similar to their own—is a kind of *communicative* competence. Care must be taken to translate technical terms into lay language, and the content of the conversation must be made culturally relevant. This does not mean adopting a cookbook approach to medicine in which a set of so-called facts regarding commonly encountered cultures can be memorized and recited as per the testable competencies model of medical education. Although people who share the same culture generally share certain understandings, immense intracultural variation has been documented. Further, it has been widely shown that many health understandings are flexible and context-dependent. Essentialist approaches to cultural competence are untenable (Fuller 2002).

In dealing with individual patients, clinicians and other health services workers will find knowledge about their clients' general cultural understandings about health and about proper forms of interaction very helpful. But it would be unwise to assume that those understandings apply across the board to all people who share in that culture; informed overgeneralization can have the same effect as uninformed stereotyping. Knowledge of general cultural patterns and common local illness categories should be seen as a starting point, not a foregone conclusion (Galanti 1997).

Health services workers should make every effort to understand patients' (or dependent patients' caregivers') present understandings of what their health concerns are. This includes how and when the condition(s) of concern came about, what might cause them, what course they might take, and what might be done to help them (Demers et al. 1980; Kleinman 1980). At the same time, clinicians should elicit information on socioeconomic factors (such as low or no income, lack of running water, or job-related time or movement constraints) that might make certain treatment courses more realistic than others. And this should be done not only with patients who differ from the clinician ethnically or racially but also with those who are ostensibly the same.

The Health System as a Foreign Culture

Communication needs to cover not just a person's complaint but organizational issues as well. This is because, to any layperson, the health care system itself is confusing and complicated. Medicine is another world completely. An initial step is to develop a practical, reliable, and valid measurement tool that can inform policy and program decisions aimed at making the system more transparent and responsive to the user.

As HSR pioneer Avedis Donabedian argues, a series of steps are necessary to improve health: (1) A health care system must be available for people to access; (2) people must access this system and (3) use available services; and (4) these services must be technically and interpersonally of high quality (1988). If these steps proceed smoothly, the likelihood of improved health is maximized. If, on the other hand, **barriers to care** exist that disrupt this pathway, the likelihood of improved health is reduced.

In a model that I generated with help from Michael Seid and other colleagues (Sobo, Seid, and Gelherd 2006; see also Seid et al. 2004), a central barrier to care was a lack of the skills and knowledge necessary for negotiating the health care system. These include the learned strategies or behaviors necessary for accessing and obtaining care and for making best use of the clinical encounter. Possession of or knowledge about where and how to find information on care availability, eligibility requirements, and so on, and facility with the culture of medicine and the health services system were key.

Functional Biomedical Acculturation

In creating the model, I labeled the skills to move within the health care system and to optimize the health care received **functional biomedical acculturation** (Sobo and Seid 2003). These skills require that people be at least minimally or functionally acculturated to the world of their health care system in a way that allows them to function within it and achieve desired ends. These skills may include, for example, those needed for gaining timely access to specialty services, making sure one's questions are answered during the clinical encounter, and ensuring that different specialties coordinate around one's care. Just as medical and other health services students must acculturate to or learn how to act in their new roles as doctors, nurses, etc., if they are to fit in and be successful, so too must lay people learn how to act as health care consumers if they are to realize their health-related goals.

Notwithstanding the emphasis on functionality and minimal skills, functional biomedical acculturation is still a much broader construct than those that are commonly used to explain or understand barriers to care. Take, for example, "functional health literacy," a construct that focuses on reading-related comprehension, which research shows to be inadequate among English speakers and even more inadequate among Spanish speakers (Parker et al. 1995; Williams et al. 1995).

Functional biomedical acculturation, however, rests on the command of a whole set of skills, not just language. Further, although the functional health literacy construct locates the barrier to care squarely within the individual, casting the patient as lacking or deficient (Williams et al. 1995), functional biomedical acculturation locates the barrier in the gap between cultures and in the health care system's own ethnocentrism as opposed to in the culture of the patient. That is, it does not rest on a blame-the-victim type deficit model. In addition, because it does not entail assumptions about assimilation that are embedded in most so-called acculturation models, the functional biomedical acculturation construct avoids sending an implicit message about the virtues of the hegemonic or dominative white middle class and, in this case, U.S. lifestyle (see also Clark and Hofsess 1998; Clark et al. 2002).

The idea that medicine is itself in many ways a foreign culture—albeit a partial one with various occupational subcultures—is nothing new in anthropological and other social science circles. But to many in medicine, it is a radical proposition. The functional biomedical acculturation construct's meta-message regarding culture as entailing more than just ethnic difference are messages that medicine needs to hear if its present interest in cultural issues is to truly increase the standard of care.

Competence: What Kind Is Needed and by Whom?

Cultural competence is a crucial component of policies aimed at reducing health inequity. Nonetheless, the concept of cultural competence is both imprecise and impoverished, at least as presently deployed. Health service providers are not the only people who need to become competent in cross-cultural exchange. Policies and programs must ensure that patients and families, too, are provided education and assistance so that they can navigate the health care system. An emphasis on skills and practices—on functional biomedical acculturation—can help us to gain insight into ways to better equip all health care consumers with the cultural competence necessary to navigate health services.

Our goal should not be to shift the competency burden to the shoulders of already vulnerable and disenfranchised health care consumers. Nor should it be to distract attention from the structural conditions that exacerbate the cross-cultural gap. Rather, it should be to raise awareness in the medical world of the essential strangeness of the system. By promoting the anthropological perspective and supporting our colleagues in achieving a critical distance (see Chapter 4), we can help create a bridge between two worlds—a strong, two-way bridge that can lead to measurable increases in quality of care.

A Methodological Bridge

The anthropological rendering of culture moves us beyond the kind of recipe collection and dissemination implicated in the cookbook medicine promoted by more simplistic versions of cultural competence. Such is reflected in blanket recommendations for avoiding eye contact with X people, not shaking hands with Y people, talking only to grandfathers when caring for Z people, and broad proclamations that people from culture A will engage in practice B. In one situation that I know of, clinicians treating a girl from Somalia for a toe problem asked about genital cutting, as if that had anything to do with the problem at hand; they did so because they had been "educated" about Somali culture. The functional biomedical acculturation construct does not support this kind of thoughtless action. It directs attention to cultural processes such as practice and discourse. Moreover, it refuses to blame the individual suffering health inequities for his or her condition. It asks us instead to take into consideration social structural factors that support poor health and poor outcomes.

Of course, not all health services colleagues have been trained to see the importance of this; because of the way that bureaucracy works, lack of vision also pervades many authorizing institutions. In my own experience, cultural cookbook-type deliverables have been requested as a product of my research quite often. My response depends on context: Wherever I sense there is room to maneuver, I gently remind or request that whoever I am working with in an organization broaden their expectations for the project at hand. I do this by providing some examples of alternative ways of approaching the project at hand. Demonstrating with examples how a broader vision of culture and meaning's role in health care can help, and pointing to how others have realized concrete outcomes improvement by taking a broader view, I have often been able to negotiate a revision in the scope of work such that the products expected of me (e.g., guideline recommendations, particular cuts of data, indicator parameters, educational message ideas, etc.) are anthropologically informed—at least minimally.

One example of this would be the creation of laminated cards describing and depicting home remedies and over-the-counter medicines that certain groups of immigrant patients at Children's Hospital may have used prior to seeking emergency care for certain symptoms (we constructed the list using focus groups). Some popular treatments interact badly with certain prescribed drugs; some may be harmful to our health (this is true generally, not just for the populations in question). The cards, which were centrally available in the emergency department's clinical area, allowed providers who did not speak these patients' languages to collect important health-related information: Patients, parents, or guardians could point at a card depicting something they had done. Because the cards depicted alternatives and training emphasized that the treatments depicted were just some of the treatments that might have been used (if any), the card system did not support stereotyping. Using the cards opened a line of communication. It demonstrated to the families, too, that their children were welcomed, valued patients.

The "here are some alternatives" approach to negotiating deliverables makes sense in regard to QI efforts, and it works to enhance the effectiveness of what might otherwise merely be bureaucratic box-checking exercises related to, for example, CLAS standards. But how can HSR keep the issues raised in this chapter in mind when designing and implementing robust research studies? Is it really possible to build a bridge between HSR proper and the anthropological vision?

To this point, our focus has been on answering the question "what." Readers are, by now, fairly familiar with what both anthropology and health services entail. The next section has more to say on "what" as we continue to build foundational knowledge regarding the field for anthropologically informed HSR, but it also begins to answer "how" by opening up the methodological black boxes of both anthropology and HSR. Once we look inside, we will find that things are in some cases much more complex and in others much simpler than we might imagine.

Methodological Theory and Practice

In Part III, we examine the theoretical basis of the methods that the anthropological approach entails. We are concerned here with **methodology**: the study of methods, including the principles behind them. We therefore also explore **epistemological** issues—issues relating to how knowledge is established and evaluated.

Chapter 7, which begins by rejecting the so-called qualitative-quantitative divide, demonstrates that many of the concepts associated with positivism as represented in the hypothetico-deductive model of science today can be and are applied in anthropologically informed research. Although Chapter 7 might be described as arguing that careful, systematic anthropologically informed work can be scientifically valid and reliable, Chapter 8 questions the notion of science itself as presently constructed in health services research (HSR). By reviewing the history of medicine and the invention of randomized controlled drug trials, Chapter 8 shows that what counts as evidence and good research design—indeed, the total definition of science from the HSR standpoint—is historically and socioculturally situated. It examines the history of debate regarding who has the power to decide on an appropriate care plan (patients? providers? payors?) and on what kind of evidence practice should be based. It also furthers the argument for the value added by taking an anthropologically informed approach to HSR by focusing our attention on questions of effectiveness—of a given care plan's impact given the complexity of real life.

Chapter 9 situates the research endeavor by exploring the various sites in which anthropologically informed HSR may be undertaken. Indeed, what Chapter 5 did for the health services landscape, Chapter 9 seeks to do for HSR. It provides insight into what to expect and how to prepare, for instance, by examining the tensions that particular sites, such as surgical recovery rooms and hospices on the one hand and employee lounges on the other can entail. It also takes a closer look at research team dynamics as well as the very need to work in teams. By the end of Part III, readers will be ready to learn about particular methods that can be applied when conducting an anthropologically informed study.

CHAPTER 7

/ Doing Science—And Other
Systematic Things

/ THE QUALITATIVE-QUANTITATIVE DIVIDE?

As James Spradley explains, anthropology's ethnographic methods help us discover or describe and delineate "folk" or lay categories and realities—the emic perspective—rather than helping us test or clarify previously conceived and ostensibly universally applicable models into which those categories and realities are meant to fit—from the etic perspective. For Spradley, the ultimate goal of ethnographic research is to "serve humankind" by eliciting "informant-expressed needs" that can be "synchronized with scientific methods" to reduce human suffering (1979, pp. 14–15).

There are certainly important differences between scientific approaches and humanities-informed interpretive approaches to scholarship, and Spradley sums up some of them here. As he implies, these two approaches also are complementary. I would go further and say that they are two sides of the same coin.

This also holds true for the data types stereotypically associated with science, on the one hand—quantitative—and interpretive inquiry on the other—qualitative. In reality, behind every quantity there is a quality. There is a subjective determination regarding what counts. The next chapter questions popular definitions of science stemming from the hypothetico-deductive positivist tradition; in this chapter we explore its accepted constructs and investigate the ways that ethnographic approaches accommodate them. This chapter is thus recommended for all readers, although those well versed in scientific concepts may wish to skim through some of the definitions.

/ TYPES OF DATA, TYPES OF ANALYSIS

Much of what anthropology does involves **primary data** (data collected in the field, for the project at hand, by and for those who will analyze it) as opposed to existing or **secondary data** (large institutional datasets put together by others, generally from administrative or surveillance systems). Although health services research (HSR) uses primary data some of the time, in the beginning it relied heavily on secondary data and this is one reason for its quantitative or numerical focus.

Qualitative and quantitative data types, and the distinction between scientific and nonscientific investigations on the basis of data type, begin to blur when one considers that the categorization of any item as an item involves making qualitative distinctions. For example, we determine the criteria we will use to categorize research participants as being rich, of average income, or poor by thinking about these categories qualitatively. We may draw the line used in determining whether a participant is in middle or old age for a given piece of research in the same way. Our cultural assumptions about when these categories begin and end are just that: cultural assumptions. They are therefore value linked and amenable to qualitative description. Even age itself, often thought of as a number, is derived from qualitative assumptions about when to begin counting (conception [however defined]? delivery of baby? delivery of placenta? first breath?) and at what time interval one's assigned number changes.

Not only do qualitative judgments determine many quantitative category boundaries—they also determine the meaning of quantitative findings once we have calculated them. That is, quantitative findings must be interpreted to have any meaning; they must be qualitatively analyzed. And meaningful interpretations are based on an understanding of the qualitative data that relate to such findings. We can say that 28% of Americans like dogs better than cats and 21% like cats better than dogs based on Crispell's pet popularity findings (1994, p. 59), but only qualitative data can help us understand the meaning of this or why it might be so. Further, to interpret the output of either qualitative or quantitative data analysis techniques, we need to know something about the ethnographic context in which the data were elicited and how the participants described each item of data as they provided or stated it.

Just as quantitative data are qualitatively conceptualized and interpreted, so too can qualitative data be submitted to quantitative scrutiny (although they must be reduced to numbers in the interim as happens, for example, when the number of times a certain theme comes up is counted and tallied, as in a quantitative content analysis; see Bernard 1995a). The qualitative or quantitative nature of the data does not, in other words, predetermine a likewise analysis (i.e., qualitative or quantitative). Figure 7.1 sums up this situation.

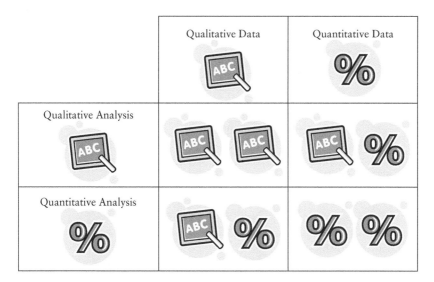

Figure 7.1 Data and analysis types (adapted from Bernard 1995b, p. 10).

In part because of the interpenetration of qualitative and quantitative approaches, many have suggested that the so-called qualitative-quantitative divide is unnecessarily divisive. Miles and Huberman (1984) write:

> In fact, it is getting harder to find any methodologists solidly encamped in one epistemology or the other. More and more "quantitative" methodologists, operating from a logical positivist stance, are using naturalistic [non-laboratory, non-experimental] and phenomenological [first-person, experience-oriented] approaches to complement tests, surveys and structured interviews. On the other side, an increasing number of ethnographers and qualitative researchers are using predesigned conceptual frameworks. (p. 20)

Werner and Schoepfle emphasize that "No quantitative study can afford to leave implicit its qualitative aspects" and go on to argue that "ethnography can be systematic and its methods explicit and replicable" (1997, p. 44).

Yet, it is safe to say that what is called "the scientific approach" rarely uses qualitative data collection and even less commonly qualitative data analysis techniques. Similarly, although ethnography can bring quantitative data and analyses into play, this is not central to ethnographic methodology. Figure 7.2 demonstrates, by overlaying the ethnographic and the normatively defined, hypothetico-deductive scientific fields on Figure 7.1, that although in reality there is a great deal of overlap, in

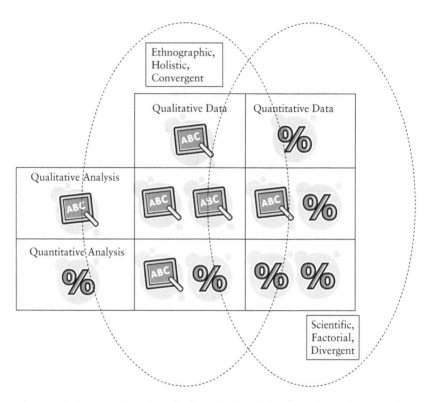

Figure 7.2 Data and analysis in hypothetico-deductive science (quantitative-quantitative) and ethnography (qualitative-qualitative); area of overlap is not to scale (underlying table adapted from Bernard 1995b, p. 10).

practice concurrence is not realized. Most activity takes place in the nonoverlapping sections of the ovals, with ethnography stereotyped as falling only in the upper left cell and science in only the lower right.

/ SCIENCE-NONSCIENCE?

Field or Lab?

One difference persisting between quantitative and qualitative relates to where data are gathered: in the field or in the lab. Ethnographic methods are necessarily different in kind from **experimental** methods because the researcher has to physically go to where the participants of his or her research live and study them in situ (in their natural setting). Everyday life is a mixture of the routine and the unusual, the predictable and the exceptional. Chance events happen that we cannot control. Experimental methods, in contrast, bring the subjects to the researcher, taking them out of their natural, rather uncontrollable settings.

The goals of experimental methods are to test hypotheses about the relationship(s) between two or more **variables** (discrete influences or states). To ensure that variables other than the variables of interest do not influence outcomes, the researcher needs to control the situation by eliminating them or otherwise ensuring that they are exactly the same across two conditions set up for a comparison. The human subjects participating often are referred to as members of the **case** or intervention group, on the one hand, and the **control** group, on the other. The first group entails cases representing the variable of interest, for example, exposure to a chemical; the control group does not, but the individuals in it are otherwise as like those in the first group as possible. **Randomized controlled clinical trials** (see Chapter 8) follow this model.

Experimental methods thus involve creating artificial conditions or posing hypothetical situations that allow the researcher to focus only on the study variables (Golden 1976, p. 16). Notwithstanding, experimental studies are high on **internal validity** but low on **external validity**. That is, the parts fit together with impeccable internal logic, but it is questionable whether they actually mirror what goes on outside the lab.

In comparison with the experimenter, the ethnographer (whose work is **naturalistic**, or carried out in a natural setting) has little or no control over variables. However, ethnographers can still build valid and reliable local causal models of cognitive and event processes by listening to how people tell them they happen. The difference to highlight here is that qualitative methods tend to focus on "case-oriented" causal processes, whereas quantitative methods focus on "variable-oriented" causality (Maxwell 1996, p. 20). That is, qualitative studies generally focus on the linkages between events or activities in a particular case or example, such as a particular individual's experience of diabetes, rather than linkages between trait variables across cases, such as income, fast food consumption, or number of clinic visits. The case rather than the variable forms the unit of analysis.

Explicitness and Systematicity

For a study to have practical application or theoretical validity, and for it to be useful in making comparisons, it is essential that its methods be explicit. The researcher must explain which methods were selected and how they were used; he or she must communicate to readers and to other researchers what was done and why; and the resulting ethnographic descriptions and analyses should be believed and accepted over anyone else's. Descriptions and conclusions should never appear as if magically spun out of thin air.

In addition to methodological explicitness, good research requires that a method is **systematically** applied. That is, the researcher must use the same data collection and analytic procedures with all research participants (or across all events or contexts). For example, if one is trying to identify problems newly admitted chemotherapy patients experience, then the same questions, preferably in the same order, should be asked of a number of such patients. Such standardization of methods means that the research can be repeated or replicated at other sites to determine whether localized, case- or site-specific theories are **generalizable**—whether they may be extended to apply to settings and populations that have not been observed (to generalize is to assume that what applies in one case applies in another).

SCIENTIFIC ETHNOGRAPHY?

The possibility—indeed, the unavoidable reality—of blending qualitative and quantitative approaches has been mentioned, as have several differences between the two: nature of data (narrative or numerical), location and nature of research (in situ or in a controlled environment) and type of focus (case-specific or on a narrow range of specified variables). In either case, some standard criteria are used to assess research quality. Although there is some debate about exactly how these can be defined so as to be broadly applicable, it is possible to apply at least some key quality indicators across the board, no matter at what point of the qualitative-quantitative or interpretive-scientific continuum a piece of research lays (Mays and Pope 2000).

Relevance

One of the first issues that should enter our minds as we try to evaluate research quality is relevance. **Relevance** refers to whether or not (or the degree to which) research adds to the existing knowledge base, either by expanding it, correcting it, or increasing our confidence in it. Funding and, later, publication often hinge on relevance.

Some assess relevance according to how generalizable findings may be; that is, can they be applied in settings other than or beyond the original research site? To some degree, this hinges on sampling methods (see below). However, it also depends on the nature of the question under consideration. Is the problem investigated strictly local or does it (or a variation on it) occur elsewhere? If strictly local, are there some things about how it is locally handled that may have global or anyhow nonlocal implications?

Validity

Another quality criterion is **validity,** sometimes termed "test validity," which in either case refers to whether variables really measure what they purport to measure. Previously, I referred to internal and external validity, which has to do with goodness of fit and is more relevant for experimental methods than naturalistic ones. But there are two problems of validity that always bear considering with regard to individual variables: First, are our variables accurate reflections or indicators of the stream of life we are trying to describe, measure, or explain? For instance, if we wanted to know about how often people ate dinner at home and why, would hamburger intake in and of itself be a valid measure? Probably not, in part because people might eat other items when out, and hamburgers do get eaten at home. But it would be a valid measure of hamburger intake. Given that, another problem of validity arises. Are our methods for measuring variance or change in relation to our chosen variables useful or effective? For example, is counting the number of hamburgers eaten in varying conditions a more useful measure for comparison than, say, their total weight? The researcher must be able to defend his or her position both in terms of selecting variables and in the manner in which they have been **operationalized** (defined for measurement or collection). The clarity of the research question is implicated.

Other problems of validity involve the more philosophical issue of whether unbiased objectivity is truly achievable. This issue, touched on earlier, is usually divided into two components: reactivity and research bias.

Reactivity

Postmodernism teaches us that the appearance as well as the psychological and cultural attributes of researchers and participants matter as we attempt to ferret out the meaning of what is going on. Certainly my own previous research experiences with inner-city black women who shared information regarding their sexual practices would have been very different had I been male or darker skinned or substantially younger or older than I was at the time (Sobo 1995). Similarly, my Children's staff badge helped me gain certain kinds of inside information from other staff members while barring me from collecting from individual employees data that might reflect poorly on their work ethic or performance.

Reactivity refers to the effect the researcher has on participants and the context in which work is carried out. In fieldwork situations, the problem of reactivity diminishes over time, so that after a year of living in an area the researcher's effect on surrounding people's behavior has (or should have) been significantly reduced (see de Munck 1998). In general, the subject's or informant's behavior is affected in proportion to the intrusiveness of the research. Bogdan and Biklen put it well: "If you treat people as 'research subjects,' they will act as research subjects, which is different from how they usually act" (1992, p. 47). Because reactivity can never be eliminated when using intrusive, formal methods, generalizations made to the real world on the basis of results from such research always are suspect.

Research Bias

Research bias refers to the theoretical preconceptions a researcher brings to bear on choice and use of methods. For example, an anthropologist who assumes that all behavior is rule-governed may infer the presence of a particular rule for explaining a behavior when no such rule is actually present. Most researchers recognize that "*all data* are theory-, method-, and measurement dependent" (Ratcliffe 1983, p. 148, cited in Phillips 1990, p. 25; emphasis in the original).

Quantitative methods attempt to minimize research bias by emphasizing the use of instruments for data collection and measurement, thereby eliminating the researcher's bias in both the data collection and analysis processes. As Kirk and Miller (1987) point out, researchers often select methods that have a high probability of substantiating their predictions or theories. Even so, there are a number of ways that researchers can minimize these threats to validity: by attending to reliability or replicability, verifiability, triangulation, and sampling.

Reliability

Like validity, **reliability**, which refers to whether a question or measure will yield the same data when repeated, depends to a large degree on the construction of a given question or measurement technique. A faulty thermometer may lead to invalid (wrong) or unreliable (inconstant) readings, just as a poorly worded question may generate invalid and unreliable answers. For instance, if we want to know how many children a woman has we might ask, "How many children do you have?" leaving her to self-report the answer. But without specifying that we mean living or surviving children (or whatever we mean), we might find a mother reporting one number when asked in one context and another number the next. Her answers will not be reliable or consistent because we have not given her a firm enough idea of what we want: Our tools are not good enough to ensure reliability. And although each of her answers may be valid in relation to her situational reading of the question, some or all may not be valid in relation to our conception of the actual question asked (number of living children, in this case). And then there is the possibility that she is deliberately trying to mislead the investigator, which will correlate positively with the sensitive nature of the topic under question or the degree to which she associates the investigator with something that she needs (e.g., medical care). Of course, if she lies in a consistent fashion, her answers will be reliable—although not valid.

In part because of explicitness and attention to reliability, another one of the hallmarks of scientific research is that it is **replicable**. Replicability means that an experiment or project carried out by one person can be carried out again by another person, which may be the case if the second person wishes to verify the findings. If I find x, and another ethnographer finds x, we are all the more sure that x is the answer to our research question. Although one ethnographer may have better rapport with the participants in his or her study than the next ethnographer, and situations change and so findings may too, in general, the replicability of a project is necessary for its verification. If the methods of a study are not replicable or reliable, then the conclusions can never be verified by an independent study.

Verifiability

For a study to be **verifiable** or its findings confirmed as sound, the definitions of concepts and methods must not only be explicit and replicable, they must also correspond to empirical referents or phenomena. Science entails observation. Introspection or rationalist thought experiments such as those undertaken by philosophers are not *scientific* endeavors: They cannot be replicated or verified.

Studies are verifiable if they specify the method of measure and the value of measure so that comparisons can be made and similar findings ascertained. For example, we may measure height either by feet or meters, or by assessments of short, average, and tall. But whereas feet and meters can be converted into one another, unless the value of tall is provided by the original researcher, there is no way to convert "tall" to feet. Similarly, socioeconomic studies that rely on class measures of lower, middle, and upper are not verifiable by studies that rely on numerical measures of class unless the former studies specify the income and other quantitative indicators used to determine class classifications.

In the first clinical research project that I was a part of—a multisite, national nutrition study—research assistants were allowed to accept "average," "normal-sized," or the like when collecting data on the volume of what was eaten. But this was not good science because what is an average- (or small-, or large-) sized apple, or sandwich, or piece of cake to one person may not be the same to another. I myself was first enlightened regarding this when, at the age of nine, I was offered a piece of cake by a neighborhood pal's mother. Happily, her normal slice was equal to four of my own family's cake pieces. Without weight or at least radius, width, and height measurements, information about any "normal-sized" cake slice is not verifiable.

Triangulation

One of the techniques that helps us verify conclusions and limits the desire we have for replicating others' work is called **triangulation**, after navigational techniques by which three points are used to steer a straight line or toward a particular destination. In triangulation, data collected with one specific method are compared to data collected with other methods. This is one way of trying to correct for the biases inherent in specific methods of data collection.

Recall our question about number of (living) children. Although the low reliability of answers tipped us off to problems with the operationalization of that variable, triangulation might have done the same for us. Let us say that a woman reports that she has three children when asked, "How many children do you have?" By double-checking her answer through triangulation (e.g., asking her sister, asking her partner, observing her), we may find that she actually has two living children. This does not mean that she was lying; she may have been answering her conception of our question. She may have had three children at one time and may have taken our question to be in relation to this total. Nonetheless, her answer would be invalid in relation to our (poorly operationalized) conception of what the question asked.

Triangulation also provides a richer and more complete picture of the study material. For example, we can legitimately obtain data on eating habits by using the following types of methods: (1) participant observation, (2) self-reports of food intake over the past twenty-four hours, (3) free lists of most commonly eaten foods, (4) Likert-scaled (e.g., never to x times a day) questions, (5) clinical assays of blood and urine chemistry, (6) and interviews concerning cooking methods. Combining two or more of these techniques will lead to a fuller understanding of people's eating practices and beliefs than data obtained from only one of them.

Sampling

Most research studies involving human participants target only a sub-segment (**sample**) of the total number of potential participants for inclusion. A probability-based random sampling method is necessary if one aims to generalize the findings from a sample population to the larger population from which the sample is drawn. In a **random** sample, every member of a population has an equal probability of being selected. For example, in a given study area, houses or people can be chosen according to a random number table. Because randomizing selection procedures for including informants into a sample increases the probability that a sample is representative of the larger population, a random sample is thus a microcosm of the larger population in terms of the relevant characteristics the researcher is interested in.

Random sampling is important for studying causal relations and variance in a population. When variance is close to zero, there is no reason to use it.

Ethnographers seldom use random samples because they frequently work with small populations such as those in classrooms or villages where there is either little variation in a given variable (e.g., all are in kindergarten) or, when there is variation, where the researcher has access to the entire population so no prediction or generalization must be made. Further, ethnography, by definition, is concerned with thick description (see Chapter 2), so breadth is sacrificed for depth. When an ethnographer has lived with a population and studied them for an extended period of time, there is some assurance that she or he knows the population well enough that his or her causal explanations and descriptions of what is typical of the community can be trusted.

Ethnographic Samples

An **ethnographic** sample is a nonrandom group of participants that help the researcher establish the range of cultural phenomena—but not the frequency distribution of those phenomena (present thinking calls for probability samples to do that). A number of strategies for assembling ethnographic (nonprobability) samples exist, but most are based around the purpose of inquiry. Most ethnographic samples are, therefore, purposive.

They are also serially or sequentially gathered. This is because of the importance in ethnography of openness to emerging issues and of the ability to continually refocus research questions as needed to get to the core of the story at hand. In fact, ethnographers sometimes move from one sample to another as research unfolds and new data needs are revealed.

Purposive Strategies

Purposive samples are created from participants or cases selected purposefully in relation to the specific purpose of the research. So, for example, if a researcher wants to learn about acupuncture, he or she might design a sampling plan to include acupuncturists or perhaps people who have undergone acupuncture. But how would the researcher determine which acupuncturists or patients to include from the entire universe of such? There are many strategies to do so, and these approaches can be linked and overlapping, depending on study needs.

One recruitment strategy would be to work down the list of acupuncturists in the phone book or to approach every patient exiting an acupuncture clinic (which should entail that clinic's permission). A purposive sample assembled this way would be termed a "convenience" sample. **Convenience** samples are assembled from the first willing people encountered. They entail "grabbing whoever will stand still long enough to answer your questions" (Bernard 1995b, p. 96). They are very useful for formative or exploratory studies in which the investigator needs to familiarize him- or herself with the field or with the general topic in question.

In a **criterion** sample, each case that meets specific eligibility criteria is selected for recruitment. For instance, said researcher might want to include all acupuncturists in the phonebook listings who trained outside the United States. He or she might want to include all of a given facility's first-time patients, or all people who are long-term patients there. A related strategy is the **theoretical** sample, in which the incorporation in your research of a particular theory or theoretical construct from the literature leads to certain recruitment decisions. A theoretical sample differs slightly from a criterion sample, which simply seeks to ensure that, from within a given population, no cases of a certain type are overlooked. However, because criterion samples entail preconceived ideas about what qualities in participants will be important, people sometimes will refer to them as theoretical.

Snowball or **chain link** samples are built using each participant as part of the recruitment team. The sample grows largely through people who know people, adding to itself like a snowball rolling downhill. If one was, for example, doing a study of methamphetamine use, it might not be easy to recruit a large enough sample on one's own. Asking each participant to tell other users about the study provides the researcher a way to tap into a socially linked chain of methamphetamine users and thus amass a sufficient (and sufficiently qualified) sample.

Another approach to sampling, still building on the purpose of a study, would be to assemble a **critical case** sample from people whose experiences promise to be particularly enlightening or data-rich, such as people who suffered from medical errors resulting in permanent harm. Related to this is the **extreme** or deviant sample: a sample of people who are extreme cases of whatever it is you are studying, such as those who are outstandingly successful in that area or dismal failures. The **disconfirming** sample assembles cases that represent exceptions to the expected rule. Disconfirming cases are very important in ethnographic research because of their potential to enhance validity. Of course, in keeping with the notion of serial sample-building introduced above, they often cannot be selected until after the initial field research period because the researcher will not know what needs to be disconfirmed.

The final purposive strategy that I will mention here is **maximum variation** sampling (for more strategies, see Patton 1990 or Kuzel 1992). A maximum variation sample is assembled from the maximum range of case types to ensure that the entire range of possible responses is accounted for. For instance, for the study of methamphetamine use, it might be important to talk to males, females, new users, hardened users, users who are minors, users with jobs, users without jobs, users who sell, etc., to stake a claim to having documented the range of responses.

Sample Size

This brings us to the question of sample size. One determinant of sample size is the size of the population that the inquiry refers to. A traditional anthropologist studying life in a village where fifty-seven people live may take as the sample all fifty-seven people. Technically, this is called a **comprehensive** sample. The anthropologist working in a city of 57,000, however, needs another way to derive a sample ceiling. One option is to use a quota. A **quota** sample's size is determined either on some theoretical basis, knowledge regarding the number of eligible people out there (sometimes termed the population **universe**), or analytic concerns. For example, a researcher who intends to undertake an intensive, iterative narrative analysis of interview transcripts may set him- or herself a quota of twenty-five interviews to avoid being overwhelmed with data.

Reasonability is key to quota construction. So are cultural numerical standards. Quota numbers normally fall in line with standardized, culturally appropriate numbering systems (e.g., quota numbers that end in a zero, such as forty, or that represent quartiles, such as fifty or seventy-five, are common). Numbers that are variations on one dozen also have been used; in the example above, twenty-four would have passed muster. But twenty-seven or twenty-three probably would have raised eyebrows. This is something one does not wish to do when asking for funding or trying to publish unless there is a rock-solid justification for it, such as when a research participant moves or otherwise becomes ineligible for continued participation.

In an ideal world, with the exception of the comprehensive sample, data **saturation** or redundancy would put a stop to recruitment. Saturation occurs when the investigator stops getting new information from participants or begins to hear the same types of answers over and over. At this point, all other things being equal, data collection regarding that topic is completed.

But the research world is rarely ideal. So, in addition to theoretical knowledge, information regarding the universe, and analytic issues, financial concerns also can lead to a particular choice for the quota. In one emergency department study I was involved in, three focus groups were held—but only because that was what the budget could accommodate. Research design textbooks rarely mention financial drivers because, in an ideal situation, research needs rather than budgetary ones should drive the design. Yet most HSR in general, and anthropologically informed HSR in particular, is not undertaken in ideal situations; monetary concerns must receive attention.

However assembled, ethnographic samples cannot be used to generalize. They cannot tell us the percentage of people in a population who are Republicans or Democrats. But they can tell us about the sample in question and they can tell us about the range of a given phenomenon; for instance, they can tell us what political parties people belong to and help us understand why people are Republican, Democrat, or anything else.

An Improbable Exception?

Having set up this contrast between probability and nonprobability samples, there are certain circumscribed circumstances in which an ethnographic sample is actually just as good as a probability sample for producing reliable, generalizable quantitative findings. In his latrine research with village health workers in Swaziland and in his maternal and child health research with Palestinian women, Edward Green (2001) collected data that, when quantified, revealed percentages that were right in line with probability-based conclusions. For instance, his figure for the number of pit latrines paralleled national random sample survey findings, and his figures for age at marriage, number of children desired, and prenatal care attendance were essentially the same as those collected by the Palestinian Central Bureau of Statistics.

As Green notes, "Some countable things are intrinsically easier to estimate with accuracy than others" (2001, p. 13). So long as we are dealing with fairly homogeneous groups of individuals who are highly knowledgeable about the domain in question and so long as the domain itself is cultural (in the sense that it is fairly well agreed on or patterned), we can be reasonably certain of our results. One need not ask a national probability sample to find out that we drive on the right in the United States; asking a few knowledgeable drivers will do. It certainly will save time and money.

Related to this, it is worth repeating here Green's observation that policymakers generally do not quote exact percentages. He notes that,

> As health planners and program directors know, it does not matter whether 45% or 50% prefer or practice cousin marriage, whether 93% or 98% attend prenatal care, or whether 22% or 24% of homesteads have a pit latrine. The first becomes "about half," the second becomes "almost all," and the third becomes "not nearly enough" for policy or program purposes. (2001, p. 16)

As suggested in Chapter 2, the role a "fact" can play in a story that someone would like to see unfold becomes more important than the exact fact itself (which is not to say in these cases that the facts do not need to be there to begin with). Green's observation that, "In practice, interviewers in sample surveys usually settle for the nearest coherent and sober neighbor, which results in sampling a little closer to the qualitative-quantitative (or purposive sample-random sample) middle ground" (p. 17) also merits attention: The very real possibility of this type of discrepancy between scientific protocol and actual research practice is something we return to in Chapter 14.

In any case, although percentages derived from ethnographic samples can be valid and reliable, a much more important feature of the ethnographic sample than this is that it can tell us both what is in the **phenomenal** or experiential, lived, perceived world of the people we are studying and how they think about this world (Dreyfus 1987). Boster (1985), Romney and Weller (1988), and D'Andrade (1995) tell us that we need comparatively small ethnographic samples (less than twenty people) to obtain confidence that members of a culture agree on the array of items or symbols or states that constitute a cultural domain or category (e.g., illness) or that they agree on the core attributes used to identify similarities among those items (e.g., signs and symptoms) and to contrast them with other cultural domains (e.g., health) (see Kronenfeld 1996).

In their discussion of Clyde Kluckhohn's *Navajo Witchcraft* (1944), Werner and Bernard conclude that "to do ethnographic sampling well ... the ethnographer must learn another culture systematically and not casually" (1994, p. 9). Thus, ethnographic sampling, like probability sampling, requires controls. We can only have confidence in findings from ethnographic samples if the ethnographer has demonstrated familiarity with that culture through previous publications and duration of stay (over a year) or, when less time is available, focuses on a particular cultural domain and has systematically established the range of elements that constitute that domain. He or she also must understand that the material presented represents a model of the culture as the informants see it—not a model of the culture itself.

Developing a Systematic Methodological Approach

It is not always possible to know, on entering the field, what data one might deem necessary at the end of the research period. In light of this, a strength of ethnographic research has been the freedom researchers have to examine concerns that emerge as important during the fieldwork experience and to discard questions developed prior to entering the field if they do not prove relevant. However, all data must be collected in a systematic way so that they are useful at the end of the day. If one encounters a new issue while in the field, it is well worth taking the time to develop a systematic methodological approach so that any information collected will actually be of use.

Further, methods for data collection are only useful if the researcher has plans for using the data collected. This point may sound simple-minded, but every year my colleagues and I encounter students and professionals with arrays of data that they have no idea how to use. Goals for analysis should be a primary consideration when planning research methods. Careful planning involves giving thought to specific analysis goals and the methods by which to collect the kind of data needed to accomplish this.

Remember that Research Is a Situated Process

The classical view of methods holds that they are part of a linear process. This begins with a research idea and a related research design, including a data collection protocol and analytic plan, and ends with findings that either validate or invalidate the idea. However, a number of scholars have argued that this view falsely represents research as a programmatic process. Martin (1982) makes the point that methods, theory, resources, and solutions are in a continuous feedback relationship, being modified by and modifying each other during a research project. Using a garbage can metaphor, Martin suggests that research is actually a messy, ad hoc affair only tidied up when put on display.

Maxwell (1996, p. 3) notes that both the classic linear and garbage can models provide equally distorted views of what actually goes on. His compromise solution is to propose a butterfly-shaped interactive model of research in which methods and validity form the empirical wing and what he calls "purposes" and "conceptual context" form the ideational wing. Research questions form the head and thorax, connecting and integrating the two wings. Maxwell's model allows for interactive feedback between the different parts of a research study while still retaining a research structure.

Linear, garbage can, and interactive models of research design all have in common the idea that methods are connected to other components of a project. In a linear model, methods are devised in regard to and follow from the question to be asked. In a garbage can model, methods and other components all "swirl about," with none taking priority over the other (Grady and Wallston 1988, p. 12). In an interactive model, there is a definite division of labor and temporal organization, but there also is the recognition that research is an ongoing process in which methods, purposes, conceptual context, research questions, and validity issues all influence and are influenced by one another. As Maxwell (1996) notes, the choice and use of methods is embedded in and interacts with other major components of a research design. That is, methods make more sense—they are more fully comprehended—when viewed against the backdrop of actual research activity.

In applied health research in particular, methods make more sense when adapted to the setting rather than to artificially controlled laboratory or experimental conditions. Such conditions poorly reflect the real-life contingencies of the health-seeking and service-providing context. The next chapter therefore examines the historic and current context, as well as some of the ramifications for knowledge, of our overreliance on the classic clinical research model.

CHAPTER 8

Epistemology and Evidence: How Do We Know What We Know?

PARADIGMS SHIFT

Thomas Kuhn (1996 [1962]) has famously argued that what constitutes good science and truth in one era (i.e., what fits the given paradigm) may be judged bad science and false in another era. Kuhn recognized that scientific paradigms shift when enough evidence mounts that cannot be explained by or contradicts the old paradigm, and that there *is* a march of science, but his ideas caused consternation in some circles when he first published them. They meant that scientific truths were, to a large degree, grounded in subjective human consensus (i.e., culture) about what is true and what is false.

Randomized controlled clinical trials or RCTs are today's evidentiary gold standard for health care. Indeed, science is more or less equated with the RCT by many in the health services and, like the moralizing rhetoric mentioned in Chapter 2 ("it's the right thing to do"), whether or not an RCT design was followed in regard to findings in question can serve as a case-closer for not only scientists but also clinicians and administrators, when one is needed for a policy decision. This overt reliance on discourse favoring hypothetico-deductive experimental science and rationality occurs in health services, despite evidence reviewed in Chapter 2 regarding the ultimate and often unnoticed importance of storytelling around or in front of the presentation of systematically collected and analyzed data. And it persists although, as just shown in Chapter 7, anthropologically informed research can—even when qualitative—be quite systematic and can address such scientific concerns as validity, reliability, bias, and so on.

Accordingly, this chapter's intent is to challenge the acceptance of RCT-style science as a gold standard to begin with. It explains how the RCT rose to prominence in the last third of the 1900s and questions its ascendancy. It does so in a way that can benefit all branches of health services research (HSR).

The focus here on RCTs and the scientific method should not be taken to imply that other approaches to health care concerns were completely quashed by science in the later 1900s. Some varied examples demonstrating the contrary include the anthropological work of Noel Chrisman on the health-seeking process (1977) and Arthur Kleinman on somatized distress and explanatory models (1981), Madeline Leininger's longstanding transcultural nursing research (2002), the demarcation of grounded theory in the context of a study of hospital death by sociologists Barney Glaser and Anselm Strauss (1965), and other efforts, many referenced elsewhere in this book. Notwithstanding, my aim here is to illuminate some of the reasons that descriptive, context-informed inquiry's strong historical roots were rather thinned in the last half of the 20th century and to show, in the end, the importance of its continued and effective application in anthropologically informed HSR.

THE SCIENTIFIC METHOD

Science is generally taken for granted in the financially wealthier nations as the ultimate authority regarding what is true and what is not. Scientific practice entails belief that the physical world can be objectively measured and known; it entails belief in what Sharon Traweek, in her study of a community of physicists, describes as "a world without loose ends. ... A world outside human space and time" (1988, p. 157). This is a world about which objective and systematic observations can be made.

For HSR and in many other scholarly practice arenas, scientific practice and progress depend on use of the **scientific method**. This consists of observing with the physical senses, hypothesizing and testing for expected relationships and predicted outcomes, then revising expectations when discrepancies arise.

Hypothesis testing often is done under controlled circumstances that help scientists focus in on exactly what they wish to observe; that is, they often do experiments or otherwise try to limit externally introduced noise ("nuisance variables"). Anthropological research, when undertaken in partnership with health services, is usually encouraged to conform to this model.

Left on their own, however, anthropologists generally prefer a naturalistic approach. They do not like to manipulate contexts because they are interested in what people actually do and say in real-life situations. Further, they usually do not take formal hypotheses with them into the field. This is because they prefer that research categories and the topics thereby examined reflect participant, not researcher, agendas.

Our dominant system of health care depends on the scientific method. Indeed, medical history has generally been constructed around the impressive and progressive accomplishments of science. Without question, the astounding progress of medical science has made life longer and better for many. However, by examining its historical framework, with emphasis on social and cultural factors (drawing heavily on Loustaunau and Sobo 1997), we gain additional perspective on these advances—perspective that comes in handy when examining alternative approaches, including anthropologically informed ones, to data collection and analysis.

U.S. MEDICINE'S EARLY DAYS

Professionalization

The philosophical foundations of colonial U.S. society were rooted in democratic and egalitarian ideals. Anti-elitist attitudes of the times supported the notion that the practice of medicine was a matter of common sense, to which all had access. Health care was generally provided within social networks and carried in oral traditions, passed down through families and friends. Isolation further necessitated self-sufficiency; rural households would have provided for most if not all their own needs, including food, shelter, clothing, and health care.

At the time, physicians could generally offer little that people could not provide for themselves. In addition, they had competition from lay practitioners of all kinds, including patent medicine companies, which sold trademarked medical preparations directly to the public, offering what were often unique explanations of causes and claiming easy cures for a multitude of ailments, from arthritis and digestive disorders to baldness and warts.

Some physicians, however, pursued a quest for control over the health care arena through the professionalization of medicine. **Professionalization** is the process whereby people with a particular skill set organize themselves such that they and only they have the right to determine standard practice within their field. Professionalization generally entails the creation of a society or association, the invention of an official news organ such as a journal, and the inauguration of cyclical conferences or meetings. It works much better for accumulating systems than for diffusing ones, in which knowledge is individually held (regarding these, see Chapter 3).

Professionalizing physicians established medical societies in some states during the first half of the 19th century and, in 1847, they met in Philadelphia to establish the American Medical Association (AMA). A reorganization of the AMA in 1902 established branch societies at the local, state, and territorial levels. Local societies had the arbitrary discretion to expel or deny membership to any physician and thus could determine membership qualifications and enforce conformity. This enabled the profession to monitor and control a widely dispersed membership.

Having a professional association allowed physicians to better organize their attack on competitive elements as well as to further develop the scientific basis for medicine and thus the legitimacy of the scientific approach. They still disagreed with and battled each other on all sorts of medical, philosophical, and organizational grounds, but the AMA provided a forum where interests could be discussed and defended as well as being a potentially unified pressure group for future political and policy endeavors.

The power of the AMA was used to raise and maintain academic and scientific standards. It was also used to further its own interests, for instance regarding the economic position of the medical profession, and to secure the autonomous right to define and enforce the restraints on and the standards of practice with a freedom known to very few professions.

The Flexner Report

In 1908, the AMA contracted with the Carnegie Foundation for a study of U.S. medical education to be conducted by Abraham Flexner, an administrator and educator. One explicit goal of the study was to standardize and raise the status of medical education. Another was to convince the public, including philanthropists, that modern medicine was a field worthy of their support.

Professional medical reformers were well aware of the need for a strategy consistent with then current historical forces. This meant offering investment opportunities in conquering disease and the promise of international status and leadership to investors (Brown 1979, p. 141). The developing U.S. hospital system, as uncoordinated as it was in the early days, would play a role to this end. The centralization of both learning and practice within a hospital setting made it much easier to maintain a particular standard of medical education with control of curriculum, training, and requirements. The system also reflected a definite pattern of class relations (Starr 1982). This was especially true in the elite private hospitals where staff members were strictly controlled and patients were either very poor (for teaching purposes) or very rich (for revenue).

The resulting Flexner Report of 1910 indexed an historical turning point in U.S. medical education. For one thing, it forced the closure of numerous medical schools that had trained women and other minorities. Further, although it supported the medical training of African Americans, this was only to care for other African Americans—not because they needed care but because they came into contact with Whites. Flexner indicated that African American medical education should concentrate on hygiene rather than surgery. He recommended that only two schools out of the seven then in existence for African Americans (Meharry and Howard) be supported and upgraded; the others he said should be eliminated (Brown 1979, p. 154).

The Flexner Report did eliminate medical diploma mills, reducing the risk of unproven, incompetent, or fraudulent treatment. However, the exclusionary race-class-sex composition of the profession that it supported, which persisted until the affirmative action programs in the 1960s and '70s, had profound consequences for the development of the health care system in the United States, some of which were indexed in Chapter 6.

Taking into account the larger context and social dynamics of the time, the Flexner Report can be seen as an attempt by the AMA not only to "attain and maintain ideological hegemony over the other sects of medicine that were still extant at the time," but also to "solidify the alliance between the capitalist class and the AMA and to establish the dominance of the researcher over the practitioner" (Berliner 1975, p. 589). Large investments are not made without hope of return, financial or otherwise. Priority areas for research and education could be chosen to provide investment opportunities with bigger payoffs and to support the class structure. Many within the AMA did recognize the dangers of alliances with strong capitalist interests, which would then have a say in designating areas of priorities in education and research (Brown 1979). Nonetheless, that is pretty much what happened. As Berliner notes, "The problems that plague the field of medicine today no doubt emerge dialectically from the attempt made in 1910 to shore up a medical system also beset with contradictions and conflicts" (1975, p. 590).

WORLD WAR II AND THE GOLDEN AGE OF SCIENTIFIC MEDICINE, OR: THE RISE OF THE RCT

By the 1940s, the power of the dominance of AMA medicine was fairly secure. However, it was World War II that made scientific medicine a national asset and an institution, serving as a catalyst for a boom in scientific research that would further define the culture of medicine. Research produced medical discoveries that lowered the military death rate and could be translated for public use. The United States emerged from the war as a formidable economic and military power; scientific medicine became associated with victory, the conquest of infectious diseases, prosperity, and leadership of the free world—scientific medicine was "American."

The 1940s and '50s were what might be termed the "golden age of antibiotics." The physicians' arsenal for combating disease overflowed with new miracle drugs, and the military metaphors used in descriptions of medical victories over disease fit nicely with the sensibility of the nation, coming out of World War II. Penicillin, which was developed in close association with military needs and objectives, proved effective against certain sexually transmitted diseases as well as battle injuries, and streptomycin was found to be effective against tuberculosis. These advances fueled the search for new drugs and their potential profits.

Pharmaceutical medicine did have challenges. As Annemarie Mol tells it in her review of the rise of the RCT (see Chapter 7) as the evidentiary gold standard for health services, "Modern states wanted to protect their populations from being poisoned by bad drugs; and where health costs were shared, the collective needed to know that the money was spent wisely" (2006, p. 406). Pharmaceutical companies had to have evidence for their products' efficacy prior to being allowed to put them on the market, and RCTs ostensibly provided this.

Mol continues: "The strange thing is that this very specific research style subsequently took over in so many other sites and situations or that it became generalized ... not just for drugs but for just about any kind of intervention" (2006, p. 406). Mol finds this "truly intriguing" because, in her view, "However well clinical trials might be able to prove or disprove therapeutic claims, and however strong their credentials when it comes to seeking evidence, they have their limits when it comes to assuring good care" (p. 406).

Improving care, Mol notes, is quite different than proving that a drug has this or that effect. Moreover, drug trials divorce various effects so that they can follow them as discrete variables (for example, in Mol's area of research these would include blood pressure at the ankles and pain-free walking distance). This disconnection means that patients and practitioners must select, or make judgments about, which effects they are willing to put up with—given a choice. But, says Mol,

> Professional care is not a matter of separating out elements, fixing [freezing] them, and putting them to use in a linear manner. It is a matter of tinkering, of doctoring, if I dare to reclaim that word from the negative connotations it has acquired and give a positive appreciation to the creative calibrating of elements that make up a situation, until they somehow fit—and work. (2006, p. 411)

We shall examine the implications this critique has for HSR protocol designs subsequently. But it is worth taking a bit more time to scrutinize the science behind medicine before we do so. This will leave us better positioned to understand how wide the angle taken by anthropologically informed HSR truly can and should be.

HOW SCIENTIFIC IS MEDICAL SCIENCE?

Medicine in Cultural Context

Medicine is (among other things) a cultural system. Partly because of this, it differs from place to place.

When journalist Lynn Payer (1988) investigated medical practice in Great Britain, Germany, France, and the United States, she found many differences. The British prescribed fewer drugs in general than the French or Germans. The patient in Great Britain was about half as likely as the U.S. patient to have surgery of any kind. Daily vitamin requirements were smaller. And British doctors were more reluctant to diagnose someone as sick based on similar signs and symptoms.

In Germany, low blood pressure was a condition requiring treatment to raise it, unlike in the United States where it was treated as a nondisease indicative of long life. Germans prescribed far fewer antibiotics and far more heart drugs than the other countries and considered the heart as greatly affected by emotions, not a pump that can be replaced.

French medicine concentrated on building up the physical and mental constitution (termed "terrain") with vitamins, tonics, diet, and exercise rather than aggressively attacking the disease with drugs and medications. The French performed very few hysterectomies compared to doctors in the United States. Treatment for psychiatric problems was likely to involve a visit to a government-approved spa, a long sick leave, or a "sleep cure."

Payer found that medical practice in the United States was highly aggressive and directed toward attacking a disease; the body was considered a machine to be fixed. Even psychoanalysis in the United States was not concerned with emotions; quoting fellow journalist Janet Malcolm's 1981 book on the practice, Payer noted that, "It rearranges things inside the mind the way surgery rearranges things inside the body—even the way an automobile mechanic rearranges things under the hood of the car" (1988, p. 150). Payer added, "Anything that cannot fit into the machine model of the body, or be quantified, is often denied not only quantification, but even existence" (p. 151).

These major differences in perception and use of medical knowledge and content persist at least to some degree, as any French, German, British, or U.S. patient will tell you when seen by a practitioner trained in one of the other named nations and those not on the list. More importantly, these differences reflect basic cultural values. As Payer wrote, the Germans, although characterized as authoritarian, were influenced by 19th-century Romanticism and saw themselves as emotional, accommodating the various facets of efficiency, spirituality, and nature—hence the focus on the heart. The English practiced an "economy" in their medicine, partly because of the way health care was financed and nationally bureaucratized, but also because, Payer suggested, the British were taught to deny the body. They were expected to exhibit stoicism and maintain a stiff upper lip (1988).

In the United States, the practice of an aggressive, heroic style of medicine, where doing something is always better than doing nothing, fits well with the national psyche or mind set. The compatibility of heroic medicine with traditional "American" values was noted even by the poet and physician Oliver Wendell Holmes, who wrote in 1861:

> How could a people [that] insists in sending out yachts and horses and boys to out-sail, out-run, out-fight, and checkmate all the rest of creation; how could such a people be content with any but "heroic" practice? What wonder that the Stars and Stripes wave over doses of ninety grains of sulphate of quinine, or that the American eagle screams with delight to see three drachms of calomel given at a single mouthful? (1888 [1861], p. 193)

These early values and approaches are still dominant, although some early industrial imagery has been replaced by computer metaphors (Martin 1994). Some treatment decisions have become even more heroic with the growth of technological possibilities, such as keeping comatose people alive on respirators.

Globalization has somewhat softened some of the differences Payer noted. For example, U.S. systems now favor health care that, following the British (and, although Payer did not mention them, the Canadians too; see below), is evidence-based. Yet patients will confirm that differences are still there, as will the continued existence of nationally distinctive regulations and policy preferences.

One could write off the differences Payer observed to a lack of understanding of the evidence; maybe some nations or practitioners have just gotten things wrong. To some extent this will be true; even choices made on the basis of what looks like the best evidence at the time practice standards are developed can later be shown to be wrong. But many medical differences are instead due to varying norms and values—cultural differences.

Take, for instance, organ transplantation. In research comparing Japanese and North American organ transplantation practices and preferences, Margaret Lock (2002) found vast differences in the general ways that members of either group understood the connections between bodies and persons and life and death.

A diagnosis of whole-brain death means that all brain activity has permanently ceased. However, the rest of a brain-dead person's body parts must be kept alive for a time after whole-brain death has been confirmed so that the organs remain useable for transplant purposes. To this end, the heart can be kept pumping and blood oxygenated with mechanical means. So far, so good.

Yet, although the notion of whole-brain death makes sense to North Americans, it remains untenable to the Japanese who, despite their high-tech reputation, have been very hesitant to embrace organ transplantation. As Lock argues, it simply does not have a good cultural fit (2002).

North American rationalism supports the equation made between the person and the mind and, by extension, the brain. But the vital essence of the person in Japan is not equated solely with the mind-brain; instead, the person infuses the body as a whole, residing in the anatomically non-specific *kokoro* (Lock 2002).

Moreover, each person is connected in important ways to other persons in his or her social network. Ancestors (the dead) remain an important part of this network, so to cut up their bodies would be disrespectful and socially disruptive. Concurrently, although North American medical practice conforms to a theory of individual autonomy—by which individuals have full rights to determine their disposition after death—Japanese practice does not: The family has that right and must be consulted. Indeed, to some degree, the family even has the right to determine when a family member is dead; doctors often wait until they have had time to come to terms with a death before proclaiming it, and thus legally creating it (Lock 2002).

Culture and Bioethics

The Japanese are not the only ones to have criticized individualistic North American bioethics. The high valuation it places on autonomous individuals does not take into account very real differences in how individuals and their families and their communities are articulated or interpenetrate. Such differences render ridiculous, for example, the extension of the typical U.S. informed consent process into contexts in which the individual is not viewed as autonomous and independent. In cultures where people overtly acknowledge that one's family or others are affected by one's research participation decisions, or where other individuals (grandfathers, for example) are the people who, culturally speaking, have the right to sign, the ethics behind our informed consent process seem critically shortsighted.

There are other problems with North American bioethics. As Paul Farmer notes (2005), medical ethics consults in the United States are often about too much care. They come into play when someone requests the right to die, for instance: the right to forgo what can be painful, expensive, overly life-prolonging care. They are not applied, however—or, are poorly applied—when the opposite problem is observed. For instance, people who cannot afford care often are denied it, despite their need. Farmer, a physician-anthropologist famous for his work in impoverished Haiti, points out that the need for health services is much more prevalent worldwide than its surfeit. Further, North American focus on the individual diverts attention from larger social-structural and political economic problems such as those related to the creation and maintenance of impoverished populations to begin with through global systems of exploitation and inequity. North American bioethics are clearly culture-bound.

Medicalization

The cultural dimension of medicine is perhaps most easily seen in the process of medicalization, through which physicians define in medical terms what may have been considered a personal or social problem and propose medical treatment as an appropriate solution. With a disease designation, medicine can act as an agent of social control. In the case of chemical dependency, for example, "medicine replaces or collaborates with the criminal justice system" (Brown 1995, p. 41). Demedicalization would occur when the problem is once again viewed as personal deviance or human weakness to be addressed by education or strong social sanctions and possibly incarceration as punishment.

In Chapter 3, I mentioned the medicalization of birth and the satire-disease called motivational deficiency disorder (Moynihan 2006). Alcoholism is another good example of medicalization when it is defined as a disease over which the sufferer has little or no control and is treated with medications and psychiatric counseling. Medicalization relieves the drinker of personal responsibility and provides a socially acceptable therapy for recovery.

Recognizing medicalization can support inquiry into the deeper sources of a problem. For example, Merrill Singer and colleagues, in investigating the seemingly self-destructive drinking behavior of a Puerto Rican subject, arrived at a wider interpretation of alcoholism as a "disease of the world economic system, and at the same time, an expression of human suffering and coping, as well as resistance to the forces and pressures of that system" (1992, p. 100).

Evidence-Based Medicine

I mentioned the rise of the RCT in the context of the contest between pharmaceutical interests in market expansion and the state's responsibility to protect the public by regulating drug approvals. But the RCT caught on as more than a regulatory tool: It acquired status as the scientific gold standard for medical evidence—a status it retains today.

The rise of the RCT proved foundational for a subsequent movement termed **evidence-based medicine** (EBM, sometimes referred to as EBP or evidence-based practice). Experts within the various health care disciplines have been studying this phenomenon, as have scholars within the social sciences. As might be expected, approaches and perspectives range widely, and I will not try to recapitulate the entirety of findings. This caveat leads me to a momentary reflexive digression.

Although acknowledging that much work on the topics I address has been done in other disciplines, the viewpoint I offer here and throughout this book is inherently that of an anthropologist. The literature drawn on is anthropologically skewed. My reliance on the anthropological literature and perspective is an artifact of my disciplinary position rather than an attempt to dismiss or otherwise discount the research traditions in other fields or the strides other disciplines have made in grappling with the questions at hand. Anthropology simply provides one perspective—albeit, in my opinion and for reasons this book explains, a quite helpful perspective—on challenges facing health care today.

EBM is medicine (or, as explained in Chapter 1, health care) practiced according to the evidence. Although EBM may have a dominative form, described below, it often is used in a generic sense that includes, or at least refers to the assumptions behind, practices such as clinical audit and guidelines-based care (described below). That is, as is true about so many of the health care ideas discussed in this book, EBM's real-life practice on the ground may be as varied as the clinics in which it is practiced. To paraphrase colleagues in one health care system where I worked, if you've seen one EBM model, you've seen one EBM model. With that caveat—and a reminder that if I am to squeeze EBM's history into just a few pages I must to some degree simplify matters here as I have for other selected topics and so will present one dominative form as typical—let us turn to the task of defining the EBM idea.

EBM's emergence figured as a reaction to the growing realization among many in medicine, both marked and encouraged by Archie Cochrane's 1972 tract on same, that tradition-based practice trumped research-based practice far too often for comfort. In part, this was because of the newness of the RCT approach, which was only just gaining force at the time. But, as is still true today, it also had to do with issues of power and the structural constraints that providers are under. For instance, as the research base grew, so did the literature, and providers simply did (and do) not have time to read it all. Further, evidence can be contradictory; what's a provider to do under such uncertain conditions?

Research was simply not being translated into practice. Concurrently, the public's trust in medicine (as other authorities) was falling, and purchasers' and payors' requirement for accountability was on the rise. Medicine was not, after all, infallible.

One response to all this was the development of clinical audit systems in the 1980s. Clinical audit takes a bureaucratic approach to health care. At first, the focus was on ferreting out unnecessary practice variations. Experts—those assumed to be familiar with the research literature and who had longstanding clinical experience with the problems in question—set standards through formal consensus processes. Clinical audits in which medical records were checked over to see whose practices were and whose were not in compliance with the standards set ensured that conformity (Lipman 2000, pp. 557, 560). **Managed care** (including through health maintenance organizations or HMOs), which began to really flourish in the United States around this time, was based on the same assumption: Factory management strategies focused on reducing overlap, unnecessary variation, and overuse as well as business valuation measures could be applied to health care.

Not all providers were happy with such managerial meddling in their healing arts. Beyond the shot taken at tradition-based practice, the devaluation of personal experience entailed in early versions of EBM also was highly problematic. The role of a provider's experience in practice is highly complex. The very nature of experience as well as the specific dimensions of experience that can be helpful for care provision is still widely contested. I must refer the reader to the literature cited in this section for a more in-depth view of the present debate, but note that experience is an essential component of professional health care provision and to wave that away was, and still is, unthinkable to many.

An alternative to imposed controls and surveillance that would still ensure that providers followed the growing evidence base emerged in Canada in the early 1990s via McMaster University (Lambert 2006). In the United Kingdom, it gained prominence when David Sackett became the director of the then newly formed National Health Service R&D Centre for Evidence-Based Medicine at Oxford (Lipman 2000, p. 561). What for efficiency's sake I shall term "EBM-proper" had emerged.

In Sackett and colleagues' own often-cited words, "Evidence based medicine is the conscientious, explicit, and judicious use of current best evidence in making decisions about the care of individual patients" (1996, p. 71). In other words, although allowing practitioners autonomy and placing value on clinical experience, this form of EBM specifically asks practitioners to use the literature. Starting from the patient whose problem the provider does not immediately know how to fix, the provider formulates a structured, answerable question and goes to the evidence base to answer that question (Lipman 2000, p. 561).

Importantly, deference to expert colleagues is not part of EBM-proper: Providers retain control over their cases rather than handing them off to specialists they find answers themselves. If senior colleagues do suggest treatment plans, junior practitioners are entitled to ask them on what evidence such suggestions are based. Even patients are empowered through this form of EBM: They are given more opportunities to share in decision-making as their providers present to them the evidence that has been discovered in the literature. The assumption that patient involvement is a good thing is based, of course, on "a culturally specific model of interaction that assumes that patients want deep disclosure" (Mykhalovskiy and Weir 2004, p. 1063).

In short, EBM-proper redistributes power within the clinical social system. It also challenges the authority of far-away health services bureaucrats in determining what the clinical agenda should be. These shifts appeal most to those most oppressed by clinical audit and dominance hierarchies—and they are most abhorrent to those whose power is under threat of being drained by them. Accordingly, as Toby Lipman shows, many of the power structures challenged in theory when EBM-proper emerged still remain strong. Established local hierarchies and related office politics still hold great sway over individual practitioners, as do resource power structures entailing financial remuneration (2000, p. 559).

Just as EBM-proper rose in part in opposition to clinical audit, something has risen to offset the threats entailed in EBM-proper. These emergences were not strictly linear; they were part of the same EBM trend, not disparate serial developments. My quick sketch of the emergence of each in this section cannot do justice to the complexity entailed. Yet I hope it will be clear that their overt goals were the same: ensuring that individual practitioners follow evidence-based standards.

Recall that EBM-proper begins with the individual patient. However, as providers' patient panels (rolls) have grown and health care systems have expanded, a population perspective has come to dominate. Guideline-based care fits much better than EBM-proper with that. For one thing, rather than being driven by unique, individual patient problems, guidelines begin from organizational ones: Analysts mine health services data bases to identify top conditions or complaints—those that are most frequently confronted by providers. In Children's Emergency Department or ED, for example, those were acute upper respiratory infection, fever, gastroenteritis, otitis media (earache), and head injuries. Accordingly, most of our pathway efforts for the ED were expended on those conditions.

Infrequent complaints generally have no associated guidelines. Although this makes sense in terms of efficiency, it can inadvertently penalize patients who present with them because treatment ideas for them may seem harder to come by than for more typical complaints. But the ramifications of this for patient-provider interaction have not been formally explored.

In frequent conditions for which there is **guidelines-based care,** providers follow a set of if-then commands when caring for patients with specific complaints. Guideline authors (generally, committees formed by professional associations) justify their recommendations with reference to not only concordant clinical studies regarding the area in question and single seminal studies but also meta-analyses. **Meta-analyses** combine quantitative findings from multiple studies and examine them using high-powered statistics. Guideline authors also refer to systematic summaries of the clinical research literature such as those created by the Cochrane Collaboration, an organization formed for this mission specifically.

Some health care groups apply guidelines as they are, off the shelf; others tailor them, transforming their action sequence recommendations into locally adapted algorithms or decision-tree pathways. Children's, for example, had an in-house pathways division when I worked there (Richardson, Sobo, and Stuckey 2003).

Guidelines and pathways are not without their detractors. Physicians frequently resent guidelines, inferring a message that their skills in determining what is best for the patient are not valued (Christakis and Rivara 1998). Excessive complexity and poor-quality evidence have been identified as barriers to adherence, as have organizational factors, such as contradicting policies (D. A. Katz 1999). Guidelines that do not mesh well with local clinical workflow patterns may not be implemented. Those that are too general in nature may actually result in increased mismanagement (Shekelle et al. 2000). Unclear or very restrictive inclusion and exclusion criteria can foster poor interobserver reliability in interpretation and implementation (D. A. Katz 1999). That is, providers may apply them differently without so realizing (Sobo and Kurtin 2003).

More important for us, at this point in our discussion, are the criteria used in guideline creation—and the criteria used in audit, and in the original version of EBM advocated by Sackett. That is: What counts as **evidence?**

What Counts as Evidence, and Who Pays?

Some of the main concerns that I and others have regarding the EBM model occur at what Mykhalovskiy and Weir term "the nexus of scientific knowledge and social action" (2004, p. 1067). For example, providers do not always critically assess the evidence that has been produced; they do not act as critical consumers. They may simply accept or reject it based on their knowledge of its source or economic and social factors that affect their practice. Evidence is sometimes accepted, once circulated, only if it embodies and reinforces existing practice preferences (Fairhurst and Huby 1998; Lipman 2000).

Another problem with EBM is the assumptions entailed about evidentiary standards to begin with. In a discussion of the parameters of EBM and the ramifications these have for the flow of health care improvement knowledge, improvement guru Donald Berwick has stated that, according to the scientific perspective, "unguided human observers are frail meters of truth" (2005, p. 315). By this he means that, to protect ourselves from unconscious and uncontrollable human biases, we must (or so the scientific community says) devise and apply formal scientific research designs complete with robust and powerful statistical methods (see also Chapter 7).

This standard has been incorporated into the filter that informs the medical publication process. That is, for a project to be deemed publishable, it must be cut from scientific cloth. This is the case even though this means that the "filter [fails] to accommodate the kind of discovery that drives most improvement in health care" (Berwick 2005, p. 315). The strength of this filter also to some degree produces and certainly reinforces demand for RCTs and the concurrent need investigators have to recruit participants for these RCTs.

As Mykhalovskiy and Weir report in a passage that validates my own experience-based impressions (and see Chapter 14):

> The patient becomes a site of evidence tied into the research reputation and career trajectories of clinician-researchers. The place of research in prestige-ranking among physicians is one motivation to constitute patients as sites of evidence. Another important set of motivations is directly economic. Individual physicians and research institutions are paid enormous sums of money to recruit, randomize and retain patients. The training of physicians in EBM may result in the perception that it is their right to demand their patients enter research studies, a demand physicians justify by the need to properly evaluate diagnostic technologies and treatments. (2004, p. 1066)

In this, evidentiary standards have important secondary effects on the shape of care, especially for diseases with no sure cure (for example, much cancer care is RCT-related).

The "Crown Prince of methods," Berwick reminds us, is the RCT or, to be more specific, it is the

> randomized, double-blind [in which, to reduce bias and reactivity, neither participants nor investigators know what the intervention is], prospective

[in which effects are measured as they happen, over time], controlled clinical trial. ... Below the RCT stood methods of less nobility, graded in their evidence value from the properly designed cohort and case-control studies of epidemiology to the lowly case series, the suspect expert opinion, and the bestial anecdote. (2005, p. 315)

Berwick uses the word "stood" in the article cited because he is crafting an argument against EBM—or at least in favor of broadening the standards for what counts as evidence (2005). Health care's fetishization of EBM has prioritized efficacy over effectiveness. **Efficacy** refers to positive results under experimental or otherwise controlled conditions, such as in a clinical trial; **effectiveness** refers to how an intervention actually works in real life, such as when real people try to take a drug as directed but find themselves awash in contingencies unplanned for. There is a third term often discussed when efficacy and effectiveness are compared and contrasted: efficiency. **Efficiency** has to do with a particular treatment's cost effectiveness. Although pharmaceutical companies vie for efficacy and patients as well as their clinicians favor effectiveness, efficiency is managed care's goal.

⫻ANTHROPOLOGICAL GOALS RECONSIDERED

Effectiveness is an everyday construct; anthropologically informed methods are useful for effectiveness studies because, as Howard Becker notes, ethnographers make observations of people operating under normal sociocultural constraints, that is, where people's actions can and do have real-world consequences (1996). Further, people's own understandings of these actions often provide far better explanations than those made up by researchers who insulate themselves from this real-world context and limit interaction to the collection of data points as per a preexisting protocol.

Indeed, many a sociocultural phenomenon has an explanation far more mundane than what researchers' theories would suggest. Take, for example, mail carriers who, despite fancy theories suggesting that they would primarily prefer lighter loads and middle-class versus inner-city routes, actually had geographic preferences: They just wanted a route that was flat (Becker 1996).

Similarly, intake staff in the emergency department at Children's sometimes failed to fasten wrist-band identifiers to children at check-in, leading to misappropriated test results and other mistaken-identity problems that compromised patient safety. We guessed the "failure to band" had something to do with work overload or even carelessness induced by low morale. However, our anthropologically informed assessment revealed that the banding problem resulted instead from ethical considerations that made sense in the here-and-now: At check-in, when the bands were supposed to be fastened, many children were scared and crying. Parents were generally scared and sometimes crying, too. Workers would set identification bands aside when they did not want to add to anyone's suffering through further interference. This finding regarding banding's undesirable immediate effects (which the safety officer acted on, for instance in framing a staff education video) would never have been made had we limited our study of the banding problem to traditional, quantitative, formally protocolized HSR methods.

/ THE IMPORTANCE OF EFFECTS

In her criticism of those who would apply the randomized controlled trial or RCT approach to our quest for better care, Annemarie Mol compares the goal of proving efficacy to the goal of improvement. The two significantly differ. This difference hinges not just on the contrast between efficacy and effectiveness discussed above but on the contrast that exists, too, between effectiveness and the **effects** of interventions—the ramifications that given treatment choices have for daily life.

This is increasingly important as chronic care replaces acute care as most common. Indeed, Mark Sullivan predicts that the "epidemiological transition" to chronic care will foster a sea-change in HSR through an "epistemological transition" that will result in the "radical realignment between the objective and subjective elements of clinical medical science" (2003, p. 1595). By this, Sullivan means that the patient's point of view will begin to qualify as important and useful evidence.

Whether care is long term or not, because of the sheer connective complexity of real-life living when considered holistically, effects should not be separated from effectiveness. As Mol contends: "Disease, illness, technology, treatment, life: they come as a package, so it would be better to study them in this way" (2006, p. 412).

Circumlocution?

In addition to being holistic and systems-oriented, the anthropological approach favored by Mol, me, and others can be described, using the language of science, as **hypothesis-generating**. We make naturalistic observations, inspect them for patterns (generally with help from those observed), and develop general ideas from these observations. These ideas are, in a way, hypotheses: They are, theoretically, open for testing.

It bears noting here, however, that most human observations are not uninformed; that is, we decide what to observe based on preconceived notions regarding what might be important. Generally, these notions come from a thorough reading of the literature regarding the people and problem in question, and they are made explicit in our research proposals. Theory, as Albert Einstein said, is not simply generated from "observable magnitudes alone. It is the theory which decides what we can observe"; without a theory, we would not know what to focus in on (Bernstein 1973). Observations are made, and they make sense, only when we have a preexisting conceptual framework to make it so.

In any case, some scholars are offended by the suggestion that anthropologically informed research is hypothesis-generating because it implies that the hypotheses should be tested using the scientific method and that anthropologically informed studies cannot stand on their own. A further logical problem is the distinction assumed when we lump anthropologically informed work with feasibility or formative work simply because it does not entail formal tests of hypotheses.

In HSR language, **formative** research is front-end work done prior to implementing a full-scale, generally science-based, research protocol. It is intended to identify potential barriers to implementation so that the research **protocol** (intervention and data collection design) can be adapted to better fit local conditions or to collect initial context information to be used in designing the protocol to begin with. When we call ethnographic work "formative," health services colleagues have a good understanding of the type of data it deals with. The terms "pilot" or "feasibility study" would work, too; "formative," however (unlike the other terms), has an explicit, alliterative opposite that all HSR-trained scholars compare it to: "summative." Research conducted using a final, unchangeable protocol is **summative**, because it sums up what happens when the intervention is implemented according to the protocol (for instance, when a pill is taken as directed or a revised hospital discharge process is put into place).

But if we take Mol's admonition to focus on effects seriously and add it to our concern with effectiveness, it is easy to see that anthropologically informed research need not be relegated to the front end as formative. It can also be substantively summative, too. The question of whether to label it as such—or as hypothesis-generating—when trying to explain it in health services circles is a political one relating to expedience, which I discuss in the final part of the book. But now, let us question the contexts in which anthropologically informed research is actually carried out and the implications these contexts have for our research processes and our potential findings.

CHAPTER 9

The Realities of Research: Where and How to Begin

Methodological discussions often begin with the ideal situation in mind. All things being equal, we think, what would it take to answer a given research question? What techniques would apply, over what timeframe, in collaboration with whom, in what setting?

However, for various reasons, the real and ideal are often at odds. Even without funding to worry about, there are practical, logistical limits to health-related data collection from human subjects. That is, research must be designed so as not to unduly burden participants, who are burdened enough already with what in the health services research or HSR context are often life and death concerns. These are par for the course in the HSR setting, although some sites entail more such challenges than others.

In addition to what in HSR parlance is sometimes referred to as respondent burden, getting involved in HSR entails a modicum of researcher burden beyond what is standard in anthropological or social science research undertaken in academic settings. This is because HSR is generally collaborative. Anthropologists traditionally go to the field alone, unencumbered by others, and write up their findings in single-authored articles and monographs, but HSR is a team sport. In this chapter, I explain the need for making collaboration work to the benefit of the research process and its outcomes after I outline some of the contingencies imposed on anthropologically informed research by virtue of the settings in which it is undertaken.

Whereas Chapter 14 discusses higher order contingencies in terms of researcher career experiences, this chapter focuses on the implications that local-level contingencies have on particular project plans. It will therefore be most helpful to readers who have not yet collaborated in team research or worked in a health services setting. Those who have done so may wish to skim the first parts of the chapter anyhow for useful suggestions regarding how to make things work when naturalistic research is preferred. However, the chapter's final section, Factory Findings, which address the validity of findings derived by a team, should be of concern to novice and maven alike.

SITE-BASED CHALLENGES

Where Things of Interest Happen

Some HSR, for example that concerning barriers to care or routine activities of daily living, utilizes community samples. But the bulk of HSR primary data collection is carried out in clinical settings. Inpatient settings are good places to study directly the myriad challenges of care provision (e.g., discharge planning). Further, in addition to clinicians and other health services workers, clinical settings have in-house populations with defined diagnoses, such as tonsillitis, pancreatic cancer, or whatever may interest the researcher. Samples from these populations can be hard to assemble in community settings. Ambulatory clinics also are good sources for data: Specialist clinics attract and serve people with chronic conditions that are in control or under maintenance (e.g., diabetes or asthma). Primary care clinics, on the other hand, can be useful for research regarding preventive care. For research on palliative care, a hospice is a good setting. And the list goes on.

The downside of research conducted in clinical settings is that patients who would be participants are generally sick or impaired. Indeed, they may be very ill or even dying. Friends and family may be distressed. For some of these people, talking to an outsider will be just what the doctor ordered, providing researchers the opportunity to at least bear witness to participant testimonies. For others, participation in a research study might cause added trauma. Even observations alone may be distressful to families and patients undergoing crises or dealing with matters that they would prefer to keep private.

Further, as noted in Chapter 5, health services settings are workplaces, too; providers as well as others who support care in whatever form have tasks to accomplish. Research can be perceived of as—and sometimes actually is—getting in the way of this.

The Need for Champions

Each health services setting has been organized by an institution, so access to respondents must be negotiated. A first task is finding a member of staff who is willing to champion the work at hand and serve as a gatekeeper—someone who can provide access to patients or whoever else is needed for a study. Although it is essential to have front-line supporters, support from leadership is crucial, too. So, for example, as noted previously, the instigators of an HIV screening program with which I was involved went first to medical directors and financial leadership. Once this buy-in was secured (chiefly by appealing to the bottom-line cost effectiveness of early identification of people with HIV), buy-in at subordinate levels could be cultivated. And, at this point, many subordinates saw the project as something leadership wanted them to participate in. Indeed, some took the endorsement too literally, assuming that they were, in fact, being judged according to whether and how well they participated. Research ethics dictate that such misunderstandings be eradicated whenever they arise.

I cannot overemphasize how important rapport with staff is to the success of the research endeavor. Most health care organizations participate in some kind of audit program, if only because the Joint Commission requires this for accreditation (see Chapter 5). For instance, patient satisfaction and experience surveys are par for the course as organizations demonstrate compliance with rules regarding quality of care evaluations. Staff members may feel as if they are under constant surveillance; some even view new computerized medical records, clinical reminders, and order entry systems as devious means by which the organization extends its bureaucratic gaze over their performance and compliance to guidelines and other standards. All those who do research must find ways to diffuse any participants' and potential participants' worries that research data collection is part and parcel of larger institutional surveillance efforts.

Critical Situations

Along these lines, trauma surgeons at one institution where I worked rejected my interest in viewing tapes of resuscitation efforts out of concern that my findings might be used against them. They felt so much performance pressure that they could not believe that a study would not result in some form of punitive action. Indeed, prior to my arrival there had been a to-do regarding the trauma-room's video camera (at that time, videos were made only for quality assurance purposes). I was not actually able to spend enough time with the surgeons to calm their fears; they were generally too busy and so was I. But, although the trauma video project never got a go-ahead, other projects did when defenses came down. This took time and hinged, in part, on good word-of-mouth from units that actually had benefited from my services.

One of the most productive relationships that I built while at Children's was with the hematology and oncology service. This was largely through the help of a pathologist, Glenn Billman, who had been at the hospital for many years and was a fan of quality and safety improvement as well as of outcomes measurement. With his endorsement and the help of research assistants trained to never overstep their boundaries with patients or staff, staff members began to feel safe with my research.

That one of my reports helped them hire another half-time interpreter certainly helped make the case for my entrance into their world. Offering their medical and administrative directors authorship on resulting publications also did not hurt (for more regarding that aspect of collaboration, see Chapter 14).

Although each site will have specific rules in place, and particular priorities, here I relate some of the hematology-oncology or "heme-onc" processes, just to familiarize readers with some of the concerns that clinical populations can have. During all heme-onc projects, it was essential for research assistants and me to wash our hands thoroughly before entering the rooms. The children being treated were immune-compromised, and we did not wish to cause further damage by bringing germs into their presence. We also had to be aware of how everyone was feeling: patients and parents or guardians alike. Were there others visiting? Was it meal-time? Was the child in pain? Asleep? Being medicated? In short, we understood that our presence was of the lowest priority for everyone involved and we adjusted our approach to recruitment and data collection appropriately.

Another unit where I was able to make inroads was day surgery. Among the issues explored there were parents' perceptions of risk for bad outcomes and of the initial intake process. Again, we had to accommodate patient, family, and service needs. Although we had important reasons for our investigations, we understood that coming in for surgery is stressful and so is being with a child who is just recovering or, worse, having problems doing so. For this reason, I chose an unobtrusive observation strategy complete with a checklist for the intake process. In the recovery room, a five-minute interview was the method of choice. This method is explained fully in Chapter 12; here, suffice it to say that parents and guardians simply could not be asked to give more time than that when their loved ones were shaking off anesthesia and they were worried about what they would need to do at home to manage their child's postsurgical care. They had more important things to attend to than our project. We also had to be very cognizant of work force needs. These limitations, of course, affected the quality and extent of data that we collected—but without making such sacrifices, the work could never have been undertaken in the first place.

Another site that necessarily entails work force–related limitations is the site of death. Limitations here have more to do with cultural understandings than the practicalities of how to deliver life-enhancing patient care with a researcher in the way. Death carries taboos in all cultures but these are exacerbated when death takes place in a hospital setting. The curative mission of hospital care means that all care is life-saving until it has specifically been declared by a doctor as "futile." Except for in hospice or nursing home care, the vast majority of patients are simply expected to live. Death in a curative facility is in some ways considered a failure. It exists as a transgression and, as such, fosters greater ambivalence then it otherwise would among the staff.

Partly for this reason, at least at Children's, approaching families directly regarding dying, death, and bereavement was not an option. The bereavement work that I helped with there was survey-based, and the survey was mailed to bereaved families after they had, in the hospital's eyes, ample time to adjust. There were also less empathetic concerns reflected in this approach, such as those related to legal risk management and worry about bad word-of-mouth that might occur if anyone took offense.

Cultural norms regarding death must be carefully navigated. However, at facilities where death is anticipated, or where most patients are grown-ups, the situation can be more amenable to research than it was at Children's. Not only might staff more easily accept projects aimed at improving the quality-of-death when death is less unexpected, but families, too, may be more approachable. The dying and the bereaved are vulnerable and there are specific ethical considerations to involving them in research. However, with proper tailoring and sensitivity, wonderful work has been done (e.g., Kaufman 2005).

Preserving Our Own Human Resources

In all of these cases and others that HSR researchers will encounter, there is another set of individuals to consider: the researchers themselves. We are reminded by Ruth Behar that "anthropology that doesn't break your heart just isn't worth doing" (1996, p. 177). But it is exceedingly difficult to have your heart broken every single day. HSR personnel must, like other health services workers, develop defense mechanisms to protect themselves from emotional upheaval—without sacrificing the humanist element of their interpretive work and the authenticity of the relationships that excellent ethnography necessarily entails.

Distancing tactics can be part and parcel of the employee mentality cultivated in some HSR organizations. Unlike in traditional anthropology, where one is expected to embrace passionately one's fieldwork and devote time round-the-clock to the endeavor, anthropologically informed HSR is generally more of a 9-to-5 endeavor (at least in theory). With a few project-based data collection–related exceptions, at the end of the day HSR personnel go home. As such, the emotion work we normally associate with paid employment (e.g., repressing one's true emotions) is sometimes quite easy to undertake, even in the most distressing situations. To demonstrate, let me give a counter-example—an example of one rare time that I can recall when work in HSR tore through my heart. Although the scene I will portray took place about five years ago, my stomach tightens and my throat chokes up even now as I try to describe it.

A new project opportunity had been presented to me by an ear, nose, and throat or ENT doc aware of my work in the day surgery recovery room. On my way through the hospital's hallways to discuss the possibilities with her in the ENT office suite, a gurney rolling out of the surgery area surrounded by half-a-dozen worn-out clinicians took me by surprise. The group's core concern, a tiny baby, lay still and small against the immense white rolling bed. There were no relatives in sight, only doctors and nurses, IV stands trundling in stride, and tubes and catheters and the other ephemera of whatever operation this little infant had undergone. The party went by in a slow cloud of silence. Having forgotten, for a single brief moment, for a reason I cannot explain let alone recall, that this was my place of daily work, I was completely and utterly undone.

This occurrence, however upsetting, was singular. Had I not developed everyday ways to defend my heart against the potential daily onslaught of trauma, I would not have been able to undertake my work in HSR, at least not in this hospital setting. Of course, anthropologists doing more traditional fieldwork have their own normalization, distancing, and general defense mechanisms, too, as portions of Bronislaw Malinowski's personal diary have infamously shown. Malinowski is remembered by many as the first true participant observer. He kept a diary, he said, as a "means of self analysis" while conducting fieldwork in Oceania during World War I (Malinowski 1989 [1967]).

/ COLLABORATION

In anthropology, we often speak of collaborating with research participants. In fact, some anthropologists call participants or subjects "collaborators" to formalize this construction regarding the relationship entailed. An increasing number of publications list collaborators as coauthors, either full-scale ("by") or in the "with" configuration. Participant-collaborators are very important; however, the collaborators that I refer to in the heading for this section are professional colleagues who we must team up with to get HSR projects done.

The Team Model

Patient Care Teams

Health care is a team endeavor. When people are sick they do not get well at the workday's end; ill health is not an eight-hour-a-day enterprise. To provide twenty-four-hour care, clinical care teams must be created. Even for acute cases successfully dealt with in an afternoon, the ever-increasing sophistication and complexity of care demands a collaborative team approach. Many recommend that staff undergo training similar to that which airline cockpit crews receive, so that they can better manage themselves—especially in times of crisis (see Kohn, Corrigan, and Donaldson 2000).

In hospitals or long-term care institutions, the team can include dozens of players. Although a clinical care team includes only those who provide clinical care, such as nursing staff, respiratory and other therapists, nutritionists, and medical and surgical docs, viewed more broadly the care team also includes parking lot attendants, intake personnel, the "techs" who do X-rays or make casts and prosthetic appliances for us, room services and facilities workers, maintenance staff, and so on. Health care organizations also have some employees dedicated to accreditation (including quality and safety) issues; a few even have a built-in research staff.

Laboratory and Clinical Research Teams

Laboratories often contribute members to a clinical care team but they themselves also are team affairs, and for similar reasons: The need for tests or "labs" does not stop at 5 P.M., and many procedures are far from instant. A fully staffed laboratory will be open twenty-four hours a day, seven days a week. Further, even for small units with limited hours, upkeep entails a number of interrelated technical steps, some complex, others mundane. A team of workers with differing capacities is called for.

In clinical research, such as the randomized controlled trials described in Chapter 8, the same is true but more so. There must be staff to administer informed consent, and once that is granted someone must ensure that the participant enrolled is properly compliant with the protocol. Someone administers medications. Someone draws blood. Someone processes blood. Someone analyzes the data. Someone writes it up for presentation. Someone prepares a report for the sponsor.

Although in small studies there can be overlap, more often, in keeping with the factorial model (indeed, the factory model) that is followed in most HSR, different individuals do different tasks. In multi-sited research, which often takes place when populations are small (such as in pediatric cancer research where, to amass enough study subjects, a number of sites must be active), the number of workers multiplies. And when this happens, so too can the number of team-related challenges.

HSR Teams

Because of its history (see Chapter 5), HSR is intimately linked with clinical practice. It is, in many ways, modeled on the clinical care and clinical research team ethics just described. Although here I write primarily about clinically applied HSR, this evolutionary footprint is found even on HSR that relies on large secondary data sets such as financial data from an insurance system; the idealized, quantitatively oriented standards of clinical science dominate.

Like clinicians and laboratory scientists, anthropologists working in health services rarely work alone. This is not just by virtue of the need for gatekeepers sweet on an anthropological project idea. It is also because most HSR is built up this way: with one principal investigator (PI) to spearhead the effort, some co-investigators to add scholarly heft or open necessary doors (they are called "key personnel" on grant applications), and a team of research assistants or associates (RAs) to collect and even analyze and begin to write up the data.

This modus operandi is very different than the traditional anthropological approach, in which one investigator does everything. In HSR, the PI need not be a complete expert to undertake a project. For example, although this would never occur in traditional anthropology, in HSR a PI may conduct a study using methods in which he or she has no facility.

It is not uncommon for an MD to spearhead a study as PI because of his or her medical expertise regarding a given condition, as well as his or her control over access to patients with such, but to have a coterie of co-investigators or Co-Is who actually plan and carry out key components of the work. For instance, a statistician may draw up a statistical plan, an epidemiologist may plan that aspect of the work, a pathologist can be in charge of, say, liver biopsies, and so on. Anthropologists can, of course, provide ethnographic services in such a set-up. And RAs generally take care of administrative paperwork (e.g., for funders, for ethics reviews) in addition to many aspects of data collection.

Usually, the PI's name goes on all publications ensuing, whether or not the PI participates in the writing process. A Co-I is of lower status than a PI, who stands as the project's ultimate decision-maker. There are other reasons to avoid a Co-I position: Money awarded for grant-funded research will be attributed to the PI, and he or she also will be the named grant-getter, no matter how much effort his or her Co-Is put into the grant proposal or other project work. This can be important in certain career tracks.

Still, the Co-Is benefit because without the PI they may have a very hard time gaining access to said population. Further, funding may be more difficult to come by on their own. And, of course, they benefit by way of the built-in community of practice that the project entails. All this is not to say that anthropologists never have their own funded research studies in HSR; they often do take the role of PI—but not always.

No matter who is PI, with the exception of some RAs, researchers in HSR (PIs and Co-Is) never devote their full time to one project. This means that they are working various parts of each week or year on a number of projects. Regardless of how many hours one's actual work week entails, organizational bureaucracies equate forty hours to 100% of a full-time equivalent or FTE employee. Given these terms (i.e., excluding weekends and evenings), researchers may spend one day a week or 20% (eight hours) of their FTE time on one project, two hours a week or 5% FTE on another, and so on, adding up to 100% time or forty hours.

A concrete example would be that, rather than having five people each undertake one project over a year's time, five people each work at 20% time or one day a week on five projects that year. This would never really happen because some people are more experienced and expert than others and so are more often leaders than followers; different people have different skill sets; projects start and stop at various times and have varying durations; and projects come in various sizes and so have smaller or larger staffing needs. In reality, then, especially when we add in the fact that percent time on one project is not actually constant throughout a given year because of the ebbs and flows of project activities, balancing percent times can be a time-consuming and creative (albeit sometimes energy-sapping) endeavor (see also Chapter 14). These costs notwithstanding, the benefits of being part of a collaborating research community can be immense.

In applied HSR, the intent is to have a direct and fairly immediate impact on service design, delivery, and outcomes. This requires a nimble, interdisciplinary team. It requires close collaboration between the investigators, the providers of services, and the end-users of the research findings. It is not something that we can do on our own, lone-ranger style.

An investigatory team of one, as is common in academic anthropology, simply does not often have the social connections in place that are necessary to see findings through to applied fruition in good time. Indeed, a number of key participants in a research project of mine regarding the actual research process in implementation science have reported that a key reason for team-making itself is the need for collaborator/gatekeeper buy-in on, and "championing" of, final recommendations and products—or, at least, acquiescence.

Factory Findings: The Mechanization of Research and Its Discontents

What Aims?

The downside of large teams and percent times that grow more fragmented as one works one's way up the personnel tree toward PI is that not everyone on a given research project knows everything about it.

I know of many cases where the named PI suffered from partial vision after becoming disconnected from a project's day-to-day workings or because of the political context in which she or he was named PI. But for RAs, partial vision is endemic.

RAs can be paid relatively cheaply to devote large percentages of time to a given project and they complete much of the day-to-day project work. Having said that, because they are generally hired only after a proposal has been funded, and are rarely brought in on investigator discussions such as those that ensue between PIs and Co-Is, they often do not have a full grasp of their project's aims. They sometimes do not understand why they must be so careful regarding data accuracy. A woman who wanted to take part in a study having to do with the menstrual cycle—a study that I was not involved with—told me that the RA taking her data altered the start date of her last period so that she might participate. I doubt the RA meant any harm; maybe she wanted to help her team reach a recruitment goal or to help the woman out because the study paid money. I witnessed similar episodes many times when, however well intended, situational logic overrides research logic in a way that, if unchecked, can lead to spurious findings (for more regarding the effects of situational logic in research settings, see Chapter 14).

Such shortsightedness notwithstanding, RAs generally develop allegiance to their project's PI, whether or not they actually have met him or her in person. This comes about through social learning and acculturation and may be especially likely when an RA is affiliated with a research unit with numerous studies. In many staff (read: RA) break-room conversations that I overheard while at one large research center, various RAs used the catch-phrase "my PI," invoking the power of that PI's curriculum vitae (academic resumé) and faculty title to negotiate a place within the RA pecking order.

No Shortcuts

Despite its compatibility with laboratory and clinical research, the interchangeable team member model as it currently stands in HSR cannot work with anthropologically informed studies. This is because of the centrality of holism and interpretation to their epistemological basis. This point is paramount. Indeed, traditionally trained sociocultural anthropologists demand research designs in which *one* researcher conducts *all* study functions.

For anthropologically informed HSR, each team member's participation should include both data collection and analysis. In some cases, data collection can be effectively outsourced to an RA, for instance, if that data will be analyzed by someone who also has collected data or by someone who has intimate, long-term knowledge of the data collection site. However, anyone participating in the analysis must, at the least, have participated in data collection activities. No shortcuts can be taken.

Furthermore, although data collection may need to be spaced out depending on what is being asked and of whom (see site-based limitations, above), it is crucial that analytic meetings are closely sequenced, time to reflect on meeting discussions and data in between meetings is provided, and researchers are not distracted by other substantive projects or data during the intensive analytic phase. Full engagement in the analytic endeavor is key to the validity and reliability of findings. That is, immersion-like conditions must be fabricated to support the degree of concentration that good anthropologically informed analysis depends on.

For example, all five of the category-development sessions undertaken for a barriers to care project that I was involved in (Seid et al. 2004; Sobo, Seid, and Gelherd 2006) were conducted within a ten-day time period, and all investigators were available to concentrate on the process. The all-hands-on-deck or total engagement approach can be hard to arrange in the context of HSR as it is organized today. Team members often do not have ample time allotted to a project to co-participate intensively. However, we knew that the success of our project depended on this and therefore, with careful planning, we managed to make it happen. The model we created was used in an intervention for children with asthma and good preliminary results have been reported (Michael Seid, personal communication, July 17, 2007, and see Seid et al. n.d.).

All this assumes that everyone involved in a given project has received ample training. RAs should have studied and practiced the techniques in question. They should have done so in a way that enables and helps ensure concordance in terms of both the data collected and the analyses applied. Thorough and fully protocolized training should be part of any research project's start-up phase.

On a related note, no project should try to do too much too fast. In recent years, applied anthropology's growth has resulted in many methodological developments promising rapid results; I describe a few of these in the next part of the book. Although new techniques have proven excellent additions to our methods toolkit, their unconsidered reception in some quarters has threatened to throw us off course by fostering a climate in which the need for intensive fieldwork gets forgotten:

> With the development of new, systematic data collection techniques that do not in themselves entail years of fieldwork, it is tempting to engage in what has become known as rapid ethnographic assessment. This involves the use of one or a few methods only; the researcher foregoes participant observation and long-term study. This may be convenient, and may even be necessary and excusable in the case of time-sensitive problems, as in the field of development or the context of a health crisis. However, it is only

truly appropriate when the researcher already has done extensive fieldwork or when we already know volumes about the population involved and the researcher has taken the time, in developing his or her study and in writing up the findings, to take existing knowledge into account. Otherwise, they might be misled as they attempt to interpret their findings, and they might mislead others with their (unsound) conclusions. (de Munck and Sobo 1998, p. 36)

One cannot grasp the anthropologically informed significance of any piece of data without a full-fledged understanding of the sociocultural context from which it has been excised. Any explanation of findings must refer back to this context; data must be situated as they are interpreted and discussed. This is one reason for the ethnographic-style content of this book: It provides readers with a modicum of familiarity with the sociocultural worlds in which they will be working.

THE ROLE OF INSTITUTIONAL REVIEW AND INFORMED CONSENT

The last aspect of the research world that I mention here is the **institutional review board** or IRB. Institutional review is a complex process that, on the surface, has little to do with methodological discussion. Still, it bears some scrutiny because without it, in many nations, research simply cannot happen. I already have noted that the IRB's role is to ensure, through proposal review and related inspection-type processes, that any research conducted under their institution's auspices is ethically designed and implemented. All of my research has been IRB-sanctioned, including that drawn on for examples in this book. So has some of the work that I have undertaken initially for quality improvement (QI).

Although IRB approval is not required for QI efforts, it is definitely desirable when external or generalizable implications are to be explored and findings disseminated (Bellin and Neveloff Dubler 2001). One can go back, after the fact, to request clearance to publish, but it is immensely preferable to work with the IRB from the start; to do otherwise in situations where publication or other forms of extra-mural dissemination are immanent is dishonest and unethical. This is the case even though IRB time-frames can cause the project to be lost.

Many IRBs meet only monthly, and applications to be reviewed may have to be in up to a month prior to that. If an IRB is undergoing internal transitions, such as to board membership, timelines can be lengthened. They also are affected when an IRB notices a point of concern in an application. This can be very helpful, as not all ethical problems will be obvious to researchers; in many cases, the added scrutiny has revealed problems that then can be fixed. Other times, IRB change requests may be a hindrance, as when board members are not familiar with the methods used or, when pressed for time, they read proposals too fast and thereby overlook data and human subjects protection plans. They also can misunderstand the nature of everyday risk and thereby treat minimal risk research, which most anthropologically informed HSR projects will be, as if they are the high risk equivalent to medical experimentation (Dingwall 2008).

Another factor affecting the time review takes is the number of IRBs entailed. The effort involved in securing all necessary IRB approvals for multi-site work or work undertaken by collaborators with diverse affiliations and thus varied IRBs is multiplicative; different IRBs can have different standards and demands in addition to differing board meeting timelines and proposal due dates. When planning a project, it is best to build in extra time to ensure that all the paperwork and approvals will be in order on the day that data collection is scheduled to begin.

Data cannot generally be collected from or about human beings without an approved **informed consent** process. Engagement in the process of informed consent usually must be documented, for instance, with the potential participant's signature on an IRB-approved consent form. To be approved, a proposed informed consent process must entail the essential steps of informing participants about the aims and methods of the project in question as well as about the risks to which they might be exposed upon participating. Further, at least in the United States, all personnel involved with a project must complete human subjects protection training to ensure that they are well aware of the general need for holding participant identities and data in the strictest confidence.

Informed consent only really works when those recruited have no cause to feel coerced (see also Chapter 8 regarding ethnocentric bias in the bioethics used to justify the process). When recruitment takes place in a clinical setting, potential participants might mistakenly believe that their continued care depends on participating. Further, because of their vulnerable position as patients or care consumers, potential participants may fear that information they share will be fed back to providers and used against them. To offset such worries, recruiters and data collectors must make clear to participants that participation really is voluntary, privacy will be protected to the extent allowed by law, and data are completely confidential. If the study protocol actually limits confidentiality, for instance if some kind of data feedback to providers is built in, participants should be fully informed of the situation.

On a related note, true anonymity may not be possible because of the need to track participants, as in a longitudinal study or when the chance of duplicate participation must be guarded against. In such cases, real names, medical record numbers, or similar identifiers may need to be collected. However, with proper planning, substitute identification codes tied to a key can be used on data collection documents. The real list of the names and the crosswalk key for the identification codes is kept in a locked file cabinet somewhere away from the data. The list should be shredded after the duration specified by the relevant IRB. Data files should be locked away when not in use.

Verbal consent can be used for projects that entail no more than minimal risk (such as the normal risks of everyday social intercourse) and in which the only document linking participants to the project would be a written consent form (see Title 45 CFR §46.117; http://www.nihtraining. com/ohsrsite/guidelines/45cfr46.html, last accessed August 22, 2008). Not all IRBs know that verbal consent is legal; those more used to clinical trials–type research may look askance at such a request. But it is worth fighting for permission to use verbal consent when risks are indeed minimal because the written consent process can be off-putting to potential participants, besides adding a layer of complexity to data storage plans.

Verbal consent is no less explicit than written consent; a script should be created and used that explains, in full, the study's aims, benefits to humanity, and possible risks to the participant. A written statement can supplement but not replace a candid conversation regarding the project, through which the participant actually gets to learn or become informed about a project in an engaged way.

Informed consent procedures have been known to be flouted by busy RAs, and participants sometimes just sign consent forms without really reading and digesting them because they either cannot read or forgot their glasses and are ashamed to say so, or they find asking questions embarrassing. Alternately, they may feel somewhat coerced into doing so because of social norms or for reasons related to dependency. But without an informed consent agreement, data cannot be collected; without an IRB-approved process, research cannot commence.

Specific Methods

The previous parts of this book have laid out the historical and philosophical underpinnings of the anthropologically informed health services research (HSR) endeavor. Its final chapter mapped the lay of the land of HSR, describing how most HSR projects are organized. We are now ready to explore some of the techniques that can be brought to bear in the quest for a holistic, systems-oriented understanding of a given HSR question. In addition to explaining some of the particular methods that I have used in this quest myself, chapters in Part IV also describe the ways that the anthropological approach has been modified in these methods to meet health services' practical needs rather than, or in addition to, purely academic interests.

The branch of HSR whose methods most nearly resemble those of anthropology is often termed "qualitative HSR" because qualitative is typically used in HSR as a marker for research that depends for data on words rather than numbers. However, as I have shown, qualitative HSR's analytic methods can be highly quantitative or noninterpretive compared to the methods of anthropology. Thus, even when HSR and anthropology seem to share a particular method, they may not use it, or analyze the data resulting from it, in the same way.

A prime example of a method that HSR and anthropology tend to deploy differently is the focus group, one of the most favored qualitative methods in HSR today. After describing the focus group method in general and reviewing its genealogy, Chapter 10 recounts and constructively criticizes various approaches to focus group research. The chapter then demonstrates, with examples, how anthropologically informed focus group data can be collected, transcribed, and analyzed.

As popular as they are, focus groups do not always suit the question at hand and they are not always logistically feasible. Chapter 11 asks how to make the most of the one-time retrospective interview format that is sometimes necessary in HSR. We consider the costs and benefits of both face-to-face and telephone interviews. Tips for keeping interviewees talking are reviewed, and a strategy for training assistants not used to thinking anthropologically is provided, along with information on note-taking conventions. Finally, we discuss ideas for drawing in anthropological theory as well as contextual information and previously published findings to build more meaningful analyses.

In Chapter 12, the importance of the situated nature of thought and action is reinforced, and ways to take context more directly into account are introduced. I describe and discuss methods appropriate for research undertaken in the context of service provision, including one that calls for as little as five minutes of people's time. I also review some informed consent–related considerations and provide instruction on coding and analysis that builds on what we have learned about these processes in previous chapters.

Chapter 13 specifically addresses the rapid-cycle improvement approach predominant in health services quality improvement (QI) circles. This chapter explores, in more depth than previously, various ways of feeding research findings directly back into the health services setting to foster improvement. Interventional sustainability also is addressed. Along the way, we revisit the traditional opposition between theory and application.

The methodological instruction in all of the chapters in this section is embedded in actual examples of anthropologically informed HSR. I have done this because methods are too often conceptualized in an abstract or idealized fashion, divorced from the real, on-the-ground, and sometimes messy or complicated settings in which they are actually practiced. To help demonstrate what goes on "behind the curtain," then, I present and discuss not just the formal steps of each method but also situational limitations, important logistical considerations, and the process of making methodological decisions in the field and in the moment.

Many of the ways in which realities in the field can limit idealized methodological designs tend not to be brought up in published research articles because authors typically aim to legitimize data and findings by demonstrating that their research methods were as flawless as possible. This does a disservice to methodological education, however. I describe some of the limitations we all face, both as opportunities for reflection on challenges to good research as well as to highlight prospects for improvement.

The real-world limits, opportunities, and serendipity involved in fieldwork leads me to a final thought: Technical proficiency does not an excellent researcher make. Howard Becker once said of a certain researcher whom he admires, "What makes his work outstanding is not that he uses some particular method or that he follows approved procedures correctly, but that he has imagination and can smell a good problem and find a good way to study it" (1996, p. 11e). Research should be systematic and methodical—but it also must be creative. Part of creativity is being able to illuminate the minutia of people's experiences—their day-to-day lives—by linking them with the larger systemic forces impinging on them.

CHAPTER 10

/ Refocusing Focus Group
Data Collection and Analysis

In health services, qualitative research is often synonymous with convening focus groups. Here we will tackle this "focus-group focus" head on. Although this book is in part a bid to move run-of-the-mill qualitative health services research (HSR) design beyond the focus group, the method does have great utility. This chapter reviews how to make the most of this method in fulfilling anthropologically informed research aims.

After describing the method and reviewing its history, we examine two focus group studies carried out in the context of HSR. I note for each the costs and benefits of specific techniques used in data collection and analysis. Each approach is good for certain goals, but some choices prove better than others when a meaning-centered analysis—one that tells the problem's story—is the main aim.

/ FOCUS GROUP PRIMER

What Are Focus Groups?

Focus groups are scheduled group discussions regarding a focal topic (e.g., food additives). They last for about one to two hours and usually have between six and ten participants. Numbers will vary with field constraints, but one dozen participants is typically the upper limit because this method relies on the quality of the discussion that the group generates. With more than twelve people, discussions can become unruly—or stilted and dull.

Focus group participants are usually unknown to the researchers. Generally, they are compensated formally (e.g., with money) for their time. Sometimes, the number of focus groups held is determined by practical matters such as the nature of the questions to be asked or the funding available for the project at hand, but ideally researchers stop convening groups only when data collected become redundant (when no new information is forthcoming).

Focus groups can be used as a stand-alone data collection method for self-contained studies or they can supplement other forms of data collection. The data they elicit can be considered explicitly formative or supplemental or the data can be more central to a study, for example, one that is specifically conceived of as a multi-method research project. As David Morgan notes, "The model here is clearly ethnography, which has traditionally involved a blend of observation and interviewing" (1997, p. 3).

Where Did Focus Groups Come From?

The history of the focus group is remarkably similar to the history of modern medicine, in that the method's military applications in World War II (e.g., regarding propaganda's persuasiveness and training materials' effectiveness) led to its formalization. From there, the focus group method was quickly adopted by marketing researchers, who saw its potential for gauging potential consumer response to particular products as well as for identifying untapped product-related needs. It fell into disuse in scholarly circles (Morgan 1997).

In the early 1980s, a number of books on the focus group method were published by marketing scholars. Further, communications researchers as well as demographers interested in public health picked up the method (Morgan 1997). This link to public health is not coincidental: Public and international health research projects involving social scientists have been key proving grounds for many now-popular applied research methods, such as those used in focused ethnographic study or rapid ethnographic assessment (see Pelto and Pelto 1997; see also Chapter 13). In any case, by the 1980s, social scientists were paying the focus group method more heed—and making methodological innovations to enhance its utility for interpretive projects.

The Unit of Analysis

For some studies, perhaps especially those with limited funds (like pilot or exploratory studies) or those with very short time-lines (as may occur in an epidemic), the key benefit of the focus group is speed. A focus group study can enroll a great many participants in little time, and focus groups can be held back-to-back if enough facilitators are available, leading to low time costs.

However, this perspective misses a number of points, including the fact that in focus group research the number of groups convened is more important than the number of participants because the group discussion is what is analyzed. Further, in anthropologically informed focus group research, having a few facilitator-investigators is much better than having an army of interchangeable staff workers, for reasons explained below (and see Chapter 9).

In terms of analytic goals, however, as David Morgan notes, "The hallmark of focus groups is their explicit use of group interaction to produce data and insights that would be less accessible without the interaction found in a group" (1997, p. 2). That is, focus groups foster, through synergetic interaction, emergent forms of information that are not accessible through, for instance, one-on-one interviews. Social interaction assists respondents in the generation of lists regarding the range of possible responses to a given hypothetical situation or the various items in a given, culturally circumscribed category (such as "barriers to care"). Moreover, social interaction helps make manifest shared, cultural norms as well as bringing to light important culturally shaped or influenced ways in which that people in groups can contest these norms. This leveraging of social interaction is one of the main features that attract anthropologists to the method.

Our focus is on the qualitative side of the analytic continuum. That is not to say that a quantitative approach does not have its merits; a combination of qualitative and quantitative can sometimes be quite illuminating. However, the very nature of focus group data—its social generation—makes it more suited to interpretation than statistical manipulation. Even when a concrete list of, say, possible responses to fever has been collected, there is no way to infer or predict from focus group data the number of people who would actually undertake one or another response. What we can conclude is what is in the response repertoire and what each type of response may refer to or mean.

If quantification is the goal, it is better to use quantitative survey methods. Surveys worded in ways that make sense given the sociocultural landscape under exploration work best. Focus groups can provide very relevant information for developing valid and reliable surveys.

Participant Mix

Our focus on emergence and interaction as a benefit of focus group research has implications for participant selection criteria and thereby for participant mix. Much focus group research specifies eligibility in regard to particular demographic variables, such as age, gender, ethnic identity, or occupation. But in certain cases, we must take all comers. This was so for my research on HIV seropositivity self-disclosure, conducted in rural New Mexico in the early 1990s when I was new to the region (Sobo 1997). Finding HIV-positive people willing to talk about their sexual relationships in this context was hard. Those who were willing and physically able to come to a group meeting were busy, so scheduling was a challenge. In sum, I could not be picky. And we all have to start each new program of research somewhere.

The resulting focus groups were definitely heterogeneous; a given group could include people who were heterosexual and homosexual, single and partnered, male and female, just diagnosed or having long since progressed to having AIDS. In this case, and despite initial disappointment because of my preconceived notions about the methodological limitations of mixed groups, heterogeneity made for very rich discussions in which people compared and contrasted their experiences. In hindsight, having unmixed groups not only would have muted this dimension but also may have led to both more self-censorship related to normative standards and less descriptive and detailed accounting.

Such information vacuums can occur anytime participants assume that certain aspects of their experiences are uniform and therefore do not merit mention. Gery Ryan told me, just before a workshop that we gave on qualitative methods at a national meeting of child health services researchers in June 2004, that he uses driving to illustrate this. He says to students and interested colleagues something like: "When you talk about driving with other people, do you mention that you drive on the right side of the road? If you taught someone how to drive, would you do so?" Maybe, if a listener or learner is from the United Kingdom, where they drive on the left. "But," he might continue, "unless there is some trigger to bring that very crucial information to the top of your mind—unless you have reason to think that such common-sense knowledge is lacking in your listeners—you will neglect to mention it."

There is great value in mixing participants in groups so that explanations or descriptions of similar common-sense assumptions will be triggered and thereby made explicit. However, for certain types of questions, it can be more useful to convene homogeneous groups. For example, female health concerns will perhaps be better addressed with all-female groups than with mixed sexes. Here it bears repeating that much of what we are told in focus groups reflects normative understandings of how things should be, not how they actually are; this tendency would be exacerbated in homogeneous groups. This is a good thing when normative understandings are exactly what is in question.

Remember that, in focus groups, the discussion is the data. As such, focus group data are essentially qualitative. But recall the review in Chapter 7 of the continuum dividing qualitative and quantitative data; they are, in actual fact, simply ideal types rather than truly mutually exclusive. In HSR, data gleaned from the interchanges between participants often get quantified during the analytic data reduction process. This can be helpful for answering some questions. But it leaves untapped the focus group method's full potential for enhancing our anthropologically informed understanding of the problem at hand. To illustrate, we now turn to examples.

AN HSR EXAMPLE

In 2005, I was invited to join in a focus group project investigating communication barriers for families with "limited English proficiency" (LEP)—particularly barriers that had potentially harmful outcomes in terms of patient safety (Bethell et al. 2006). The tendency to adapt a method to suit one's disciplinary needs is commonplace and, just as I do this for anthropological purposes, so too do other researchers adapt methods to serve their disciplinary foci. This particular well-run project was headed by a policy researcher with no anthropological background but a wealth of other experience. In context, the project was a success and it provided data that would probably never have been collected using an anthropological design.

The Protocol

The study entailed, among other things, five focus groups conducted in South Florida (two groups and a total of eight LEP participants) and Southern California (three groups and a total of seventeen LEP participants). All participants had a child aged zero to seventeen who was hospitalized within the prior six months at a study site. These parent focus groups followed what researchers call a "panel" design; participants in an initial focus group were slated to return for a second focus group approximately one month later. However, only twelve Round 1 parent focus group participants also participated in the Round 2 focus groups.

Although the loss rate here is on the high side, it is definitely not out of the ballpark in qualitative HSR. It is, to a large degree, a function of the lack of relationship building that is characteristic of this type of research as well as a lack of ethnographically informed foresight in determining where groups should meet. (For an illustration of a typical HSR recruitment protocol, see the next example; I also write more about focus group locations below.)

The first round of parent focus groups included four phases: (1) introductions and open-ended discussion on how participants define good or poor quality hospital care; (2) a discussion about specific communication problems participants have witnessed or experienced, with the express aim of identifying their ultimate causes; (3) a card-sorting prioritization exercise to identify key problems perceived by participants and discussion of results that focused on sixteen communication-related problems or issues identified through a literature search prior to the focus group meetings and printed on the cards; and (4) discussion of how health care organizations should address the issues raised by the focus group participants.

During the follow-up focus groups in Round 2, the open-ended dialog and card-sort exercises were repeated and differences from Round 1 results were discussed. Parents commented on findings from a related set of provider focus groups. They also reviewed a draft survey on hospital quality, safety, and communication designed to collect information from LEP parents.

This is a twist on what is known as **cognitive interviewing**: a valuable method in which a respondent walks the researcher through the decisions she makes as she does an activity or fills in a questionnaire (Aday 1989; Sudman, Bradburn, and Schwartz 1996; see also Chapter 13). It often is applied informally and naturalistically in participant observation, for example, when shadowing key collaborators. In this case, one can learn not only what a participant would theoretically do but what his or her actual actions were; one can also learn more about the real-life context of his or her decision-making. This was how we learned, for instance, about the causes of missing identification bands in Children's Emergency Department, referred to in Chapter 8.

After reviewing the survey, participants in the LEP focus group engaged in a mock money-spending exercise in which they were asked how they would spend $100 across different issues identified in the survey's questions. In addition, participants commented on whether and how the survey might be valuable, shared ideas for the most efficient, effective administration techniques, and discussed dissemination of findings.

As is typical in focus group research, discussions were audio taped, transcribed, and translated. Rather than discuss the analysis now, I shall focus on the way that each group was run—not because they were run poorly but because they were run differently from what an anthropologist might have expected.

Pitfalls

First, anthropologists typically schedule about four closely related questions per focus group and listen intently to interactive patterns as well as to the substance of the discourse. However, the LEP project's focus group process was highly formalized, permitting little participant-participant interaction and demanding quantification at certain stages through the rating, card sorting, and budgeting exercises. Such formalization is common in HSR focus groups. Many are run by moderators who apply a very directive approach and rely on highly structured elicitation activities. Participants generally acquiesce to assertive moderators, keeping silent regarding ideas that do not overtly fit such a moderator's data-limiting approach. In addition, when formal exercises occupy most of the focus group's time, time that might be spent in open-ended, interactive discussion among participants is necessarily eclipsed. As a result, transcribed discourse like that for the LEP study can be very thin compared to that found in more anthropological focus group research.

Because the protocol had to be followed (the San Diego site was added after the fact), rather than suggest modifications I saved my energy for the analysis phase. I argued (and saw inserted into project reports and publications) that many of the challenges reported by our Spanish-speaking LEP sample were not necessarily related to English skills but were more or less par for the course for all health services users. As Chapter 6 maintains, many of the problems that we blame on culture actually stem from other concerns. There is a vast literature demonstrating that English speakers themselves report communication challenges when trying to navigate today's health services. Some from the study in question reported: receiving different opinions from different doctors; a lack of communication between a hospital doctor and one's regular doctor; and a sense of being coerced into agreeing to tests and procedures (Bethell et al. 2006, p. W3–6).

The methodological clincher here was the sample make-up. We recruited only LEP participants. Had we recruited a control sample (i.e., English-proficient but otherwise equivalent individuals), my point might have been more obvious to project team members. This highlights one pitfall of all but the best-financed focus group research: a general lack of comparative data.

ANTHROPOLOGICALLY INFORMED FOCUS GROUP METHODS

Prior to the LEP work, I had been engaged in a project to develop a model of barriers to care as parents see them (Seid et al. 2004; Sobo, Seid, and Gelherd 2006). The project assumed that parents perceive of and organize barriers to care differently than health services researchers. It used focus groups whose participants were recruited from among those who participated in a school-based, district-wide project that a colleague had overseen. The focus group sampling frame included parents who reported their child having a chronic health condition, spoke English or Spanish, and had consented to further contact ($n = 246$). Children with chronic health conditions require more health care than normal; we assumed that their parents would be a rich and efficient source of data to understanding and developing strategies for overcoming barriers to care.

The study design called for quota samples of ten English- and ten Spanish-speaking adults from this group. Given that each parent had extensive experience in health-care seeking because of the children's conditions, and given the particular focus group methods that we would use (see below), a sample size of twenty was deemed sufficient for eliciting the depth of information necessary for our purposes.

However, had there been a way to build flexibility into the budget for this work, some mention of saturation or redundancy allowing for an expandable or contractible focus group number would have been inserted. Another shortcoming was our failure to return to the population to test the validity of our findings. Again, this had more to do with the structure of funding than our methodological proclivities. Further limitations to this study will be discussed when we explore the analytic protocol (for more on how organizational factors can shape the research processes, see Chapter 14).

Recruitment

Potential participants each were assigned a computer-generated random number and contacted in the random number order by telephone, or mail if there was no working number, until quotas were reached. The study was described, and potential participants were invited to participate. To achieve our quota of ten Spanish- and ten English-speaking participants, we cumulatively attempted to contact twenty-seven English speakers and thirty-two Spanish speakers, or fifty-nine (24%) of the 246 eligible adults. Of these fifty-nine individuals, twenty (34%) had moved, leaving no further contact information. Of the thirty-nine actually contacted, six (15%) refused.

We scheduled the thirty-six consenting individuals for focus group participation, knowing that some would not actually attend. Thirteen (33%) never showed up, even with repeat appointments. When twenty (51% of those contacted) had participated, we reached our quotas and recruitment efforts ended. I include this information here only to give readers some idea about what to expect when recruiting for formal studies fitted to the HSR framework such as this one. The figures reported are quite typical.

Data Collection

The key difference between this study and the LEP project had to do less with sampling and recruitment than with how our focus groups were run. After informed consent was procured, discussions focused on three major questions or topics: (1) families' experiences in general with the health care system; (2) barriers to access, use, and receipt of quality care; and

(3) strategies families have used to overcome these barriers. This "funnel-based" forum (Morgan 1997, p. 41), with its broad beginning and narrower ending, allowed for free discussion while ensuring an acceptable degree of comparability across groups. All were audio taped.

Three focus groups were conducted in English, three in Spanish. On average, the groups each included three participants. Although we had planned for more, this turnout was fine: Smaller groups sometimes generate less normative rhetoric, and with fewer speakers there is more time for in-depth discussion regarding particular experiences than is possible with large numbers of participants. Although little empirical research has been done, Morgan endorses smaller groups when participants are highly involved in the topic at hand, and when researchers desire a clear sense of each participant's experiences (1997, p. 42), as in this particular project.

The focus groups were conducted by a pair of facilitators—a moderator and a recorder—both trained in health promotion and education. A focus group **moderator** is in charge of getting and keeping people talking, whereas a **recorder** is in charge of practical matters (e.g., taking back-up notes in case the tape recorder fails, making incentive payments). Our moderator was purposefully nondirective so as to generate as much experience-based narrative data as possible and encourage "sharing and comparing" among the participants (Morgan 1997, p. 21). The discussions were as participant-controlled as possible, given their focused aims. Facilitators adopted techniques designed to bring forth information that participants themselves deemed important, and to expose understandings existing below the level of surface (superficial, official) talk (Campbell and Gregor 2004). For example, the moderator adopted an "interested listener" rather than a dictatorial role (Quinn 2005, p. 41). She sought to avoid collusive conversational turn-taking and gap-filling (in which implicit meanings are assumed to be shared; Campbell and Gregor 2004).

Preparing Transcriptions

Our project manager transcribed these audio tapes verbatim in English or Spanish and she and her co-facilitator translated the Spanish transcriptions into English. The two workers reviewed each other's transcriptions for accuracy, playing each tape again while proofreading every transcript. If time and money are short, a random spot check system can be devised whereby 10% or more of all transcription work is reviewed. If all work is accurate, the rest is assumed so; if the work has problems, then resources must be found for a full review and, as may be necessary, for retranscription or retranslation.

In a more typical HSR study, transcription and translation would likely have been contracted out. If so, we would have paid for a process known as **back translation**, whereby non-English transcriptions are translated into English by one contractor and then back into the non-English language by another. The new non-English transcription (the back translation) is checked against the original transcription so that errors can be identified.

Another difference between our study and the HSR standard was that, rather than waiting until all the data were collected, we transcribed in between focus groups. Listening to the tapes alerted the co-facilitators to questions that might be clarified by participants in the next focus group, if appropriate. Transcribing so soon also meant that, if an audio recorder actually failed, it would be discovered early and study workers could then draw on recall to paraphrase what participants had told them. Or, if a tape was sporadically muddy, they could make notes from memory if possible.

Any paraphrasing or filling-in would have been enclosed in square brackets, also called box parentheses, which look like this [ ]. Such brackets always symbolize the fact that whatever they contain was not quoted verbatim but was instead filled in by the transcriber [like this]. Any uncertainty regarding what is in the box must be indicated with a question mark [like this?] or [?]. Specific conventions can vary. The key is consistency and full compliance with whatever conventions have been devised and agreed on.

Linguistics and other fields interested in discourse or narrative have complicated notation systems capable of delimiting to the nth degree how much a voice is raised or softened, the exact duration of a pause, whether a speaker drew breath and for how long, if a final consonant was dropped or an extra r added, etc. The fullest transcription possible is desirable so that the fullest possible record of what transpired will be available should another scholar with, say, linguistic interests wish to analyze the data. Having said that, in the unlikely event that money is no object, a simple verbatim transcription—one including every word that was uttered—is all that is required for most anthropologically informed projects. So, although "Yeah" offered on its own to mean something like "I agree" must be noted verbatim, background or "back channel" feedback (the "yeahs," "uh-huhs," and "mm-hmms" that people offer each other as encouragement to keep talking or because it is socioculturally expected of them) can be ignored.

Meaning is not just in words, however. It also is conveyed in how things are said. So raised or lowered voices, slow or fast speech, big silent gaps, etc., are of concern and should be noted. This can be done using square brackets (e.g., [speaker pauses]; [speaker laughs]; [yelling now]). We do not use ellipses (...) for pauses because they are so frequently used to indicate cut text in actual quotations.

The high potential for confusion even in just ellipses demonstrates again that it is crucial to keep a list of all transcribing conventions being used. In addition to those conventions already discussed, this list may include: header information (for instance, project title; time and date of audio-taping; number of participants and relevant demographic data; duration of focus group; moderator's names); how to refer to the moderator or facilitator when his or her voice is heard (I use initials followed by a colon); speech interruptions (I use a double hyphen at the end of a line to indicate that a speaker was cut off by the next speaker); and overtalk, or two or more people talking at once (I use boxed comments). Even something apparently trivial as how to denote uh-huh" and "uh-uh" should be noted. Likewise, a spelling list should be created for words like "yeah" and "gonna" (or "gunna"?). Consistency now will protect against later confusion.

Data Analysis

I designed a qualitative content analysis protocol to analyze the focus group transcriptions. The various techniques drawn on for the analytic design are commonly used in anthropological discourse analysis for identifying, interpreting and grouping, and ordering themes (Ryan and Bernard 2003; Strauss and Corbin 1998). The protocol included triangulation through the inclusion of all involved researchers; this was to offset possible concerns regarding subjective bias—but also, and moreover, we did it to enhance the analytic process and product.

A key goal of the analysis was to derive a socioculturally contextualized schema for organizing or categorizing the barriers to care. A schema is a generic or prototypical experience-based or learned mental model of reality or some part of it. Schema-oriented analysis goes beyond simply counting (quantifying) terms or phrases. It aims to characterize the variously connected frames of reference that participants use to order their perceptions and understanding of the concepts (in this case, barriers) represented in those terms or phrases. These can be derived by carefully and systematically attending to the narrative contexts in which particular concepts are mentioned (Bernard 1995b; de Munck and Sobo 1998; Glaser and Strauss, 1967; Patton 1999; Quinn 2005; Strauss and Corbin 1998).

Systematic Listening

The initial step in deriving the parent schema was to listen, systematically, to all focus group tapes and carefully note or list all barriers specified by participants. Such listing may be termed "data extraction" if a translation for HSR traditionalists is necessary, but because we did not seek to divorce data points from the situational context in which they were derived, it might be considered disingenuous to speak so.

Before lists were made, the focus group moderator and recorder had been listening informally between focus groups. When appropriate, they would present the subsequent focus group with some of the barriers mentioned by the previous group, to elicit feedback. Through this modified form of "subject review" (Basch 1987; Patton 1999), focus group participants provided input into this part of the analysis process.

When all focus groups had been completed, our key group of three listened systematically to the tapes following a formalized protocol: At least two researchers listened to each tape to extract data, and the focus group moderator (also the project manager) listened to them all. While listening, we took careful notes on all barriers mentioned, bearing in mind the situation-specific contexts in which they were brought up (i.e., the narratives or story lines that they were part of). We compared like incidents and looked for negative cases or cases in which barriers were surmounted or mitigated. We attended to repetitions, metaphors and analogies, key words, speech transitions and linguistic connectors, indigenous categories or typologies (e.g., ideas expressed colloquially), and speech events, such as reasoning or depiction of causal chains as well as evaluations, shifts from past to present tense, and false starts and hesitations (Hill 2005; Quinn 2005; Ryan and Bernard 2003).

Ethnographic Contextualization

Transcriptions of the tapes were available for reviewing context information when needed. Moreover, everyone involved in the analysis had been working in child health services settings and with similar populations for some years. This gave us the requisite experience to understand the scenarios being reported and to comprehend their significance in terms of access to quality care. This is crucial: Anthropologically informed research must interpret data in light of and position findings against the everyday experiences of stakeholder populations. Locally patterned thought and action and the present-day and historical local and global reasons for those patterns must be accounted for.

Without on-the-ground experience, our analysis would have been sorely handicapped. We would have had no point of reference for interpreting how and why x or y was being construed in the transcriptions as good, bad, or unremarkable. We also would have been in the dark as to which suggestions for action that were generated on the basis of the research would be considered practical enough for implementation.

Data Management

We used a standard word-processing program to store and organize the transcriptions as well as to store and organize the category data (i.e., the barriers lists). Although specialized computer programs can be invaluable for content analyses in which word and phrase counts are paramount, especially when data sets are very large and coding schemes complex, and they can help analysts organize data, they cannot themselves infer meaning or draw the kinds of semantic (meaning-related) connections that are necessary for in-depth qualitative analyses. In addition, standard word-processing software currently offers robust word or phrase search and even code search capabilities, for example through indexing functions.

The goal of the research was to identify the range of barriers. Therefore, the fact that some items were redundant because they had been noted by two or more of us, or had been mentioned more than once by focus group participants, were of no consequence to the analysis. In any case, the number of times something is mentioned in a focus group is not necessarily an indicator of its deep significance. If research aims to determine how many people believe x or do y or how often a group mentions z, the focus group method is not the one to use.

The lists of barriers were merged at the end of each tape review session. The final, merged list contained 320 barriers, all at various levels of specificity. That is, at this early stage in the analysis, individual participant viewpoints and modes of expression still infused the barrier data.

Model Creation

Efficient Generalizations

Purists would argue that focus group data are not generalizable, first because of the contrived group dynamic but second, and more important, because statistical inference to the larger population is not the point. In both examples, samples were created using randomization; this supports the argument that they are representative. Notwithstanding this, our focus was descriptive, not predictive. Still, if we take generalizability to mean that a theory built up from our data can help us make sense of what is going on in similar situations or with similar persons, as Joseph Maxwell shows qualitative researchers do (1992, p. 293), then generalization is appropriate.

To reduce the barrier data so that such generalizations might be made efficiently, we reviewed the merged list repeatedly to identify potential categories into which the specific barriers might be grouped. Category validity was ensured through a team approach in which all research team members individually considered and then together discussed and arrived at consensus regarding barriers and categories and their definitions. In keeping with the anthropologically informed focus on meaning and experience, much of this discussion centered on the situation-specific contexts in which the various contested barriers were encountered and the story lines that they were part of. For example, a respondent's concern over the time clinical appointments take makes a particular kind of sense when viewed in light of the fact that she had to take all of her children with her to a single child's appointment because there was no one to care for the others after school if she was not home from the appointment by that time. This meant taking them all out of school for the day and bringing them with her on multiple buses to get to the clinic. Complicating matters even more was her husband's expectation that their home would be clean and dinner would be on the table that evening when he returned from work as well as the fact that the family relied on a school lunch program for the children: No school meant no lunch.

After two review sessions, and three work sessions lasting an average of two hours each, the discretely listed barriers were sorted into twenty-seven categories. To arrive at that point, we created several sets of 320 numbered cards, each with a specific barrier listed. We met together and named the potential categories that emerged from our repeated reviews of the barriers cards (not an a priori or previously conceived list). We each then separately sorted our barrier cards into piles representing the potential categories. Potential category contents were compared and discrepancies resolved through discussion in which negative cases and rival hypotheses regarding categorization were explored. This took place category by category: After one potential category and its contents had been agreed on, sorting for the next was begun.

We might have done this quantitatively, in an automated fashion. We could have painstakingly coded the data using index tags in word processing or qualitative data management software, and then run searches or queries to determine the frequency of item co-occurrences, or how often word or phrase x was uttered in the provenance of y (after determining, of course, how near two words or tagged phrases needed to be to count as co-occurring—within twenty-five words? within 250?).

Leaving aside the fact that this technique inevitably omits some relevant co-occurrences (when, for instance, a verbose speaker mentions the second of the two terms 251 words later), it can be a useful approach to take if time and money allow it. It is useful, for instance, if a data set is massive—which focus group data sets normally are not. More often, its utility stems from the fact that a given research team is, for whatever reason, not truly engaged with the qualitative nature of the data. This can happen when teams are put together in a piecemeal, piece-work fashion, or when members are otherwise not supported in taking a hands-on, start-to-finish approach to collection, transcription, and analysis that includes an emphasis on the iterative review of transcriptions in order to appreciate contextual meanings and connections.

This hands-on type of engagement plus the use of checks and balances—in this case, the fact that we had multiple analysts with extensive background in the problem who would question each others' interpretations—made automated searching unnecessary to our project. It is true that our analysis would have been more robust had we included other methods or types of data and so the capacity for triangulation, and a participatory research component whereby participants themselves sorted and grouped the items would have been ideal. Still, we were engaged with the data. We knew what the participants said; we knew their stories and were equipped to derive key categories without computer assistance or interference.

Deliverables

Throughout our analysis process, the list of potential categories was revised. Categories were reviewed to ensure that each existed at the same level of contrast. Some were further subdivided; others were collapsed. In the end, twenty-seven final categories were created. At this point, the barriers within each category were inspected and any that were similar were collapsed so that each category's itemized barriers list was as succinct as possible. From the twenty-seven categories, questions were generated for a barriers to care questionnaire (the BCQ; for more details regarding BCQ development and for field test results, see Seid et al. 2004).

In tandem with that, a process-based conceptual model of parents' experiences of barriers to care was generated. This part of the analysis sought to identify patterns and linkages and to build a theoretical model from the ground up (Glaser and Strauss 1967; Strauss and Corbin 1998). The model sought to capture the experience of trying to access health care, so the categories were arranged bearing in mind the temporal sequence of the clinic visit, the basic spatial parameters of the experience, and the cyclical nature of health care utilization. I generated the model's figure prototype between our work sessions. It was refined, with group feedback (including review of negative cases and exploration of rival hypotheses regarding the connections proposed), as the categories solidified. Thus, its creation (like the creation of the twenty-seven categories) was based on an iterative and intersubjective process of reflection on the focus group findings (including negative cases) and of rival hypotheses regarding the connections proposed.

In an ideal world, participants rather than analysts would have constructed the model. Yet, considering the financial and logistic limitations of the project, we were pleased with what we were able to deliver—and it certainly has not gone untested.

In the model derived (see Figure 10.1), parent-identified barriers were grouped into the following temporally and spatially sequenced categories: necessary skills and prerequisites for gaining access to the system, realizing access once it is gained; front office experiences; interactions with physicians; system arbitrariness and fragmentation; and outcomes that affect future interaction with the system. The research demonstrated that by applying anthropologically informed discourse analysis techniques to formative qualitative data, our knowledge of the parent experience could be enhanced and a more powerful definition of barriers to care could be developed. Based on our work, including not only this model but also the BCQ so derived (Seid et al. 2004), my collaborator has since developed an intervention for children with asthma and good preliminary results have been reported (Michael Seid, personal communication, July 17, 2007; and see Seid et al. n.d.).

The BCQ represents a typical deliverable in the context of focus group research undertaken for HSR. Focus groups also are commonly used in the health services to generate recommendations, guidelines, or educational media aimed at patients or particular classes of providers. For instance, a focus group might be convened to develop ideas for a poster intended to promote hand washing among medical staff members. In a project that I am just beginning, focus groups will probably be used to generate data on what types of alternative or complementary care parents of children with autism may be interested in receiving.

In these examples, focus groups are convened as direct means to ends. When used in HSR proper, however—that is, for research as opposed to quality improvement (QI)—focus groups are more often conceived of as formative or as eliciting intermediary, building block data to underwrite the development of summative quantitative research tools, as was the case with the BCQ. Where does that leave the process-based model (depicted in Figure 10.1)? It was actually unique because, although it added value to the BCQ, and will certainly inform future research on barriers to care and the parent experience of these, it was initially derived as an anthropologically interesting end in itself.

Alone, such products often are not deemed important enough by the powers that be to justify research spending. However, making focus groups as anthropologically informed as possible by striving to generate models such as the one just described helps ensure that resulting surveys or questionnaires as well as more immediate deliverables such as posters or guidelines or care process changes truly reflect the cultural context of

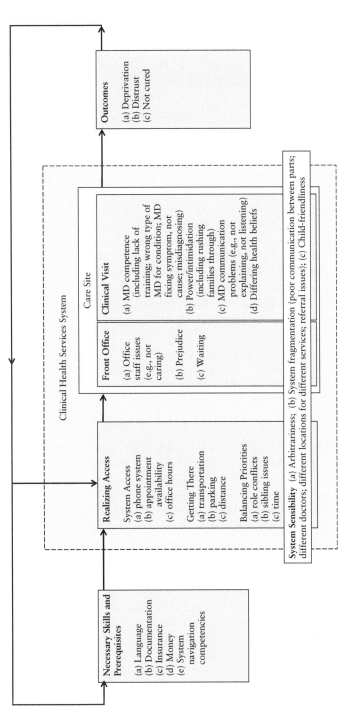

Figure 10.1 Process-oriented, experientially based conceptual model of parent-identified barriers to pediatric care (reprinted, with permission, from Sobo, Seid, and Gelherd 2006).

the actions or ideas implicated. They yield information, then, that is not only more valid and reliable but also more useful in improving health services. This utility, when demonstrated, paves the way for more funding for anthropologically informed HSR projects.

KEY CONSIDERATIONS, LIMITATIONS, AND IMPLICATIONS

In HSR, focus group research and qualitative research are often synonymous. However, work done in the HSR tradition tends to push focus group data toward the quantitative end of the continuum and often so highly formalizes the focus group process that the types of interaction that anthropologically informed scholarship depends on cannot and do not emerge. To counter this tendency, a more open-ended, nondirective approach to data elicitation is recommended, with fewer facilitator-determined form-imposing questions and more participant-determined content. Ample time for discussion is imperative if participants are to do more than simply identify or highlight superficial aspects of the topic in focus.

Recruitment within the HSR model poses another challenge. The projects described recruited participants from among people otherwise unknown to the investigators. Recruiters were often research assistants getting hourly pay rates with little vested interest in the project in and of itself. Additionally, participants often had to go out of their way to take part.

Short of embedding focus groups within a larger (e.g., ethnographic) study entailing long-term relationship-building, making participation as easy as possible is absolutely essential. Focus group meeting places should be located in safe, easy-to-access areas convenient to participants, such as community centers, rather than at hospitals or health care centers that are difficult to find one's way around in and more difficult to get to—even with one's own car, in which case they can also be hard or expensive to park at. Locations should not be intimidating, as when using a library or educational setting for a study of the impact of illiteracy on medication-taking. Locations should not be potentially stigmatizing; for example, in the HIV seropositivity self-disclosure research, even though HIV/AIDS resource centers were available, they were not ideal because some potential participants could not afford the social risk of being seen entering or exiting one of those.

Another barrier to beware of has to do with funders' expectations that a certain number of focus groups will be conducted. If possible, build in flexibility so that more or fewer groups might be convened as needed. Also remember to build in, if possible, some forum in which participants can review the analysts' findings (the panel design mentioned in regard to the LEP study is one way to do this, but new samples also can be drawn).

This brings us to the last focus group related consideration we have space for here: the analysis. It is tempting to count the number of times a topic comes up, which leads to a quantitative content analysis. However, unless participants are representative of a larger population, having been selected randomly and so on, there is no justification for numbers-based inferences. Further, even the simple descriptive function of theme counts is questionable: As we already have established, some of the most important details may not be overtly stated or they may only be stated one time. These are some of the reasons that conclusions drawn just from number of mentions can be misleading.

They also miss the best bit of what the focus group method offers. With nondictatorial facilitation, participants' discussions are generally much too rich to stop at counting up parts. An analysis based on iterative reflection undertaken with a holistic orientation can bring to light important information that can make a big difference in the quality of care. An example from the second focus group project illustrates this.

Among other things, we documented some of the workarounds or strategies that parents had developed to work around barriers and thereby optimize their children's care and the contexts in which they used them. For example, regarding asthma inhalers, parents shared advice like this: "Always make sure you tell [the clinician] to put at least two or three on a prescription, so you don't just go and get one inhaler for ten or twenty dollars, which your co-pay is. You can get like three inhalers under the same prescription, so some doctors, you have to tell them that is what you want. They go, 'Oh, oh I see.'"

Once providers know this, they can offer such prescriptions automatically and in a nonjudgmental fashion when medically appropriate (although this workaround may not work with all insurance plans). Routinizing this offer is helpful to patients or parents who would feel stigmatized if made to advertise their poverty through a request, or to those who simply would not know to ask. Shortly after this analysis, I received a similar, money-saving offer myself from a physician serving my son at the institution where we undertook the barriers to care project.

What Next?

The benefits of focus group research for describing the range of possible responses to a particular issue as well as for revealing important points of convergence or contention through group interaction are great. However, there is much more to anthropologically informed HSR than focus groups, as the next few chapters show. When reading about these other methods, continue to bear in mind the general process described here for attending to contextualized meanings; it is an essential analytic strategy that serves as a basis for handling many of the other forms of discourse-derived data that I will be describing.

CHAPTER 11

/ Making the Most of
One-Time Interviews

As H. Russell (Russ) Bernard has noted, "Unstructured interviewing is the most widely used method of data collection in cultural anthropology" (1995a, p. 208). As opposed to focus group data, which reflect the social interactions of focus group members and are helpful for typifying a process or cataloging the range of responses to a certain type of situation or items in a specified category, interview data can yield extensive and nuanced case-based information.

Traditionally, anthropological interviewing has differed from interviewing in other fields because it takes place within the context of long-term participant observation in which the researcher gets to know study participants intimately over time and participants come to be teachers or mentors. This broader ethnographic process not only enriches the interview itself, but also allows triangulation with a myriad of other data sources, each of which provides a multiplicative double-check on the larger story being fashioned. That is part of the value added by being there (see Chapter 4 and Figure 1.1).

Thus, the quality of the researcher-respondent relationship is key to successful interviewing. Reflecting on this in the context of their ethnographic work, rehabilitation scientist Mary Lawlor and anthropologist Cheryl Mattingly remind us, "Gaining trust is not a mere matter of method or of 'being nice,' but a developmental process that requires time to build" (2001, p. 148). However, although some exceptions exist, anthropologically informed health services research (HSR) often lacks this time dimension because of the immediacy of health needs being served as well as the traditional HSR preference for research that entails time-limited contact with subjects. Anthropological health research that does take time often gets published not in HSR journals but in anthropological journals; it reaches more anthropologists than anyone else. This is not a bad thing, but it does limit the clinically related impact of such research.

A number of texts describe the traditional anthropological interview process in detail; Spradley's (1979) is a classic. This chapter instead covers situations where one-time only interviews are all that are possible—situations in which long-term relationship building with participants is not an option but, to get high-quality data, trust must be established anyhow. It begins to explore the basis for such trust (a topic developed further in Chapter 12). It touches on training, for instance in interview facilitation or elicitation techniques. It reiterates the need for ethnographic-style immersion to allow for the best possible interpretation of data—and acknowledges the possibility that such immersion may not be directly possible (see Chapter 4; see also Van Dongen 2007). And it introduces some simple field note conventions that support subsequent analytical work.

/ FACE-TO-FACE, SEMI-STRUCTURED INTERVIEWS

While discussing the continuum of ethnographic immersion in Chapter 4, I outlined the methods I used for an HIV education and prevention study among inner-city women in Cleveland, Ohio (Sobo 1995). I did focus groups, surveys, and interviews at two service sites. I loitered and observed at each site while waiting for women to interview. But I did not do any real participant observation. I did not sit in on clinic visits. Moreover, I never went home with any of the participants and, although I lived in Cleveland, too, my neighborhood was very different from theirs. Nonetheless, my perspective was holistic, and I was interested primarily in cultural aspects of HIV/AIDS risk denial; to expand on from Brink and Edgecombe again (2003), anthropology's "signature" was in the work.

In 1999, I designed and oversaw a similar study of families with children with Down syndrome—a study that depended on interviewee accounts rather than participant observation. The study team and I visited some of the sites and participated with some of the groups that served families with children with Down syndrome. The final segment of the study involved repeated in-home interviews with select mothers of children with Down syndrome. But, again, short of having or adopting children with Down syndrome ourselves, full-scale participant observation was impossible.

Notwithstanding, over the course of our studies we were able to produce a number of insightful papers and presentations. How could we do so with such limited options for immersion? We did so by tailoring our interview and analytic processes to *participant*-prioritized issues so that anthropologically informed insights could be gained. In describing these processes, I draw heavily on Erica Prussing's write-up of our work (Prussing et al. 2004; see also Prussing et al. 2005).

Project Origins

The project in question grew out of concern among some physicians that parents of children with special health care needs were using complementary and alternative medicine (CAM) for their children without sharing this information with the children's MDs. In the case of Down syndrome, specialized therapies included growth hormone therapy, "cell" therapy (which involves repeated injections of freeze-dried or lyophilized cells derived from the fetal tissue of sheep and/or rabbits), piracetam (a cognition-enhancing drug, FDA-approved for use with Alzheimer's disease but not Down syndrome), neurologically based programs such as body movement patterning, and targeted nutritional supplements.

These therapies have been criticized in studies and editorials by clinical researchers and providers for lacking empirical support and for having the potential to cause harm as well as for their potential to unfairly exploit the hopes of parents. So, after a review of the literature addressing pediatric CAM use in general and the literature on families' experiences raising children with Down syndrome and other disabilities, we undertook a small interview-based research study. We aimed to explore parents' perceptions of the extent and quality of communication about CAM with pediatricians, elicit parents' recommendations for improvement, and formulate new research questions. Those new questions led to inquiries into the learning curve for functional biomedical acculturation (see Chapter 6) and, among a subset of later recruits, a longer term study involving four home-based interviews per participant.

Data Collection Methods

When the Down syndrome project started in 1999 we did not have a long-term relationship with the "Down syndrome community" or extensive experience with the topic, so we had to start by building up community trust before attempting in-depth or longitudinal research. In considering which methods to use, we also had to be sensitive to the fact that families with children with special needs have far less time for research participation than other families because of the additional time demands they face. Because of this, and the fact that the population is not extensive, focus groups would have been very hard to organize. And, although focus groups would have been fine for determining the range of experiences parents could have communicating with clinicians about CAM, we saw added value in collecting parents' individual narratives.

Case-based data would yield longer, richer, more detailed accounts of specific clinical encounters and other relevant events. These, in turn, might lead us to useful insights into any culturally relevant patterns of thought and action that typified a turn to CAM or communication with clinicians about it. Bearing all this in mind, we developed a limited, one-time interview approach in which we asked parents themselves to educate us on the basic issues involved in their CAM use and communication decisions.

The initial interviews took place in our offices. In some research, however, participants prefer a home visit. This may be the case when they are ill or when their visit to you will be difficult logistically or socially (i.e., it might be stigmatizing; see Chapter 10 regarding where to hold focus groups). Homes are not always ideal sound-wise; there may be distracting noises as well as other distractions, such as children or interruptions when phones ring or friends come calling. Participants may feel under pressure, too, as if the interviewer is a guest. However, it may be important to see a participant in his or her home, whether to gain a better sense of context or because the research protocol demands it, for instance if a medicine chest or kitchen cupboard inventory is called for, or if the researcher needs to observe the participant as she or he goes about a particular activity in the home. Alternately, the home might be ideal simply because a participant cannot leave it.

If the participant comes to the interviewer, as was the case for the present project, arrangements should be made to secure an appropriate space for the interview. A comfortable private room with a door that closes is essential, and it is always nice to provide interviewees with a drink or other refreshment if possible (if visiting a home, bringing something is a nice touch, too). Other helpful steps include meeting participants at the designated transit stop or parking location and ensuring that parking is easy and free or always providing them with specific mass transit or taxi instructions and vouchers. When possible, reimburse participants not only for time interviewed but also for travel time and gas or fares as needed.

Keep Them Talking

Our interview followed a **semi-structured** format. It included a series of **open-ended** questions to elicit parents' descriptions of, for example:

- knowledge of Down syndrome prior to their child's birth and now;
- perception of how their lives have changed through the experience of raising their child;
- types, age of onset, duration, and financial costs of CAM therapies used, if any;
- reasons for CAM use or non-use;
- perceptions of the effectiveness of CAM therapies used; and
- degree of information about CAM shared with their child's pediatrician.

The semi-structured format somewhat standardized the information gathered, making cross-case comparisons possible. More importantly in terms of what anthropologically informed interviewing has to offer, it gave parents the opportunity to raise topics and concerns that interested them, and to do so in their own words. That is, although the semistructured format marked out some territory to be covered, because questions had open ends the parents themselves determined what was relevant, making the findings more likely to reflect their concerns than those of the researchers.

Interviews lasted for an average of 1.5 hours. How did the interviewer, Elizabeth Walker, keep interviewees talking when their relationship was really that of strangers? Adopting a nonevaluative stance and demonstrating humility and the sincere belief that the respondent is the expert or teacher are key steps to successful interviews. And so is remaining silent while maintaining an expectant, hopeful, nonjudgmental facial expression the **silent probe**. In anthropologically informed interviews, transcriptions of what was said should have very little to attribute to the interviewer. However, if silence goes on for more than six or so complete seconds, echo probes also can be used. **Echo probes** entail repeating the last word or phrase that the participant offered, with an upward or questioning inflection, and serve as a request for clarification. Another technique is to simply say "Tell me more about that" (regarding these and other probe techniques, see Bernard 1995a).

Data Analysis Methods

Researchers must get permission to tape and transcribe each interview. Although some projects send tapes out for transcription, I find that transcribing is itself helpful for analytic purposes; every listening and thinking opportunity helps. Further, self-transcription helps ensure against transcribing errors, as when one word is mistaken for another by a transcriber not familiar with the terms used in the interviews (for some ideas regarding transcribing conventions, see Chapter 10).

Analytic methods were reminiscent of those described in Chapter 10. Although all members of the team participated, Walker's family moved out of the area and so Erica Prussing took the lead in examining the key themes in parents' accounts by analyzing parents' illness narratives: the stories they constructed to explain the meaning of the illness. Prussing was able to do this because the interview structure was open-ended enough to allow parents to do more than simply recount the events involved in communicating with their pediatricians or check yes or no as to whether they did this or that (regarding team turnover, see Chapter 14).

With an interested interviewer willing to let them take the lead, parents had been able to frame their descriptions within broader stories about their roles as highly engaged caregivers and advocates for their children.

And because Prussing was attentive to these broader stories or narratives in the analysis, she was able to give voice to the parents' perspectives in her research write-ups. These features typify the anthropologically informed difference. So did our ability to tie findings from this small project into the larger program of research that I had been developing.

Because we were aware of the disability literature and were able to dovetail this work with other research being conducted in our research center—such as the barriers to care work and my own small study of the club foot clinic, where infants born with clubbed feet were treated—we were able to see how parents' stories fit within the available cultural frames that all parents whose children have special health care needs may from time to time draw on. We also brought in our knowledge of other overarching cultural narratives such as regarding informed health care consumption. Had we not been exposed to these other communities or literatures we would not have been able to glean so much from the interview transcripts (regarding narratives, see Chapter 2; regarding the club foot clinic work as well as informed health care consumption see Chapter 12).

Lessons Learned

What did we learn by taking an anthropologically informed approach to the interviews? First, parents who used CAM specified that they did not do so to "cure" Down syndrome itself but to enhance their child's well-being. Prominent goals involved enhancing their child's development, such as improving attention, providing appropriate neurological stimulation, and facilitating learning.

But perhaps more important was what we learned about the major barrier to parent-pediatrician conversations about CAM: Pediatricians were assumed to be disinterested in or even hostile toward CAM unless they overtly proved otherwise. Had we not made specific attempts to encourage trust, ask open-ended questions that allowed interviewees to frame their own descriptions, and invite broader social issues into the discussion, it is likely that this understanding of CAM use as existing within a broader narrative of caretaking and well-being would not have been identified. Had interviews focused solely, and more quantitatively, on the medical efficacy of CAM use, for example, we would certainly have missed these broader motivations and issues.

Based on our findings, we recommended that pediatricians initiate conversations about CAM as part of routine clinical care. These recommendations referenced then-recent articles that offered strategies for creating a nonjudgmental climate for conversation and ideas about how to help families evaluate claims about CAM efficacy. In other words, we did not simply toss our findings out to clinicians; we also provided some tools to help them apply the lessons learned.

Importantly, the Down syndrome work took place at a time when Children's Hospital (the host site) was developing an integrative medicine program and many physicians on staff championed CAM in certain circumstances. In this CAM-supportive context, we also were able to leverage lessons from unexpected CAM-related findings that emerged during a pharmaceutical medication administration project that we conducted with families in hematology and oncology or "heme-onc" (where cancer was treated); that heme-onc study plus strategies for doing interviews when care is actually being provided will be reviewed in the next chapter. Here, we now turn to one-time interviews by phone, which are useful when it is impossible for interviewer and interviewee to get to a mutual location, whether because of physical limitations or financial ones.

TELEPHONE INTERVIEWS

When interviewees are not available in person, phone interviews may be a valuable data collection method. They do offer specific challenges in part because the technology results in greater anonymity and no visual cues—for example, body language cannot be used. Yet, they also can be surprisingly useful. I never would have known this had necessity not intervened during a 2001 evaluation of the culturally oriented outreach and enrollment activities of California's Healthy Families/Medi-Cal for Children (HF/MCC).

What Is HF/MCC and Why Did We Need Our Telephones?

HF/MCC provides low- and no-cost health insurance to low-income children. I developed and oversaw the incorporation of a telephone interview component into the evaluation after the planned quantitative analysis of program records faltered because of missing, invalid, and unreliable data. The protocol was published to serve as a model for use within other evaluation efforts (Sobo et al. 2003).

I will talk here about the protocol, providing project-specific details. But remember that the same telephone interview techniques can be used whatever the topic of inquiry if adapted accordingly. Here, as in all sections of Part IV, examples are given to illustrate concretely, rather than by me just saying "Do this" or "Do that," the steps one might take to implement a method.

California's Department of Health Services (DHS) oversees the HF/MCC outreach program. A critical challenge for HF/MCC was to inform the families of eligible children about the availability of the coverage and to actually enroll the children. In December 1999 and January 2000, seventy-two community-based organizations (CBOs) were awarded contracts to provide, to the communities they serve, so-called culturally appropriate outreach and enrollment services. DHS wanted to know if enrollments were facilitated through the CBO efforts and, if so, which types of efforts were most effective. Data to answer these questions were thought to be easily available from documents that DHS provided.

In reality, the data were neither easily accessed nor reliable. For example, there was no uniform format for CBOs to record number and type of outreach strategy. Additionally, numbers contained in the materials provided did not reflect actual enrollments, in part because CBO staff members were not filling in enrollment applications correctly. A bias toward underreporting was discovered, as were problems related to discrepant reporting timeframes.

The evaluation team was challenged to find a way to evaluate CBO success without the use of reliable quantitative data and in light of some competing agendas identified during the initial data retrieval and abstraction process (e.g., rewards for applications completed rather than for actual enrollments). I therefore developed a qualitative telephone interview protocol for collecting narrative data from front-line CBO staff. It required training project staff to administer the interviews, transcribe and reduce them in interview notes, and analyze the resulting data.

Training Needs and Methods

We had not planned on interviews and my time was otherwise engaged. So I invited two staff research associates or RAs (both with MPH degrees) who had participated in the initial quantitative data abstraction portion of the project to undertake the interviews. Although neither had done phone interviews before, let alone qualitative ones, they were extremely familiar with the project and the issues relevant to insurance outreach and enrollment programs. And our department had a commitment to fostering professional growth. So I devised a plan to train them for the task ahead.

Prior to conducting the telephone interviews, the RAs received training consisting of a directed reading regarding interviewing (Bernard 1995a, ch. 10) and two two-hour skill-building sessions under my tutelage. These included interviewing practice via role-play and training in rapid rapport building and elicitation methods. For example, the RAs learned to explain to any reluctant interviewees that their views were important because they were the experts from whom we wanted to learn. They also learned to use both silence and the so-called echo probe when an interviewee finished an answer (see above). A further skill-building session was undertaken after pilot interviews had been conducted by the RAs and reviewed by me.

I have since adapted this training regimen for numerous other projects. This project was conceived in a rush, but whenever possible more training time is taken. For instance, in a cancer-related study described in Chapter 12, the RAs and I had four group meetings over a one-week period followed by one-on-one practice and coaching sessions. Although more time is always ideal, an intense (even daily) meeting schedule helps support learning and recall.

Also, trainees on other projects generally read more than just the one chapter mentioned above, including readings tailored to the project at hand. For instance, in the cancer project we also read up on ethnography in nursing (using Hodgson 2000) and in a project on medical travel or tourism that I am presently engaged in we read up on open coding (Strauss and Corbin 1998, ch. 8) and various other forms of text analysis (e.g., Bernard and Ryan 1998; Seidel 1998). This book, too, supplies helpful training materials; chapters may be used on their own to help train RAs for particular projects that readers may plan.

Setting up the Interviews

Subject-wise, the CBOs' front-line staff members were to serve as key informants for what was by then being called the "qualitative arm" of the child health insurance study. **Key informants** are people who, because of their occupational or other status or role within the community in question, are strategically placed to provide information of interest to the research team. About two weeks before the data collection phase (while the RAs' interviewing training was taking place), a letter was sent from DHS to all CBO contractors informing them that the evaluation was occurring and that telephone interviews should be expected. The letter also confirmed the constructive intent of the interview while assuring anonymity and encouraging freedom of speech.

Interviews were conducted at interviewees' convenience, both out of respect for interviewees and because this increases interview completion rates. Although some contractors found it convenient to be interviewed on the initial contact call, most preferred to schedule an interview appointment; thus, most telephone calls were followed up with a fax confirming the telephone interview appointment and describing what to expect.

If an individual could not be reached, a message was left. If the call was not returned, another call was made; nonresponders were called at least once each week during the interview scheduling and calling period until contact was made or the interviewing phase ended.

Nonresponders

Because the data collection phase was very short, the sample of interviewees (n=48) was necessarily a convenience sample. A follow-up **nonresponder analysis** demonstrated no statistically significant differences between those who were reached and those who were not. The analysis compared the responder and nonresponder organizations on the following background characteristics: location (rural vs. urban); type of organization (government vs. nongovernment; for-profit vs. not-for-profit; school based vs. non–school based); type of mission (health vs. nonhealth; ethnic vs. non–ethnic affiliation; religious vs. non–religious affiliation); whether the target population was of immigrants or nonimmigrants; and number of applications completed and enrollments accomplished. Although not central to the study's aim, this type of analysis is useful because it helps answer questions or complaints regarding possible sample bias.

Data Collection

Data collection spanned ten working days and was punctuated with two quality assurance and pre-analytic brainstorming or, in some vocabularies, "hypothesis-generating" review sessions. Intermingling data collection with phases of theorizing allowed us to account for or incorporate data that other studies might simply discard at the end as irrelevant to the original intent or hypotheses (see Bernard 1995a).

The **interview schedule** (in this context, schedule means topic or question list) was piloted with the first four contractors interviewed. Small adjustments were made in the logistics of conducting the interviews, note-taking conventions, and the use of subtopic probes (see below), but substantively the interview schedule was unchanged and these interviews were included in the final analysis. When a population is large, or notable changes are instituted, pilot interviews generally are discarded as incomparable.

Interviews generally took forty-five minutes to one hour. The interview schedule included seven focused questions designed to collect data on front-line barriers and enablers as well as best practices and lessons learned (see Table 11.1). Because of the nature of the project, the questions were written in collaboration with and approved by the DHS; they reflected DHS priorities. Yet we were able to word them so loosely that there was still room open for interviewees to determine the parameters of their answers. I include them here as examples of what such interview questions might look and sound like.

All questions were prefaced with suitable introductory statements and RA tools included short probe lists to ensure that all related topics deemed relevant to the evaluation had been covered. For example,

Table 11.1 Interview questions (see Sobo et al. 2003)

1. What steps did your organization take to get the project off the ground?
2. What are all the things you have to do to enroll a child? Can you list the steps for me, and tell me where in the process you were most likely to get stuck and why?
3. What particular steps led to successful outreach and enrollment? Why did these activities or strategies seem to work the best?
4. What activities or strategies turned out not to work, or were less effective than you thought they would be? Why?
5. What other obstacles were there to doing effective outreach and enrollment, and what steps did you take to overcome them?
6. What adjustments have been made to the scope of work as time has passed, and are changes in your organization's approach to the project expected in the future? Why?
7. Is there anything important that I haven't asked about? Would you like to add anything here?

the initial question was prefaced on the interview form with: "First, I'd like to ask about start-up activities." The focused, open-ended question itself ("What steps did your organization take to get the project off the ground?") was followed by a list of subtopics that included: enough time, determination of enrollment goals, hiring problems, staffing levels, staff training, supervisor-staff relations, and value of past experience. These subtopics and their definitions were agreed on through discussion between evaluation team members as the data collection form was developed and during initial training.

If the interviewee did not bring up all of the listed subtopics voluntarily, the RA doing the interview would probe for information regarding them. All RAs would thereby collect information on each of these aspects of start-up. At the same time, by keeping the questions open-ended, other information—information deemed pertinent by interviewees if not by the evaluation team—could be obtained.

Data Analysis

In part because the analysis needed to be done quickly, rather than to tape and transcribe entire interviews and then perform an analysis, the RAs began the analysis during the interviews. However, as noted in Part II, anthropologically informed analysis tends to co-occur with data collection in any case, largely because of the reflexive, iterative nature of interpretive work. This is another reason that, rather than speaking of **interviewers** above and **analyst** below, as I did in an earlier draft of this section, to show how in anthropologically informed HSR one person does jobs that in traditional HSR are divided between many individuals, I decided in the end to refer to the RAs here simply as RAs. In the anthropological research tradition, data collector and data analyst (and research designer and paper writer and the like) should be one and the same.

Note-Making and Form Format Conventions

Note-taking and preliminary analysis conventions developed specifically for this project facilitated transformation of data at three distinct levels of removal so that the analytic process that generally follows data collection could be streamlined to fit the timeframe of the project. The triple-level note-making and analyzing conventions allowed for (1) direct quotations, (2) paraphrased material, and (3) investigator identification of patterns or hypotheses. All were distinctly labeled during note-taking so that errors of attribution would not occur: RAs distinguished paraphrased material from direct quotations by using quote marks on the latter; they designated their own hypotheses (and distinguished these from paraphrased material) with an initial question mark in the left margin. Paraphrasing was simply noted, with no distinguishing marks. However, I now recommend the use of a designated paraphrasing symbol (such as a P or a dash) to ensure that a note-maker did not simply forget to mark the segment in question with quotations or question marks.

Notes for each question were taken on separate pages of the data collection form. At the top of each page was one question and its front matter and probes (see above). Each page also had space at the top for entering the organization's (and key informant's) identifier; this was for tracking purposes, so that if pages were separated we would still know which answers were whose.

A face page should include space for other required study information, such as the date, start time, and end time. I recommend using military or nautical time; if not, A.M. or P.M. must be circled on the form. I require use of a leading 0 for single digit time entries (e.g., 01:07) and I use four cells (interrupted at midpoint by a colon) to make time entries easy.

Question Response Summaries

After interviewing and note-taking (i.e., preliminary "abstraction" of the data) was completed, the RAs separated the data collection form's pages; that is, they separated the questions. This was a key reason for the form's one-question-per-page format. Another was to ensure ample note-taking space; not doing so is a common error.

Working on their own, the RAs reviewed and re-reviewed every interviewee's answers to each of the seven questions. Because data already had been reduced through the note-taking process, rather than formally coding each page or answer set—and see Chapter 12 for details on how we might have done that—for this project the RAs simply looked for patterns in the responses. They also sought to document the range of responses to the situations discussed and any myths or misconceptions that might be held by the interviewees. One downside to this method is that connections between answers to the seven different questions might be missed, but we were protected against this by having each of the RAs review all of the questions over an intensive short-term time-frame rather than parceling the questions out, one by one, to disparate analysts or to analysts who did not collect data.

After each RA had prepared summary sheets individually and for each question, the sheets were shared and compared. Any differences in interpretation were to be resolved through discussion between the RAs. However, agreement was high: Summary sheets emphasized the same points and no substantive differences were noted. A final composite summary statement was prepared for each question. The composite documents formed the basis for the findings report; original interview notes provided illustrative quotations and stories as warranted. The findings accounted for the lion's share of the final report that was delivered to DHS and were the basis of the majority of the recommendations made.

Benefits of the Telephone Interview Protocol and Limitations

The inclusion of the telephone interview component immensely enriched the picture that the evaluation team formed regarding the costs, benefits, and challenges of CBO-based outreach and enrollment efforts, thereby enhancing and increasing the value of the recommendations regarding best practices and strategies for culturally appropriate outreach that we submitted to DHS. Although our RAs had little initial qualitative research experience, the structured training and data collection methods I used facilitated their productive contribution to the project. Moreover, the addition of the "qualitative arm" allowed us access to context-related data that would otherwise have been unavailable to us. This included information regarding the context of CBO work, such as how confidentiality strictures meant that CBO staff members could not track the progress of individuals' applications or how they sometimes had to work without contracts. It also included information about targeted families, such as how eligible families sometimes refused to be enrolled because of their erroneous but apparently widespread belief that enrollment would jeopardize their immigration status.

Properly executed, telephone interviews can provide the kind of rich narrative data necessary for illuminating complex, dynamic processes and various stakeholder groups' views. Further, the use of focused, open-ended questions firmly guides interviewees to speak to the topic of interest while allowing them to organize their answers in terms of their own priorities as well as to talk about aspects of the topic in question that are important to them. These often include aspects that investigators do not think to ask about, not having gone through the same experiences as interviewees; the exasperating need for each of one client's children to enroll in a different program because of the differing status of each child's biological father is a good example.

The benefits of telephone interviewing notwithstanding, data gleaned from interviews such as the ones just described and, to a lesser extent, from one-time face-to-face interviews, are not easy to interpret because the picture presented to investigators during such interviews is necessarily partial. For one thing, with one-time interviews, time for discovery is limited. Leads cannot be followed up. For another, social desirability factors and concerns over presentation of self on the part of interviewees may lead them to highlight or ignore particular topics; repeat interviewing and triangulating data collection would mitigate this. A contrasting view is that one-time events minimize the perceived need to self-censor. A method seeking to capitalize on this is described in the next chapter, which also reviews observational methods.

CHAPTER 12

/ Collecting Data as
Care Happens, Or: The
Importance of Being There

Although data collected retrospectively, in regard to hypothetical scenarios, or from a distance can be useful, data collected in context has more value. There is no substitute for being there. On-site presence enables us to experience a given location, sometimes allowing us to participate in the activities, sounds, smells, sights, and so on that constitute that sociocultural arena. We also can talk to people while they undergo events of interest, such as a patient undergoing chemotherapy or a clerk admitting patients. In real-life situations, research participants have immediate access to their personal observations and feelings. They can describe processes in real-time, as they engage in them. The fog of recall bias does not apply.

There is another benefit to on-site interviewing. In terms of patients in particular (or their parents or guardians), interviewing in context also allows the researcher a special short-cut to developing trust. When we enter a doctor's office as a patient, we trust or hope that the clinician has our best interests in mind as well as the training, experience, and expertise necessary to help us. Patients share intimate and sometimes embarrassing details in the hope that providers will do the right thing with our information (see Sobo 2001). Patients often extend this type of trust to others who step in when a consultation or procedure is ongoing. And, I would argue, based on what I have seen, patients are quite likely to extend trust and hopeful openness to an interviewer who has legitimately entered the scene.

Even so, as the preceding chapters have demonstrated, there are certain contexts in which our research can be intrusive and, to execute it in such situations, we need to be sensitive to all else that is unfolding. This would be the case, for example, when observing and interviewing a woman in labor. We must adapt the data collection methods to suit situational needs. In this chapter, speedy methods and those entailing what is sometimes called a "low respondent burden" are highlighted. The need for extra assurances of confidentiality when working with vulnerable, hospitalized populations also is reinforced.

In this chapter, perhaps more than elsewhere in Part IV, one of my key goals is to demonstrate the value of analyzing findings from any given circumscribed project in light of a larger understanding of context, as when a project is part of a larger ongoing program of research or when it is ethnographically embedded. The implicit need for on-site observations is explicitly examined toward the chapter's end, where in addition to describing observational techniques I provide a concrete and personal example of how immersive, participant observational experience informs and can catalyze analysis.

I would never pretend that deep relationships are established in the time-limited interviewing circumstances I will first describe. I cannot recall any of these projects' participants' names just now, whereas I can name plenty of people who worked with me for longer periods of time in Jamaica nearly twenty years ago. However, because of the situations entailed, and because I had already worked in the hospital where these projects took place for several years and therefore had a store of experiences against which to contextualize them, I have more faith than I otherwise might in my claim that data collected anonymously and quickly can be meaningful—and helpful.

/ THE FIVE-MINUTE INTERVIEW

The Risks of Care

One arena where only the fastest protocol would be permitted (for reasons reviewed in Chapter 9) was the discharge room in Children's day surgery unit, where recovering patients were reunited with their parents or guardians and given time to "wake up." The location was relevant to the hospital's increasing concern with patient safety. According to the Institute of Medicine's landmark report on patient safety (Kohn, Corrigan, and Donaldson 2000; and see Leape and Berwick 2005), every year, between 44,000 and 98,000 deaths result from adverse events in hospitals. In other words, hospital errors result in more deaths than car accidents, breast cancer, or AIDS. Some of these errors, of course, take place in day surgery.

The Institute of Medicine's findings had received a great deal of popular press. I was curious about how this and related reports had affected the public's perception of medical services. The literature suggested an increase in health services' interest in "harm reduction" and "responsible health care consumerism." I wondered if these ideas also infused parents' discourse regarding their children's safety in hospital. More specifically, I wondered whether the risks that parents worried about (if any) were the same as those highlighted by hospital risk management departments and considered in ongoing patient satisfaction survey work. If not, what were they? And where did they stem from? As I describe the project that ensued, I pay special attention not only to method selection and implementation but also to the coding and analysis process (transcription was dealt with in Chapter 10). The model described can be generalized to any anthropologically informed research involving transcribed narrative data.

Research Design and Recruitment

For quality improvement purposes at Children's, and in tandem with a patient satisfaction initiative, thirty-five parents' (or guardians') self-reported perceptions of their child's chances for experiencing a medical error during day surgery were collected during rapid open-ended interviews in the discharge room. Although focus group data would have been informative regarding the range of worries parents might have had, and individual interviews conducted outside of the day surgery setting would have yielded rich and interesting case-specific data, for this project I decided to collect data as near to the event in question as possible. Respondents would thus be able to directly reference situational knowledge, and their discourse would reflect immediately salient issues without the bias introduced by memory decay.

Because the majority of patients and families at Children's spoke English or Spanish, all English- and Spanish-speaking parents whose children came through surgery without complication were eligible to participate. Permission for the project came when I was on leave, so Leticia Gelhard, who had worked with me on the barriers to care project described in Chapter 10, conducted all of the interviews under my oversight. Although the arrangement was not ideal, it was better than risking the project's loss to a subsequent change in day surgery management's priorities or those of my own unit's director. And Gelhard had already proven herself an excellent worker. Although not discussed in publications, research-related decisions often hinge on pragmatic considerations such as these (for more, see Chapter 14).

The project's sampling method was purposive and based on convenience. Recruitment was slated to end when saturation was reached with a minimal sample (i.e., when no new data were forthcoming for several interviews and after at least ten English- and ten Spanish-speaking parents were interviewed). In this fashion, twenty English- and fifteen Spanish-speaking parents were interviewed over the course of three days (August 26–29, 2003). Being in the discharge room for extended periods of time in close sequence was ideal in terms of the interviewer's ability to observe the scene on the unit.

Nurse Betty Lapinski or, when she was unavailable, her designee, identified eligible parents for the interviewer and facilitated the interview process by informing all nurses that the project was taking place and by allowing Leticia Gelhard to spend time in the discharge room. The room was longer than wide, with an alcove to one side; the main furnishings were movable visitor chairs and the patients' rolling beds. It was relatively quiet except for the low hum of nursing activity and murmuring parents alert to their groggy, recovering children's needs and feelings.

After potential interviewees had had time to reunite with their children—generally one-half hour after each child had been wheeled into the discharge room—the interviewer approached them and asked if they would be willing to volunteer to talk with her about their worries for about five minutes. Informed consent was verbal (see Chapter 9). Only one parent refused, and this was because the child in question had special health care needs and the parent felt it necessary to focus fully on the child.

Although conducting the interviews directly postoperatively and only when operations had good immediate outcomes introduced a recall bias, it also diffused the surgical team's ethical concerns about highlighting parental anxiety pre- and peri-operatively (before and during the operation). Because the window of time parents spent in the discharge room was ideally limited, and to disrupt clinical work as little as possible and thereby ensure the project's continued welcome in the surgical area, the interviews were brief—very brief: five minutes, in fact.

The Five-Minute Method

The immediate goal of the **five-minute interview** is to get a respondent talking and to encourage her or him to talk for five full minutes after asking a single, focused, discourse-opening question. The question can be followed by silent and echo probes as needed (see Chapter 11 and Bernard 1995a) but it is, ideally, the only question asked. Not much more should be done, although nods of approval and other encouraging body language are fine. Especially with such limited time, it is essential that the interviewer not lead the participant or inadvertently silence or talk over her or him. Although people frequently begin a five-minute interview response by saying they really don't have anything to say, with proper encouragement many participants have no trouble filling air time.

The five-minute method is an adaptation, for rapid assessment purposes, of the "five-minute speech sample" approach developed in psychiatry (Gottschalk and Gleser 1969). It does not allow for wholly participant-determined interview content or for the type of extended discourse analysis or ethnographic discussion that less time-limited projects based on repeated and lengthy interviewing can produce, but the five-minute-interview does allow investigators to collect data quickly when time is short and action or immediate utility is prioritized.

As such, the method allowed every parent present when Gelhard arrived on site to be interviewed. This can be important politically: Experience at Children's has shown that families excluded because of a researcher's time constraints often see this as unfair and even prejudicial. It also can be important in terms of perceived data quality. Especially when findings are damning, clinicians can be quick to infer bias. In my experience, clinicians can interpret a dependence on parents willing to commit to lengthy interviews as biasing a sample, which would make the findings irrelevant to their practice.

These concerns notwithstanding, the adapted five-minute method was proven, through this project, as able to support a deep understanding of a very narrow area. Because the method and the questions it is appropriate for are so focused, especially with the interpretive edge that several years of experience in the setting in question provides, one does not have to talk to a parent for very long to elicit important and actionable qualitative information.

How were five minutes of discourse elicited in this specific project? Gelhard asked: "Please tell me: What worried you about your child's operation?" If another probe was needed, she asked, "What are the risks of the operation?" and/or "What are all of the things that could have gone wrong?" My goal in making the questions and probes so open-ended was to elicit perceptions that we never would have thought to ask about ourselves. The question and probes were modified as needed during data collection to elicit the type of detailed information required. For example, in some cases, to help kick-start a narrative, Gelhard asked the parent what questions she or he had asked during the preoperative assessment or preparation meeting, when the surgical consent forms were signed.

Each five-minute interview was audio-taped back-to-back, with only an identifier number (e.g, "interviewee x") and the date and time dictated as each new segment began. Gelhard transcribed the tapes and translated as needed.

Coding and Analysis

I analyzed the transcripts using an intensive, iterative process much like that described for the focus groups in Chapter 10, except that I worked alone for the most part: Gelhard had been seconded from another project and she returned to that by the time I got back to work. I had been reading Gelhard's field notes on an ad hoc basis throughout the data collection period and queried her whenever questions arose regarding data quality or clarity (see Chapter 11 regarding field note techniques).

Before I began the formal analysis, Gelhard fully debriefed me regarding her interviewing experience. I then reviewed the transcripts to identify salient themes and generate theories regarding how these themes fit together, taking Gelhard's notes into account as needed. The process I used is modeled on "open coding," which is part of the **grounded theory** approach described in Strauss and Corbin (1998) and Glaser and Strauss (1967).

In opening code, an analyst reads the text in question with the aim of identifying and labeling variables. "Essentially," writes Steve Borgatti, "each line, sentence, paragraph etc. is read in search of the answer to the repeated question, 'What is this about? What is being referenced here?'" The labels, or codes, he says, "are the nouns and verbs of a conceptual world." As Borgatti goes on to note, pushing the analogy, adjectives and adverbs, too—properties of the noun and verb categories—can emerge as important themes to be labeled (http://www.analytictech.com/mb870/introtoGT.htm; last accessed June 16, 2008).

An important factor in this emergence is that texts are read much more than once. In addition to iterative (repeated) reading, the analyst approaches the text recursively, so that the interpretation draws strength from itself. One insight feeds or builds on another when, for instance, something noted during the fifth reading of a given passage reminds the analyst of something that he or she failed to notice in a previous reading.

As is commonly done in this type of analysis, to document my process and ensure that I did not forget or misconstrue particular insights or links that I had made, I took careful notes regarding what I was thinking about a given passage and exactly why I thought it might represent a particular concept or theme. I also wrote notes on the situation-specific contexts in which these themes were mentioned or offered up (i.e., the narratives or story lines that they were part of).

Further, I used the same theme identification and verification techniques described for the focus group analysis in Chapter 10. For instance, I compared like examples across cases and looked for negative cases that might disprove budding hypotheses. I also attended to repetitions, metaphors and analogies, key words, transitions and linguistic connectors, interviewees' own categories or typologies, and particular linguistic activities such as reasoning or depiction of causal chains as well as evaluations, shifts from past to present tense, and digressions (Hill 2005; Quinn 2005; Ryan and Bernard 2003). By thinking through the logic underlying such communicative techniques or shifts, the investigator can advance the analysis—whether transcriptions are from long or very short individual interviews or even focus groups.

In this case, to further document emerging findings, I listed the themes in a table format with sample exemplifying quotes. As a check on validity, Gelhard reviewed these for relevance and consonance with her experiential appraisal of the interview data. The list was much like a formal data dictionary or "codebook." These documents list the exact code names, definitions, examples, and coding rules specific to each theme—which, having thereby been operationalized as codes, now can actually be referred to as such.

Code names (names for each theme) come from a number of sources. Some names are drawn from the context in which the concept commonly arises in a text. Others are just terms that participants use themselves, such as children referring to "shots" or nurses referring to "frequent fliers" (i.e., patients seen frequently). Technically, when used for code names, such terms are called "*in vivo*" codes because of their living source (Glaser and Strauss 1967; in medicine, *in vivo* refers to processes taking place inside an organism).

Whatever they include, qualitative codebooks are fluid objects in the early days of their inception. They can change throughout the coding and analysis phases, albeit more slowly as time passes: New codes emerge and others are revealed as needing honing or even as irrelevant to the questions at hand.

Because open coding requires researchers to "open up the text" (Strauss and Corbin 1998, p. 102) through repeated and very close readings and to compare exemplars and search for negative cases, "by the time one identifies the themes and refines them [into codes], a lot of the interpretive analysis has been done" (Bernard and Ryan 1998, p. 609). Indeed, in the day surgery study, the lion's share of the analysis was finished by the time I created the theme-and-quote table mentioned above (themes from which are shown in Table 12.1). This expedience was supported by the fact that the data were so limited but also by my method of coding not at the fine-grained level necessary for most grounded theory projects but rather at a coarser level. That is, even as I noted specific types of fine-grained examples, higher order categories were developing. These coarser grained categories, rather than the lower order specific examples, were what I represented in my code names. When multiple coders work together, specific instructions must exist regarding granularity or initial codes may come in at too many different levels of specificity for a tight analysis.

More typically, and especially in larger studies, codebooks initially focus on fine-grained themes and, in fact, it is this kind of theme that the term "open code" more accurately refers to. It is only after the fine-grained (open) codebook has stabilized that a formal phase of coding the relationships or links between fine-grained "codes" by grouping them into coarser grained "categories" might occur (much as we did for the focus group mentioned in Chapter 10). This process is part of what scholars in grounded theory term "axial coding" (Glaser and Strauss 1967; Strauss and Corbin 1998). In addition to assembling open codes into groups, axial coding also involves relating categories to each other; it often entails graphic depictions or models because axial links can be very complicated and complex.

Category creation can be done with cards as we did for the focus groups, or it can be done through direct interaction with the texts. If a team is working on the analysis, each member's potential categories must be compared and all agreed-on categories must be strictly defined for future application. Potential category contents, too—their subsidiary code sets—must be compared and discrepancies resolved through discussion in which negative cases and rival hypotheses regarding code categorization are explored.

A holistic perspective on the data is assured when each investigator has taken part in deriving or inducing the open codes and categories; in this way, each has intimate knowledge of the codes that might be chosen for any given category—knowledge that can be useful in discussion and decision-making. As well, to promote analytic integrity during category development, it is good to have on hand a list of all codes on one page of paper as well as copies of the transcriptions being analyzed. Each analyst should also have his or her code-making notes handy. With these materials, investigators can check any code's original contexts for meaning-related information as needed, which should be frequently in a grounded theory type approach. Each can support his or her interpretation with direct reference to his or her notes, or the text. Disagreements that may arise are resolved through discussion.

The detailed description of the relationships between categories (including subsidiary codes) and their experiential context as well as the broader cultural context in which this experiential context is embedded form the substance of a given anthropologically formed textual analysis. Importantly, in light of the expected analytic emphasis on context, protocols that entail neither relationship-building with participants nor actual fieldwork—that is, protocols like the one we followed in the day surgery study—are only useful when a broad literature on the topic in question already exists and when deployed by individuals with prior experience in the area of inquiry (Pelto and Pelto 1996). That background and experience provide the necessary context for interpretation.

In analyzing the relevance of the categorical themes identified in the day surgery project, I took into account four years' experience working in Children's Hospital and some actual participant observation in the surgical unit, during which I had the opportunity to experience worry about my own child's risk for medical error first-hand. I bore in mind also my previous work on risk perception (e.g., Sobo 1993b, 1997, 2001). Had

I not had this background experience, the analysis plan would have been unjustifiable—at least from the anthropological perspective.

Findings

Our focus in this text is methodological; however, I wish to discuss the findings of this particular project at length to demonstrate how helpful anthropologically informed research can be—even in limited data collection contexts (for a full account of the project, see Sobo 2005). Although there are exceptions, and our experience in day surgery may have been extreme (in part because it was our first foray in there), limited data-collection contexts are common in research that probes the experiences of patients, families, and health services workers.

The research under discussion resulted in very little data, quantitatively speaking: We had thirty-five interviews, each lasting five minutes more or less. In other words, we had about 175 minutes of narrative data to transcribe, which is equivalent to only about two formal, in-depth, one-on-one interviews (these normally do not last over one and one-half hours because of fatigue, although interviews undertaken in the less formal context of participant observation can last all night).

In light of the minimal word-count of the data set, the richness of the analysis is telling. It demonstrates what can be done with proper preparation and effort if data are collected in a context well known to the investigator and the investigator is able to adopt and move between several socioculturally situated perspectives (see Chapter 4 regarding this need and the benefits of the category boundary reconfigurations that may be so induced).

Importantly, the interpretation is framed against what were, generally at that time, compelling issues in health services: the devolution of harm reduction strategies to patients and families, for example, via safety tips aimed at health services consumers (http://www.ahrq.gov/consumer/20tipkid.pdf; last accessed August 22, 2008), and health consumerism itself, as exhibited in the increasing demand among patients for particular health care goods and services. But it also considers theoretical issues at the core of medical anthropology, such as risk perception, power relations, and embodiment. In this, the analysis formed not a free-standing exercise but part of my long-term professional program of study, just as it became the impetus for a follow-on exploration of how parents and providers negotiate day surgery consent processes.

The Sample

To situate the present findings, we had collected basic demographic-type data from the respondents: parent gender, child gender, child age, number of siblings/offspring, procedure, and—as add-on questions after

Gelhard realized their potential importance—whether the parent took a facility tour prior to the surgery and whether the child had had surgery previously. Most participants were female (mostly mothers) with more than one child (2.2 for the Spanish speakers; 2.4 for the English speakers). There were no significant differences between the demographics collected for the Spanish- and English-speaking subsamples, although the children in the Spanish-speaking sample were slightly younger (their average age was five years as opposed to six). Most procedures undergone were high-volume procedures, such as tonsillectomy, or relatively minor or noninvasive ones.

Presenting Qualitative Data in Tabular Format

The major themes identified in the transcripts through my analysis are summarized in Table 12.1. I include this here to demonstrate how findings may be summarized for audiences that expect reports to have tables. Sometimes, such tables actually have a relevant embedded quote or two (e.g., Prussing et al. 2004). However, although such tables, with or without quotes, do provide a handy way to lay out the emergent themes, they can never replace detailed descriptions of the contexts in which excerpted quotes were spoken and an exposition of what they mean.

Descriptive Findings

Many of the children in question had had previous surgery (44%; $n=27$ because this was an add-on question). And most were undergoing procedures that most parents saw as low risk. One parent explained,

Table 12.1   Major themes regarding day surgery risks to children: parents' perspectives (reprinted, with permission, from Sobo 2005)

Worries or fears
1. Children's fear and non-cooperativeness
2. Anesthesia risk (learned from urban legends, and the consent form)
3. Inherent risk due to nature of children (e.g., size, potential allergies)
4. Complications (e.g., bleeding, incomplete removal, wrong-site surgery)
5. Postoperative complications (e.g., pain, bleeding, vomiting, infection, fever)*
6. Care plan uncertainty
7. Powerlessness to control child's safety

Reassuring considerations
8. Comforting clinical practices (e.g., intake Q&A opportunity; ID checks)
9. Prior experience (i.e., previous operations)
10. Routine, minor, or low-risk surgery
11. Medical necessity
12. Trust (e.g., good reputation of Children's)

*Worries about fever and infection were slightly more common among Spanish-speaking interviewees.

"Tonsillectomy is typically a routine procedure, so I really wasn't concerned" (102). Even participants whose children had not had surgery before could say, as one parent did, "My nephew and niece both had it done, and two friends, their daughters just went through with it. So [there was nothing to be worried about]" (105).

The numbers in parentheses are interviewee numbers. I am providing them here because doing so or using pseudonyms is typical in any extended presentation of narrative findings. Here, interviewee numbers designate language spoken. Because the first interviewee happened to be an English speaker, English speakers' numbers begin with 1; Spanish speakers' numbers begin with 2; the final digits simply relate the recruitment order.

Many parents worried about their children's emotional well-being and whether they would cooperate, partly because of hunger (children generally fast prior to surgery) but also partly because of unfamiliarity with the surgical setting. As one parent said, "Our biggest worry is that he, his, that he gets to calm down so he doesn't get scared. ... He is terrified of masks and when the doctors have masks on, that stuff scares him" (112). One explained, "If you don't explain well to them what is next, what are the steps then they don't understand and start to cry and they don't want to go in" (202).

Some parents wanted to stay with their children in the belief that they might calm them. One wanted "Just to be able to watch him. ... Maybe a room where we can see in ... with a window or something ... I wouldn't know what they were doing at all to begin with, but just being able to watch him, if something was going wrong, I would know immediately" (117).

Parental disempowerment was clearly felt by some when speaking to clinicians. As a Spanish speaker told us, "Your mind goes blank when the translator gets there. It is traumatic or actually you feel powerless, you feel useless" (211).

The primary thing that parents thought might go wrong had to do with anesthesia. As one mom said, "You hear of other kids, you know suffering of having problems with it so it is always in the back of your head. ... Some kids can die under anesthesia, they get too much, they have brain damage. Those kind of things" (106).

Parents referred to stories heard on the news and through the grapevine to justify the fear of an anesthesia administration error, and this would generally be because of too much, never too little. But they also referred to information they learned during the intake process and when signing the anesthesia consent form: "If you read the risk sheet even up to even death, so that is why it was really scary for me" (108), one parent said. Another remarked, "When you go to sign the document that says there are so many things that can go wrong you just worry that those things will happen to your child, that is what scared me the most" (121). For example, "On the paper it says that there could be people that won't wake up from the anesthesia, that is my main worry" (201).

Accordingly, there was some worry about the degree of experience brought to bear on their child: "It does say that there might be some residents or students who might be administrating the anesthesia and we wanted to make sure that we have the actual anesthesiologist doctor do that instead" (119). Another parent said that she worried "if they knew how much anesthesia to give a baby" (211).

Although these two parents referred, at least indirectly, to physician skill levels, most believed that errors might occur because of the children's physical immaturity, natural diversity, and as-yet uncharted natures; children are not typical adult patients with established health histories, so anesthetizing them is inherently risky. "Since it is the first time that she gets any, I didn't know how she would be" (205), said one parent.

Unknown allergies were often blamed: "Being at his age you never know if he is actually allergic to anything yet, he might not have had that drug that he is allergic to, so you always worry. ... When he is four years old he hasn't had a life yet to know if he is allergic to anything, so and we would never know" (107).

Of the other worries mentioned, one was wrong-site surgery, but not many parents mentioned this. One who did said, "You hear all the time where he goes in for his tonsils and they castrate him or something" (107).

The more generic fear of complications was mentioned more often. One parent feared "just [that] there is something that goes wrong that is not typical" (107); another worried that "They don't take everything out and they have to come back to the hospital" (215). A somewhat related fear was that "The surgery would be more complicated than they thought and they wouldn't be able to fix the problem" (113). Parents of a child with cerebral palsy said, "We're always nervous" (112), and they related this back to the unexpected complications during the child's birth.

A substantial proportion of parents feared postoperative complications such as bleeding, vomiting, or infection, sometimes coming in the form of fever. These fears seemed more prominent among the Spanish speakers.

Going home also was a concern to some. One man worried that the instructions they were given were not correct (213). Another asked, "Is he going to be sore, we know this, he is going to be grumpy. ... I'm wondering, will his car seat hurt him, because we have to buckle it right here [i.e., over the circumcision], I am worried about that" (120). One said, "The thing is, how am I going to move him, moving him. ... Not knowing how to hold him" (204). Along these lines, preoperative questions regarding how long the procedure would take, whether the waiting room was comfortable, whether siblings could come (child care was a problem for some), and how parking worked also were mentioned, although not commonly, perhaps because of the expressed focus of the interview. Children's does offer a facility tour so that families can familiarize themselves with the premises prior to an operation, but none of the parents we asked took that tour; only one remembered being offered it.

Despite the worries that parents had, and the few indirect references to physician skill, the parents rationalized taking the risk of having their child undergo surgery in two ways. One way was to consider the benefits to be gained. "No, I needed, she needed this done; she couldn't breathe" (118), said one parent. "I was more worried about the problem that she had" (209), said another.

Most commonly, they praised Children's and Children's staff, referring to the hospital's or their doctor's reputation, whether mythic or real, for providing safe, high-quality care, or to the opinion of a respected individual. For example, one father said, "I know that the doctor is a good doctor. The wife really like him" (107). He also said, "If anything atypical happened here this was the staff to deal with it" (107). Another parent said, "We heard some good things about Dr. [Smith] from some other parents" (101). One parent explained that whatever went wrong would be "not really at the hands of the doctor, because they are well-recommended doctors" (204).

Another method of risk refutation was by selectively calling out disconfirming evidence—that is, evidence that Children's was indeed safe and not a risk-ridden place. For example, one parent noted, "It put me at ease seeing them checking and checking and checking" patient identification and instructions (107).

As a final position, faith entered the picture. "You trust in God I guess to make sure everyone is—make sure that the doctor is doing his job" (107), one parent offered.

Explication

Double Dependence

Elsewhere, I have discussed narrative patterns of risk rationalization in relation to elective eye surgery (Lasik), which I explain as due to the otherwise culturally problematic nature of exposing oneself to unnecessary medical risk (Sobo 2001; see also Chapter 2's discussion of the wisdom and monogamy narratives). The Lasik narratives were thereby linked to culturally prominent themes regarding responsible medical consumerism.

Why bring up this comparison here? Because of the light it sheds on the limited data we had formally collected. Just as each individual interview conducted in the field under traditional anthropological conditions is made sense of in light of other evidence gathered, our knowledge of the broader cultural context in which outpatient surgery is undertaken can help us pry meaning from the findings. In other words, understanding and analyzing the data as not only locally but also more generally culturally embedded can bring extremely rich qualitative insights out of even limited amounts of data. In that sense, in addition to comparing cases that occur within the context under investigation, it is helpful to apply the comparative method of ethnology, in which findings from one sociocultural group are compared to findings from another so that understanding is increased. We do this implicitly any time we study a given group because we always gain insight by comparing them with us; here, however, the comparison is explicit and it is supported in the first instance by pointed similarities: Each group has undertaken a form of day surgery.

Lasik is almost always elective; it is undertaken for cosmetic or lifestyle reasons. But the pediatric day surgeries on which the postoperative interviews focused were medically indicated (i.e., they were recommended by a doctor on the basis of medical need). One therefore would not expect to see declarations of responsible consumerism in the data from the five-minute day surgery interviews. Yet, the findings just reported show how wrong such an expectation is. It is wrong at least in part because it does not take into account the important variable of patient dependency, which is doubly determined in the case of medically necessary pediatric care. It is related to social structural arrangements that position patients as dependent on the medical system as well as to cultural constructions of children as dependent and vulnerable beings.

The Lasik patients chose their surgeons and generally paid on a fee-for-service basis, thereby acting as informed consumers, whereas pediatric day surgery providers are generally assigned through a referral system and important insurance regulations apply. In other words, despite the assumption of their free will and ability as consumers to take personal responsibility for their consumption choices, pediatric day surgery patient parents have little say as to where the surgery will be performed or by whom. They are in a structurally dependent position in relation to providers (use of the term "consumer" in health services is, in this sense, deceptive).

Moreover, although the Lasik patients were adults, the pediatric day surgery patients were children—minors, understood as dependent on their parents to have their best interests at heart. The cultural construction of children as inherently vulnerable—a construction that infuses much scientific research and many social services programs—has been critiqued as involving the "mistaken concretization of essentializing concepts" (Frankenberg, Robinson, and Delahooke 2000, p. 586; essentialism holds that specific kinds of people have specific, inherent traits—traits that are part of their essence). Vulnerability's ascription to children in the contemporary Western world is historically and culturally determined. In practice, Ronald Frankenberg and colleagues argue, vulnerability is situationally and relationally determined. It is contagious rather than the property of individual (children's) bodies: When children are present, certain types of vulnerability can be produced in adults as well.

For example, day care providers are vulnerable to accusations of negligence or abuse. In regard to the present project, the parent of a child in day surgery may feel vulnerable to social approbation if parental role expectations are not well executed—or are deemed (e.g., by day surgery staff or providers) as such.

Careful Consumers and Good Parents, Or Constrained Consumers and Dependent Parents?

As noted in Chapter 2, people are keen that others, and they themselves, see them as fulfilling cultural expectations. Thus, for reasons that may have to do more with cultural expectations for parenting and for responsible consumerism than medical necessity, parents in the present study rationalized or refuted the risks their children were subject to. They referred to the routine nature of the surgery, the hospital's good reputation, the clinicians' professionalism and training, and previous pediatric care experiences that had good outcomes, whether for their own children or children they knew or knew of. In offering such declarations, parents affirmed their existence as "good" parents—careful parents who would do all they could to minimize their children's exposure to potential harm—and good consumers—informed consumers able to make and exercise wise choices regarding care.

Accordingly, they rationalized the potential for medication-related harm as related to neither the clinicians' lack of skill nor to their own lack of consumer acumen but, rather, to weaknesses intrinsic to childhood physiology. In keeping with the essentializing notion of the vulnerable child mentioned above (Frankenberg, Robinson, and Delahooke 2000), children's bodies were understood as immature and, as such, vulnerable to stimuli or exposures that would not harm adults (e.g., because of "weaker" livers). Further, in contrast to the stable, mature body of the adult, the child's body is still in flux (see also Castaneda 2002). Each child's body and its patterns of reaction (e.g., allergies) are therefore to some extent unknowable—even for clinicians.

Although U.S. popular culture offers countervailing images of children's physical resilience, plasticity, and compensatory ability (Castaneda 2002), parents did not mention these. Rather, they focused on concealed, unanticipatable vulnerabilities. This figuration, in which the body is its own worst enemy, may be related to popular understandings of the immune system in general and auto-immune responses in particular (including those implicated in cancer and HIV/AIDS), in which the body becomes the cause of its own destruction (Lupton 1994; Martin 1994). This type of thinking, which deflects attention away from social and political-economic causes of ill health mentioned in Chapter 6, may be particularly virulent in the United States, where individual rights and responsibilities are paramount and both success and failure are linked to individual circumstances, including personal choices (Leichter 2003).

This focus also may reflect the recent increase in—and media coverage of—allergic reactions in children. As Rous and Hunt note in relation to contemporary children's allergy risk management regimes, often instituted at schools in response to parent demands, "Allergies are important exemplars of risk: they are complex in their etiology, often unknown until they manifest themselves in some catastrophic incident, and they are unequally distributed" (2003, p. 829). In this, they resonate well with the cultural construction of children as vulnerable and defenseless and the pervasive notion that environmental dangers surround us.

These now include even peanuts, once an innocent mainstay of the childhood diet. Peanuts exist instead now as treacherous hazards not only in their own form but also as particles which, dispersed throughout the food supply, pose a hidden threat to life (Rous and Hunt 2003). They are not allowed in many child-centered spaces, such as at Children's own child-care center. In the hospital proper, latex was off limits, even in balloons, again because of the allergic potential.

The focus on children's potential, hidden vulnerabilities may have the benefit of increasing comfort levels in regard to provider-driven procedural risk, deflecting responsibility onto the child's own (immature and defenseless) body, making provider-driven errors less of a threat. But this benefit is perhaps at the cost of increasing the sense of powerlessness reported by some parents—for example, in handing the parent role as the child's protector over to the surgical team when the child is taken away. And although it can only be inferred through our knowledge of the inconsistency between the high expectations that the health services have of consumers and the actual lack of options generally available, powerlessness related to one's limited ability to express so-called consumer choice (i.e., to act as a wise consumer) regarding health services also might have been intensified. The relational nature of vulnerability (Frankenberg, Robinson, and Delahooke 2000) is clear here.

Rationalization or Refutation: Whose Perspective Is Prioritized?

The tension between wanting to do all that one can do to minimize one's child's risk for harmful medical error and the actual options one has in doing so is an important factor underwriting risk rationalization. It also calls to question the propriety of using the term "rationalization" to describe the discursive processes at work. Risk rationalization entails justifying a risk as rational by demonstrating that the benefits of taking that risk are greater than the costs. Often, this involves appealing to cultural logic or to ideals, as regarding role expectations. However, sometimes parents in the five-minute study actually *refuted* the risks prioritized by the health services system by appealing to information gleaned from experience or other sources—information that competed for authority. In either case, the positioned nature of risk calculation is clear.

This does not imply that once a parent arrives at an opinion on a given risk that she or he necessarily sticks with it or that it is completely consistent with other opinions he or she holds. The increasingly public diversity of expert opinion and related anxieties about information's reliability (Rous and Hunt 2003) as well as the constantly shifting landscape of risk (Green and Sobo 2000) leave opinions subject to change. Still, parents' surgical risk narratives should tend to follow the same basic patterns, highlighting the same themes on an as-needed, situation-specific basis.

The risk management department perspective and the hospital safety agenda was not generally prioritized by the parents. Further, the risks they were concerned about were not limited to children's physical well-being but included social risks as well. Health services research (HSR) is usually so highly structured that it prevents respondents from expressing their major concerns, doing little to enhance our understanding of patient perspectives. And quality improvement efforts framed solely in terms of the risk management agenda will suffer the same shortcomings, limiting health care's ability to provide patient-centered care (Huby et al. 2007). The data from this study demonstrate the value of throwing off those reins by offering participants an opportunity to set the agenda.

Action Implications

Because the research took parent perspectives into account, a patient-centered action task list could be developed; however, the parameters of the task list were ultimately provider-centered despite the stated focus on parent views. As would be standard practice in many health service organizations, they were fitted to the risk management concerns of the year in question. Still, the action agenda, devised by key members of the surgical team on the basis of findings presented by the author at a group meeting, was created using the themes from the research as an organizing framework (see Table 12.1).

Themes relating to ongoing practices that decreased parents' sense of vulnerability were singled out for use in staff education to promote the continued or increased application of those practices. For example, "comforting clinical practices" was to be highlighted in education relating to patient identification bracelet checks (which help avoid wrong-site surgery and the like).

Themes relating to vulnerabilities were used to guide patient information efforts. For example, in response to "children's fear and non-cooperativeness" team members suggested measures that would lead staff to encourage families to take the facility tour and to assure parents that they need not feel embarrassed if their children cry or resist. In response to "anesthesia risk," team members decided to try to provide parents with actual hospital data on the number of deaths from anesthesia (none). In regard to "powerlessness," team members decided that encouraging use of the safety tips referenced above might help parents feel empowered as adjunct care team members. And an initiative to begin discharge instruction in the pre-operative assessment meeting was developed, so that parents would not have to wait until the actual time of discharge to learn about the child's home care plan and expected recuperation pattern.

Because of risk management priorities, the group decided to ignore the question of surgical consent timing. They did, however, suggest making copies of the consent form available on check-in, so that parents might at least have the opportunity to read the form before being asked to sign.

It was clear from the interview transcripts that the preoperative assessment meeting is very important for parents in terms of information exchanges that may modify their original risk perceptions, and most of the items on the action agenda centered on this period. Moreover, to augment findings, the team agreed to permit me and my staff to observe preoperative assessments; observations took place in summer 2004. I mention the project here only to demonstrate how trust is built with teams over time and to show that no project is an island; each piece of work can be discussed as if discrete but, in fact, each exists as part of a larger, unified, and evolving applied anthropological agenda.

Recap

The findings just explicated were gathered using a five-minute-interview method that I adapted for use in HSR contexts where research is focused and data collection possibilities are limited: The method allows interviewers to collect data quickly when time is short and action or immediate utility is prioritized. Provided that its limitations are fully understood, it can provide researchers with a deeper and more actionable understanding of a very narrowly focused area than traditional HSR methods.

There are limitations to the work one can do with the method, and limitations of the present study are good indications of what those may be: the predetermined agenda, the limited time spent with each participant, the fact that children and other relatives may have been within hearing range, necessitating the interviewee's self-censorship, the timing of the interview, which in this case may have introduced an outcome-related as well as a recall bias, and the dependent position of the parent and child patient in relation to Children's staff and the possible perceived need for impression management. Still, findings from studies that use the five-minute interview method can, as did the day surgery work, have important implications not only for health services quality improvement but also for theoretical questions, which in this case concerned health-related risk and vulnerability.

/ SHORT, SEMI-STRUCTURED INPATIENT INTERVIEWS

The five-minute method is powerful but it is not the only way to get data when patients are in care. Some patients are in care for a long time and, in most cases, the lulls in care giving can be exploited by investigators looking for a good time to talk or sit in with parents and families. Indeed, we used patient free time in heme-onc (hematology and oncology) to learn from parents (and guardians) of children with cancer about medication safety and other concerns. In this case, we also were able to do more observational work than we did in day surgery because the unit was in the main part of the hospital, with more access points, and because the social links with heme-onc partners were not as new as they were in the day-surgery project. Both the medical safety officer who suggested the project (Glenn Billman) and I were already personally known to the heme-onc directors. In addition to illustrating the short interview design and implementation process, this example illuminates the value of research design flexibility for incorporating participant priorities into the research. It also provides some easily transferrable specifics regarding team training that complement those already reviewed in Chapter 11.

Why Heme-Onc?

Our work in heme-onc focused initially on medication administration errors. Such errors are not limited to heme-onc patients. However, pediatric cancer patients are extremely vulnerable to medication errors. This is because of their frequent hospital and clinic visits, complex and frequently changing medication protocols, highly toxic medications, and use of multiple care providers at multiple sites. Medication administration problems can have serious health consequences as well as cause significant disruptions to the delivery of care.

Therefore, we had great cross-organizational support. Heme-onc medication administration errors involved not only the pharmacy but also nursing (including for discharge planning and education), chemotherapy scheduling, the ED (the Emergency Department, through which many unplanned-for readmissions took place), and quality management (e.g., in terms of safety). Importantly, we were particularly interested in at-home errors to start with. The fact that employee culpability could be interpreted as only indirect lowered the organizational defensiveness level appreciably, easing our entrance onto the heme-onc floor.

The project team, which consisted of me, three RAs who would do the lion's share of data collection and analysis, and the medical safety officer (an MD), worked very closely with the heme-onc directors (an RN and an MD) as well as with three social workers interested in the project and the parent liaison (herself a parent whose child had had cancer). The heme-onc directors would be reviewing and approving the project's designs and reviewing the data generated. Their leadership and involvement was pivotal. It would ensure that the data collected were relevant and actionable. It also guaranteed heme-onc's buy in, which helped ensure that heme-onc would actually act on actionable recommendations.

The project design was ethnographically oriented; that is, it had as its ultimate goal the production of an evocative written record of a given set of experiences. The project intended to identify what parents perceived as worrisome medication-related care processes and describe what it is like for parents to have their children involved in them.

Participants' Role in Writing the Research Plan

Originally, this project intended to assess only parental perceptions of their ability to safely and confidently administer medications at home to their child. Because we were more interested in identifying the range of perceptions rather than in quantifying adherence to particular practices or thought patterns, we planned to convene parent focus groups. Many parents stayed on campus for the duration while a child was receiving treatment. We thought that parents whose children were actively in treatment, asleep, or otherwise engaged would be happy to have something to fill their time and glad to have other parents present as co-conversationalists when asked to share their viewpoints in the focus group setting. All willing parents of a child with cancer in Children's care would be eligible to participate.

Recruitment for the first group took place in September 2001 in the parent lounge of the outpatient clinic; a heme-onc parent liaison served as the recruiter. A convenience sample of four women (all English speakers) was assembled from parents resting in the family day-treatment (outpatient) waiting room. Two RAs met with the group in one of the treatment rooms. The discussion lasted about thirty minutes; parents were forthcoming but also eager to get back to their children. The focal questions were: (1) Are your child's medications confusing? If so, how are they confusing? and (2) What were your challenges when you adminis-tered the medication on your own?

We also asked if they had heard about our medication coordination program. This program asked parents to bring (all) home medications to the hospital when checking in so that staff could physically review their medication regimen with them, looking for inconsistencies between what they were taking and in what doses and what the medical record indicated should actually be the regimen in use.

But home medication was not what the parents wanted to talk about. The general sentiment was that their children's medications were no longer confusing, once they had gotten into the routine of giving them. Major concerns about administering medication revolved not around potential errors but simply getting children to take it.

None of the parents had heard of the medication coordination pro-gram by name. When we explained to them what it was about, two of the mothers remembered seeing the yellow flyers encouraging people to bring in all their medications at every visit. However, neither thought it applied to them. In any case, these parents were very resistant about bringing in their medication because it would disrupt the routines they had established. Further, how would they bring in medicines requiring refrigeration?

A hallmark of anthropologically informed research is its responsive-ness to emic or insider concerns. These findings demonstrated to us, as they should have to any investigators open to the emic point of view, that we were barking up the wrong tree. Another indication that the project was misconceived was that the parents were not that easy to recruit away from their children. We switched the focus of the study from the outpatient to the inpatient setting (where parents have more free time). We decided against focus groups in the inpatient setting, however, because parents who were visiting their very ill children rarely want to be pulled away from them, even to help with quality improve-ment. We also expanded the project's scope based on the focus group feedback. Further, we added a question on use of complementary and alternative medicine (CAM) because of the hospital's emerging interest in integrative medicine; some CAM modalities might interact negatively with pharmaceutical regimens.

Our experience in heme-onc demonstrated the benefits of responsiveness and flexibility in the field. Allowing participants to help drive the research design had actionable implications that would not have emerged had we stuck to the original plan.

Our redesign was facilitated by the fact that this project was undertaken for quality improvement purposes, although permission was granted, retroactively, to disseminate information about the project and, in particular, our methods when we realized the potential value of that. Without the need to conform to a preapproved protocol, we were free to be flexible regarding our methods. If we had wanted to change from focus groups to interviews and to ask additional questions for an IRB-approved research study (i.e., one with ethics board approval; see Chapter 9), we would have needed to request permission and demonstrate that risk levels for participants were unchanged. Unless, that is, we had had the foresight to build ample room into the project protocol to make such changes. This might have given the IRB cause for pause, but there are ways to write such protocols; one way is to simply ask for somewhat more permission than you may need so that if you do need to do more focus groups or to add on interviews or, say, a survey, you have the ability to do it quickly and without adding to the IRB's or your own paperwork burden. The trick is to do this in good faith and with good reason.

Developing Interview Questions

With heme-onc directors' input, an interview data collection form was designed for use with the parents. This form consisted of a number of highly structured, closed-ended, quantitative, demographic-type questions such as are typical in survey research, and four open-ended questions regarding the medication administration process. Not intended for statistical manipulation because the sample would be small and nonrepresentative, the demographic information would allow us to precisely describe the sample from which data were collected. But the meat of the study would concern answers to the four questions. These are shown in Table 12.2, which also indicates some of the conventions we used on the interview form to foster consistency in how the interviews proceeded. One of the open-ended questions was embedded at the end of a structured (yes/no) question so that it might only be asked when applicable (see Question 2).

Before inspecting the questions, recall the telephone interviews described in Chapter 11 and how a training regimen was developed to ensure that the RAs could do the job properly, letting participants speak

Table 12.2   Open-ended interview questions (reprinted, with permission, from Sobo et al. 2002)*

1. Please think about the medicines (CHILD'S NAME) has been getting here at the hospital (today/yesterday). Which parts of the medication process worry you, and why?
2. Have you had to give (CHILD'S NAME) any medicines at home?   Y   N
   - IF NO, GO TO QUESTION 3.
   - IF YES: When you first got those medicines for home, did a doctor or nurse review them with you?   Y   N
     - IF NO: We want to make sure that all your medication questions are answered so please ask your physician about a medication review. GO TO QUESTION 3.
     - IF YES: How was the review helpful to you when you went to give the medicine/s by yourself at home?
3. Some people supplement hospital care by doing other things for their children's health, such as using chamomile or Yerba Buena or mint tea, or Echinacea. Are there herbs or home remedies or other forms of healing such as acupuncture, massage, or spiritual healing that you have ever used for (CHILD'S NAME)'s condition?
4. This interview has focused on (CHILD'S NAME)'s medicine. But I know there are lots of other things that may concern you. Thinking back on your child's experiences here or at home, what would you have liked Children's to have done differently?
   PROMPT: Were there things about the system, or things the staff did or did not do, that worried you?

*Capitalized words are interviewer instructions. They are not to be spoken aloud. If words are enclosed in parentheses, a substitution or selection is indicated as follows. For capitalized words, substitute the appropriate word depending on context. For lower-case words divided by backslashes, select the appropriate word. In Question 1, for example, during morning interviews say "yesterday." Explicit instructions regarding word choice were provided in a specialized, detailed interviewer guide.

freely. We did the same for this project. So, although open-ended questions are generally not scripted, because our RAs were inexperienced in open-ended interviewing techniques, we scripted ours. When probing would probably be necessary, the probe was scripted, too (see Question 4); otherwise, probes were discussed in the interviewer guide and left to the interviewer's discretion. This ensured interviewing consistency between RAs and increased interviewer efficiency.

After final modifications to the data collection form were made, a Spanish-language translation was created (and back-translation was used to affirm its validity). The translation was done by one of the RAs who is bilingual (Spanish-English) and had been responsible for the bulk of English-to-Spanish translation work for Children's in-house research unit for the two years prior to the instigation of the study in question.

Training the Team

As noted, none of the three RAs helping with this project had previously participated in quality improvement work of this nature. This was not on purpose; rather, it had to do with the limited availability of resources for this work and a concurrent desire to expand RA capabilities through good mentorship. However, a specially designed, focused interviewer training itinerary for the RAs that was based on what I did for the telephone interviews (see Chapter 11) sufficiently prepared the RAs for the limited task at hand. It included four sixty- to ninety-minute group meetings over a one-week period and involved the creation of an explicit interviewer guide (see Table 12.3).

Table 12.3   Interviewer guide excerpts

Interview #:
> This is a consecutive number (1 through x). Pre-number your forms. Fill in the interview # on every single page. This way, if a page becomes detached, we will know which interview it belongs to.

Consent:
> Consent is verbal. Remind the interviewee that s/he can opt out at ANY time.

Start and finish times:
> Expressed in hours and minutes. Use leading zeros so all spaces are filled in (e.g., 00:34). Fill in a start time only after consent has been given. Fill in the finish time at the end of the interview. Afterward, calculate and enter the time total. Do not round.

Interruptions:
> If the interview was interrupted for more than a minute (e.g., while the parent tends to other business), make a note at that point in the data collection form and record the duration of the interruption in minutes. Afterward, subtract that time from the total time of the interview (make a marginal note by "total time").

Format signals:
> ALL CAPS indicate interviewer instructions that are *not to be read aloud*.
> ALL CAPS in parentheses are to be replaced with the proper term.
> For 2 or more terms in parentheses, select the most appropriate term to read out loud.
> *Do not* read pick list or answer options aloud unless absolutely necessary.

Probes:
> Review Chapter 10 in Bernard (1995b) and make sure you know about and can apply the various probe techniques.
>
> *Silent probes:*
> Silence is very effective, as are any *encouraging sounds* (uh-huh) or body *gestures* (nods) that you can make.
>
> *Clarification probes:*
> Ask participants to "*tell me more about that*" whenever you can. Don't assume that you know what they mean; always get clarification.
>
> *Final probes:*
> To ensure that each question is *fully* answered, always ask for more information. Move on only when more information is not forthcoming. For example, if a participant lists chamomile tea as a supplement to hospital medicines, finishes telling you how it works, and then falls silent, ask if there are other supplements s/he can think of. Do not take silence as the indication to move on until you have made your *final probe*!

continued

Table 12.3   *(Continued)*

Question order:

> If the interviewee provides information for a question before you ask that question, simply go to the question and make notes as appropriate. Feel free to skip that question later if you feel *certain* it was *fully* answered.

Entering data:

> Make sure that the form is *hole-punched* prior to entering data
>
> Fill in all blanks; use leading zeros as needed (e.g., for time) or NA
>
> All questions: Always try for more specifics than the participant at first offers

Notation conventions:

> For our purposes, verbatim note taking is not necessary. However, if an interviewee provides a wonderfully expressive statement, be sure to write it down. Distinguish actual quotes from paraphrasing and from your own thoughts by using the following conventions:
>
> - *Verbatim quotes*:   enclose in quote marks ("like this")
> - *Paraphrasing*:   begin with 'P' or '-' (-like this)
> - *Hypotheses*:   begin with '?' (?like this)
>
> Make sure to begin a new type of notation on a new line.

Group meetings were supplemented the following week with one-on-one meetings with me. During these meetings, each RA's interviewing technique was critiqued and tips offered. The RAs also met informally with each other at least once weekly after data collection got underway and formally with me and the medical safety officer on a weekly basis. The purpose of these meetings was to discuss each week's progress, troubleshoot interviewing techniques and situations encountered, and debrief the group regarding recent interview impressions. In short, the purpose was to stay connected as a team.

Interviewee Recruitment

We discussed sampling in Chapter 7, so I will not say much here except that we set a quota for the interviews of twenty parents. The RAs partnered with three heme-onc social workers to facilitate the identification of parents that we could approach. All English- or Spanish-speaking parents of inpatient children with cancer were eligible.

Arranging interviews in an inpatient setting can be difficult, but our protocol provides one example of how this can be done. To initiate interviews, the RAs paged the social workers and asked for the name(s) and room number(s) of any inpatient(s) for that day whose parents were present and could be interviewed. During the interview phase, the name of only one otherwise eligible parent was withheld because of safety concerns related to that parent's history of unruliness.

Once a patient's name was obtained, an RA would go to the Heme-Onc Department and explain to the front desk clerk that, as part of the medication administration performance improvement initiative she would like to see the named patient's parent. The front desk nurse would then page the patient's nurse for final approval for the interview. If, for any reason an interview was at that time felt to be inappropriate (e.g., because of clinical needs, or if a parent was concerned with comforting his or her child at that moment, or if the parent had gone home or to work), an interview was not initiated.

On average, only four interviews per week could be completed. There were several reasons for this. First, the episodic nature of cancer care meant that a child underwent many cycles of hospitalization. Within as little as two weeks, the RAs were being referred to the same parents for interviewing. Second, parents were not always approachable because of the ongoing clinical needs of their children nor were they always available (i.e., many parents work or have other responsibilities, especially in the daytime). Third, the RAs were only available on a part-time basis.

When they did have a parent to approach for the sake of patient safety, the RAs washed their hands before entering a patient's room. Upon entering, the RA would recite the scripted introduction and offer the parent the option to participate in or decline the interview. Confidentiality was assured and appropriate data protection procedures were put into place.

Data Collection

Parents who agreed to participate in the project were invited to sit and talk in the hospital's gardens or elsewhere, away from their child's side. The purpose of this request to relocate was to provide each parent with the option of moving to another site so that she or he might speak freely without concerns about being overheard by the child or a care team member. But—and this is telling in regard to the types of challenges on-site, prospective HSR can entail—none were willing to do so. We accommodated participants' wishes. Coupons for cookies from the cafeteria were given as a token of our appreciation for their willingness to help us.

Although specific spaces were provided on the data collection form for demographic-type data, narrative data were written onto the large blank areas left on the form's pages below the scripted open-ended questions. In part because the project was a form of rapid assessment, but also because it is a valid way to do research when detailed or linguistic-style discourse analysis is not the goal, rather than to tape and transcribe entire interviews and then perform an analysis after the fact, RAs began the analysis during the interviews themselves, as we did with the telephone study (see Chapter 11 regarding the conventions used, or see the bottom row of Table 12.3).

Analysis

Quantitative data were entered into a computer spreadsheet as collected. We used SPSS for Windows (Version 9), but any spreadsheet package, such as Microsoft's Excel, would do. Spreadsheet data entry enables an interviewing crew to review basic information regarding the sample during the data collection phase. When the data collection phase ends, frequencies can be calculated as needed (but with small convenience samples, statistical testing is not indicated).

Qualitative data were reviewed on an ongoing basis by both the RAs and me. I also checked interview notes on an ad-hoc basis throughout the data collection period and queried the RAs whenever questions arose regarding data quality or clarity. The RAs reviewed their notes after each interview and developed hypotheses as more interviews were collected.

Formal analysis was delayed until all interviews were collected, and proceeded much as the telephone interview analysis did (see Chapter 11). Each RA examined her interviews on a question-by-question basis to identify themes and generate hypotheses. The examination consisted of reading and rereading the participants' answers, with an eye to identifying salient themes and implications, both explicit and suggested. Summaries of these analyses were written up, separately, for each of the four open-ended questions. This technique is in contrast to the case-by-case way that the day surgery and Down syndrome study transcripts were analyzed. Disconnecting questions from cases does do violence to any cross-question connections that interviewees made. However, it was justified by the fact that the present project entailed a firmer prior grasp of the domains of interest to participants than the day surgery or Down syndrome work did. Having a remit to answer certain circumscribed questions for a funder might also lead to this kind of analytic design.

After completing the question-by-question content summaries, the RAs submitted them both to me and to each of the other RAs for review. We then came together to compare notes and discuss findings. Each RA supported her interpretation with direct reference to interview note contents, which were available to all of the other interviewers. Disagreements were resolved through discussion and a group summary was prepared, discussed, and handed off to me for finalization. After reviewing all twenty interviews iteratively myself, I incorporated the RAs' conclusions along with supporting data into a final report, submitted to heme-onc and members of Children's leadership team. Limitations to the project were similar to those discussed for the five-minute interview work in day surgery mostly centering on limited time spent with each participant and their potential self-censorship.

Major Findings

The reason for discussing this study goes beyond its helpfulness in illustrating particular interview-related techniques. It also demonstrates the value of subverting the tradition of following a protocol as planned and waiting until all data are collected to analyze findings by instead responding in an anthropologically informed fashion to initial participant testimony as it was collected. Had we not done just that, any findings that might be reported here would maybe speak weakly to our original research agenda but they would certainly not tell us anything of value about participants' real concerns. At a minimum, being anthropologically informed means being open to emic orientations and being willing to report on those rather than clinging to initial research questions.

In brief, overall, the inpatient medication process did not worry parents. They acknowledged that things might go wrong but felt that, as one parent said, "They don't intentionally want to harm my daughter." Note the similarity between this trope and the themes that came up in the day surgery analysis.

What did worry parents were the side effects of potent chemotherapy medication and the pain that their children were in. Seven of the families, or one in three, reported some CAM use. The most common CAM modalities were vitamins, massage therapy, and brewed tea— specifically, mint and chamomile. The main reason for using CAM was summed up by one parent who said, "It seems to make her feel better and that makes me feel better." The build up in the child's body of toxic chemicals also may be at the root of much of the CAM use. One parent intended to use milk thistle for protecting (cleansing) her child's liver. ("The kidneys are flushed out with water but the liver cannot be cleansed that way.") Another, with the caveat that "I probably shouldn't tell you because I might get in trouble," told us in reply to the question about CAM that she sometimes did not give her child required medication because the child's little body "could not take it."

Only after mentioning their worries about the side effects of prescription medication did parents mention concerns about timely medication delivery. Sometimes this dovetailed with worries about shift changes. A father reported a nurse prerecording in his child's chart that the next dose of medicine had been given, without telling the next nurse that she had done so. The next dose was thereby nearly missed.

Moreover, parents specifically commented on the perceived breakdown of communication between nurses and nurses, doctors and doctors, and doctors and nurses. For instance, a child needed surgery and the surgeon was ready to do it. However, a new doctor wanted to do more tests and delayed the surgery. The primary doctor was not informed of this until the mother called and told him. In another case, a child was prescribed an asthma medication. The nurse told the parent to administer the medicine when the child was symptomatic when, in fact, the drug should have been administered on a regular basis. When the doctor realized the nurse's error, he told the family not to listen to the nurse. Parent faith in the quality of nursing care was thereby undermined, as was nursing's authority.

Regarding discharge education on medication administration, one parent said that it would be helpful not only to see what the actual medicines look like, but also what the actual doses look like, so that parents might have a more realistic idea of how much to give. Another suggested that nurses tell parents a drug's pharmaceutical name, taking care to teach them how to pronounce it. This is common practice now but back then we were just coming to understand these needs.

Another unanticipated finding was that, although most parents found the formal medication review process helpful, the nurses' approaches to these reviews were inconsistent. Some parents received types of help or information that others may not have. The reasons for this were unclear. We suggested a standardized medication review protocol to ensure equity across families.

But we also guessed that nurses might be trying to tailor the review to the perceived needs of the parent. If so, the fact that some parents requested more in-depth reviews suggests that the nurses' efforts at segmentation were failing. This led us to suggest in the study report that the nurses needed a tool for assessing parent information preferences. We also suggested, on the basis of the finding that English-speaking parents were much more likely than Spanish-speaking parents to be asked to bring in medications (two in three, as compared to one in three), that more translators were needed. Heme-onc used our recommendation to secure one. And in regard to the preferences assessment tool, see Chapter 13.

/ OBSERVATIONAL RESEARCH

As noted at the outset of this chapter, there is no substitute for simply being there. Interviews conducted in context can be extremely illuminating, especially when combined with setting-related background knowledge. But if interviewing is impossible or ill-advised, as it is for instance when gatekeepers have failed to see the value of a study, or during a resuscitation, what can be done? Formal observational methods help fill the gap.

Observations are a mainstay of traditional anthropology. Interviews allow us access to what people say they do, but observations can provide information on what people really do. They permit insight into context that simply is not available with experience-distant methods. They are helpful supplements even for context-based interviews. They should be used often in anthropologically informed research because of their concretely descriptive and contextualizing function. Among the key benefits of an anthropologically informed approach is the fact that on-site experience can underwrite insight. The chapter's final example reinforces this lesson.

Observing can be an intense undertaking when done for research purposes, because of the constant need for vigilance. Depending on context, one might see or hear things that are distressing, as in an emergency department intake bay. And observing can be very tiring when observations are beginning and one does not know what to look for: Everything seems potentially important—which, of course, it is.

Good open-ended or unstructured observations are assisted and in some ways created by good note-making techniques. The conventions described in regard to telephone interviews can be used effectively (see Chapter 11). But as important as how you write is what you write. To begin with, each set of notes should contain specific context information. Where are the observations being undertaken? At what time? What is the weather like?

Notes also should be rich. A common error is lack of detail. For instance, to note there are books on a shelf is not to note much, unless one also describes what kind of books. Comic books differ from children's books, which differ from novels, textbooks, medical reference guides, and the like. New books or books with unbroken spines can mean something quite different than a shelf stocked with old, dusty, or well-worn texts, just as cloth or leather-bound volumes may mean something different to those bound in paper. For open-ended field notes, the more detail the better.

Field notes should have breadth in addition to depth. When starting a field stay or observational data collection phase, especially one without preconceived questions, it is best to write down everything. In truth, everything will not be important in the end. But at the outset, it is hard to know which observations are trivial and which are not. So it is best to start large. It also pays to write down the obvious, just in case this has hidden meaning that will be revealed down the line. As the field phase progresses, attention naturally narrows and key themes emerge. At that time field notes, too, may become more focused.

Structured or Systematic Observation

An adjunct to open-ended observation is systematic observational activity. Especially for projects with circumscribed scope, but also after the researcher has been on site for some time and familiarized him or herself with the ebb and flow of action, systematizing the observational process can make it more manageable and productive. A good anthropological researcher will never cut him- or herself off from the opportunity to witness and follow-up on an unanticipated or infrequently occurring special event that will help generate extreme insights. But still, if seen as a tool and not a barrier to such deviations, systematic observations can generate a great deal of data.

In systematic observations, data collection tools or instruments (forms) are designed to help observers make the most of their time in a given location. Such tools generally include checklists of strictly delimited observable actions and checkboxes through which the observer can indicate whether or not they did happen. Sometimes, observations are timed so that, for example, the observer scans a room every five minutes (or one, or ten, etc.) to see if the activities on his or her list are being undertaken. Other times, observers follow specific individuals as cases, checking off actions and noting the time of their occurrence.

For instance, in a study of health services staff hand-washing practices, one would perhaps observe when a clinician enters a room, when (if) he or she approaches the sink, and what techniques he or she uses in hand washing (if at all). The proper techniques are well described in the safety literature, including requirements for the water's directional flow down the hands to the fingertips and the duration of proper washing. Hand-drying activities also would be part of the observation (are fresh towels used or an old rag?). So too would whether people wash in company or alone. When they wash with others, what do they talk about, if they talk at all?

One also might note, in a nonwashing situation, whether the patient requested that the clinician wash his or her hands. How the patient made the request also can be noted. For instance, a patient may request hand washing by questioning whether it has been done or with a direct request to do it. Asking about hand washing is one of many safety tips that health services organizations have passed along to patients, in part devolving responsibility for seeing that it takes place.

Clearly, developing a well-conceived hand-washing observation form will be essential for a sound observational hand-washing study. Categories will need to be definitively defined or operationalized so that any two observers watching the same scene would come away with their checklists filled in exactly alike. Some real forethought is required.

I am working now on a workforce project detailing politeness. Consider the process of handing in lab orders to a clerk. How can we tell if the order was asked for politely or not? Gut response is something I do trust in the seasoned observer, but to generate checklist data from naturalistic observations we need to quantify "politeness." What behaviors would be observable? How could we delimit them so that politeness's presence or absence could be determined?

To operationalize politeness, rather than simply engaging in self-reflection, it is helpful to quickly interview health care workers themselves. For instance, one could sit by a clerk station and ask, after each request has been put in, "Was that polite?" A confederate could wait outside and interview each requestor similarly. In this fashion, qualitative experiential data can be converted to checklist data fields.

To keep this research on the qualitative end of the continuum, or at least anthropologically informed, it is essential that participants inform the analysis of what the data actually mean, too. It also might be wise to ask, in the particular context in which the politeness question has been asked, why it really matters. Important insights about organizational issues can thereby be generated and used to inform the analysis.

There are a number of important considerations for doing systematic observations that I have not mentioned here, such as timing of observations, reduction of reactivity in those observed, and the need for ensuring that seasonal or other forms of patterned variation (such as by weekday or time of day) are taken into account. For an excellent review and discussion of these, see Bentley, Stallings, and Gittelsohn (1994).

Participant Observation

Participant observation is often impossible in HSR, for reasons outlined in Chapters 4 and 9. Patient care cannot be compromised by, for example, me playing at medicine. However, if the topic under study is operational or administrative rather than clinical, there often is more room to maneuver or to insinuate oneself into a participatory position. For instance, it is feasible to work as a full participant observer in a hospital cafeteria. Helping chop carrots or wash dishes is not going to be too disruptive (of course, proper clearances must be attained; related tasks such as attending and participating in the same hygiene training that all new dietary workers undergo can be a learning opportunity).

I have not yet worked in a hospital kitchen but while at Children's I was a participant observer on an employee leadership council study that focused on ways to enhance employee morale as well as (or by way of) increasing employee participation in organizational governance

(Sobo and Sadler 2002). More recently, under the auspices of a very large integrated health care system, I have been researching research, working to understand particular HSR processes behind the scenes (so to speak; one person's backstage is another person's front).

At another level, my entire HSR career can be seen as one long participant observation engagement. And, added to my employment in HSR, I experienced several productive unplanned stints as a participant observer at Children's when my family was among those served. This was the case for acute care in the emergency and urgent care departments and for chronic care, in orthopedics. I also participated for six weeks in the weekly club foot clinic.

The anthropologist who contracts an illness in the jungle incorporates the indigenous medical treatment process into his or her ethnographic take. Likewise, I incorporated these family experiences to enhance my ethnographic perspective on Children's as an organization, employees' and patients' experiences with the organization, and health services in general. The club foot experience was, although painful in some ways, a boon to my ongoing research with the Down syndrome project.

In brief, I had to bring my club-footed baby to the hospital every week for the first seven weeks of his life for treatment. Concurrently and subsequently, he underwent surgery and was treated for a number of orthopedic conditions, including with devices and physical therapy. I took this opportunity to talk with other families and clinic staff members and to watch and learn. My family's experience, though definitely not major in the big scheme of things and incomparable with the experiences of the families in the Down syndrome study or other families whose children have major special health care needs, enhanced my understanding of what the Down syndrome families and other families with children with special health care needs go through. It enhanced my ability to build, for providers as well as parents, a conceptual model of how such families perceive the task of optimizing their children's health care and to make recommendations of how to enhance their experiences with health services and otherwise better support them.

Cross-Project Comparison

One reason for focusing on special health care needs children is that they account for most pediatric health services system usage. Further, and for this reason, such children are particularly vulnerable to suffer from shortcomings of the system. Sometimes, because the children generally require ongoing interactions with the system, chain reactions ensue from what on their own are small problems, leading to otherwise preventable disasters, whether in terms of a child's physical or mental health or family well-being.

Much of my work has focused on the parent experience and what this can tell us about improvements that are needed in the health services system. By the time of my participation in the club foot clinic, the Down syndrome project first introduced in Chapter 11 had been augmented in a number of ways, including with a longitudinal, focused study tracking four families with newborn infants who had received a Down syndrome diagnosis. Its focus had shifted to how families learn to navigate the health care system for their children who need it. Findings had been fed back into the system through various channels.

Kimberly Dennis had collected and analyzed qualitative interview and home-visit data from the four families enrolled in the longitudinal part of the project. In reading her report (2004), I could not help but to keep noting the ways in which my own family's experiences seemed so similar. I felt awkward doing so, because our experiences were relatively benign. And yet, I reflected how the content of my club foot clinic participant observations could be organized quite easily using the overarching categories that had been identified in relation to the Down syndrome families.

By juxtaposing the experiences of two groups of parents, I was able to develop a "noncategorical" model of parental coping—a model generalizable to all categories of children with special health care needs—and one that can be understood and applied by health service workers. Key variables are: (1) initial classification, (2) care coordination, and (3) stigma management. The contents of each domain are shown in the graphic I developed to disseminate the model (see Figure 12.1).

I mention and include the figure here not so much for the findings it conveys (for those, see Sobo 2007) but rather to emphasize the fact that findings must be presented to potential end-users in a format with which they are comfortable if they are to absorb or act on them. The providers I had been working with liked figures, as do the editors and peer reviewers for the journals they read, so that is why I made one. It was later revised to satisfy a theoretically inclined audience of social scientists (see Sobo n.d.).

The model depicted in the figure for the clinical end users provides a map of the territory with which those involved in the care of children with special health care needs contend. As such, the map can help its readers orient themselves to the territory relatively rapidly and thus to enjoy earlier navigational success than those who must forge their own way in the dark. The figure's economy demands that it be explained when presented; doing this in person and telling data-derived stories regarding its components makes it that much more powerful for fostering change (something we examine more closely in Chapter 15).

I do not hold that without my own family's foray into extended orthopedic care I would never have come to the same conclusions. However, that experience did catalyze the comparative process that would have

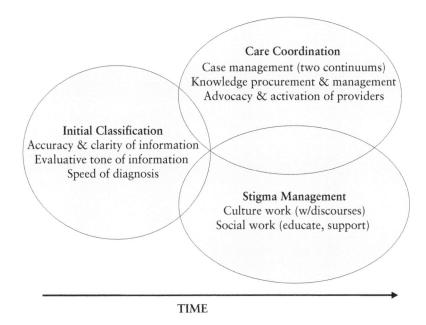

Figure 12.1 Non-categorical model of parental coping in managing health care for the disabled or chronically ill child. The model depicted is dynamic; interactions in one sphere affect interactions in the other spheres, and experiences accrete interactively over time. For some conditions, a number of subsequent, subsidiary diagnosis phases are entailed (reprinted, with permission, from Sobo 2007).

been necessary for it to have happened. That is, if I had conducted several disparate formal studies of families whose children had several disparate chronic conditions, and then reflected on similarities and differences long enough, I would have eventually seen the light. But participating myself in the club foot clinic and subsequent related orthopedic assessments while reviewing the cumulating Down syndrome findings made the comparison viscerally obvious. People sometimes ask how I can use so freely my own experiences in conceptual modeling, interpretation of data, theory-building, and even teaching. My answer regarding the non-categorical model is that it would have been negligent not to.

CHAPTER **13** / Making Rapid
Improvements

Applied health services research or HSR aims to produce actionable
results. As Chapter 9 explained, having an impact requires excellent
teamwork. The team must be nimble; it must be able to accommodate
politically necessary as well as scientifically called-for changes, whether
to the planned-for protocol or personnel or even the overall project
emphasis. The team also must have strong social connections within the
site to be affected.

In addition to the need for social network building that immediate
implementation requires there is an inherent need for speed. However,
the short cycle time often required in this type of work presents important methodological challenges. This chapter shows that, with careful
forethought and preparation, rigorously designed research can be carried out rapidly and results can even be used in real time to inform and
improve the services under study.

/ THEORY VERSUS ACTION VERSUS PRACTICE

There is a longstanding scholarly tradition of classifying research as
basic or theoretical on the one hand, and applied on the other, with
basic research informing theory and applied research informing action.
This oppositional scheme ignores the existence of a continuum, denies
that a particular project could in fact be a bit of both, and evades the fact
that action is always theoretically informed in some sense and vice versa.
Excellent examples of these facts are seen in HSR, which is historically
service oriented. HSR only rarely has entailed developing knowledge for
only knowledge's sake, as the old saw goes; knowledge is always sought
with benefit to some population or entity in mind, such as the state,
the taxpayer, the health care organization, the service provider, or the
patient. Recall that HSR emerged in the same political context as did
Medicaid and Medicare; its initial function was accountability related—
it was "applied."

However, knowledge not coupled tightly to action, whether that action consists of new policies or improved interventions, is not, technically speaking, applied. It may be said to have applications. And others may, eventually, pick it up and use it for action. But, in and of itself, it has limited ability to improve health services—until action is undertaken. So, the timing of action is crucial to the applied research designation.

This may sound like hair splitting. But the definition of applied anthropology is currently in question, with various other appellations competing for priority. To appreciate this, consider an alternate tag: "practicing" anthropology. The label's sound evokes the materialist notion of praxis, or theoretically informed action. Praxis refuses the theoretical-applied distinction. At the same time, however, the practicing label also can evoke providers' construction of research not labeled as such as antagonistic, or at least in opposition to, practice (clinical service; recall the discourses referenced in Chapter 5).

In the HSR context, most people just call research with direct applications "applied" research, and for this reason I will stick with it here. One lesson of this book is that, when in Rome, culturally competent linguistic choices are probably (so long as they are ethically defensible) the most efficient and effective choices to make. Talking past research partners by using unfamiliar or esoteric word choices will backfire in any attempt to foster the increasing acceptance of, and desire for, an anthropologically informed HSR. So will ignorance of health services' immediate agendas, most of which revolve around system optimization through some form or another of improvement.

/ CYCLES FOR IMPROVEMENT

One method frequently used for improvement in health services quality management groups is **Rapid Cycle Improvement** or RCI, also known as the Shewhart-Deming cycle (Berwick 1996; Davidson 1993; Langley, Nolan, and Nolan 1992). A version of RCI called "Plan, Do, Study, Act" or PDSA has been promoted within health care by the Institute for Health care Improvement (IHI). IHI and its leader, Donald Berwick, have been very influential in health care quality improvement (QI). Essentially, PDSA consists of realizing a problem and then: (P) designing a plan to address it; (D) doing or implementing the plan; (S) studying its effects; (A) acting to revise it as needed; and so on in a series of PDSA cycles. It is often depicted graphically as a wheel or spiral. Because it repeats, it also is known as a form of continuous quality improvement or CQI.

If I may continue despite the alphabet soup we have just entered (remember: "When in Rome"), the goal of RCI using the PDSA method promoted by IHI is to permit "inductive learning—the growth of knowledge through making changes and then reflecting on the consequences of those changes" (Berwick 1996, p. 620). PDSA is, in many ways, akin to applied anthropology research in which theory is built inductively from or "grounded" in data (Glaser and Strauss 1967). Hypotheses or theories are developed and tested continuously over the course of a given project. Change is evaluated and findings are fed back into the project, for example, as modifications to a part of the protocol or in the development of a new hypothesis or theory to be tested.

In health services, PDSA is traced largely to William Edwards Deming, who (with inspiration from Walter A. Shewhart) promoted RCI while assisting with postwar industrial reconstruction in Japan. Both Deming and Shewhart (and Joseph Juran, also part of this CQI circle), participated in the Hawthorne Western Electric factory studies of the 1920s and 1930s—studies that were central in the creation of organizational sociology, social psychology, and anthropology.

RCI, using PDSA or another variant on the Shewhart-Deming theme, is designed to be fast. It entails short-term goals, achieved with constant incremental improvements. It requires study and reflection but differs from traditional research as HSR conceives research because protocol revision midstream is expected and encouraged, whereas in HSR that would be seen as compromising methodological integrity. In this, it is akin to the anthropologically informed approach, which values local needs and can accommodate them through built-in flexibility.

/ WORKING WITH WORKAROUNDS

Perhaps because it is so complex, and decisions made in one realm can have numerous unintended effects in another, health care is infused with workarounds—practices that people invent to offset inconveniences that institutionally imposed structures or procedures may entail. For example, taping a self-locking door's bolts back so that the door does not lock is a workaround; it helps busy workers move back and forth between rooms with expedience. Although in the short term this workaround has benefits for those who have imposed it, it may also compromise security or safety, which the automatic lock was installed to protect.

Understanding workarounds often opens the way to rapid improvement. It allows an organization to benefit from worker wisdom regarding a need to streamline processes and, at the same time, provides an opportunity for managing the risks that workarounds may unwittingly entail. It depends on being open to emic accounts. One of my recent projects entailing a workaround concerned an HIV screening intervention. It uses computerized clinical reminders to spur screening test offers among patients identified, by a computer algorithm, as being at risk for HIV. The organization that hosted the study has a wonderfully computerized patient record system, so all providers use the computers at office visits. Proponents of the HIV screening program sought to capitalize on that. The HIV screening program was justified by internal data suggesting that less than one-third of the system's patients who could be identified as at-risk for HIV infection had actually been tested for HIV infection.

Importantly, the HIV screening program was really a pilot project being tried out at various sites in the system. As part of my research, twenty interviews with providers using the clinical reminder were undertaken (this was more efficient than observations would have been; for one thing, the reminder comes up for some providers only one or two times weekly, if that). When I analyzed the interview data, which had been transcribed verbatim, I realized that providers who were successfully using the reminder were doing something special. They were presenting the HIV screening test offer that the computer told them was indicated for that particular patient as if it was simply routine. This never would have been discovered without using open-ended interview methods that allowed participants to talk about practices that *they* deemed important.

The health care system in question was not actually trying to routinize screening tests (as the algorithm's very existence shows: Routine screening would not have required it because everyone would have then been made a test offer whether or not risk factors existed). However, presenting the HIV screening test offer to targeted patients *as if* routine effectively encouraged patients to consider the offer rather than to react out of hand in a negative fashion because it lessened the test's potential stigma. Symbolically routinizing HIV screening also helped providers manage scarce time effectively.

What were some of their strategies in play? Clinicians either sandwiched the offer between other less stigmatizing and in some cases really routine tests or procedures or they pitched the test (however indirectly) as part of the standard visit process: "If you broach it as if it's a general blanket that the [organization] does for everybody, there's no connotations taken with it." In a slightly different twist that was so unique it bears mention, a provider interviewed during a mid-course feedback evaluation on which I was consulting after the HIV screening program's full-scale regional rollout said that she presents the reminder as if the lottery has been won: as if it is the patient's lucky day because the health care system has selected her or him for a test offer.

These normalization practices were workarounds of a type; they were methods for making the system work better without changing it. Because the HIV screening program was an implementation project rather than a research study per se, we were able to feed information about selected successful strategies for making HIV screening test offers back into the project, such as the sandwiching tactic mentioned above.

We were able to offer project-bolstering suggestions because we asked providers what they were really doing rather than what they were supposed to do and we made them feel comfortable with telling us through our nonjudgmental phrasing and body language. As the next example shows, patients and families often have things to say too that, when really listened to, can fuel improvement efforts.

PATIENT INFORMATION AND INVOLVEMENT PREFERENCES

The Problem: No Profiles

In the hematology and oncology (heme-onc) research described in Chapter 12, I noticed that nursing care quality might benefit from a quick and easy way to gauge patients and particularly parents' communication preferences—that is, their desire for information and involvement in care-related decision-making. Given accurate information regarding parent communication preferences, education messages can be tailored so that the minimum standard message is communicated at the level desired. Additional messages can be communicated, as possible, in keeping with parent preferences. Similarly, decision-making opportunities can be tailored to parent involvement wishes.

This was perceived not just as a worker or patient satisfaction issue. Proper at-home medication administration is particularly important among pediatric cancer patients and their parents because pediatric cancer patients use many highly toxic pharmaceuticals. They are extremely vulnerable to medication errors, which can have serious health consequences, cause significant disruptions to the delivery of quality care, and entail considerable financial costs. If we could figure out a way to help nurses gauge preferences, we could work this into the succession of PDSA cycles that the interview study was part of.

A literature review had previously revealed that pediatric cancer patients and their families are immediately responsible for many at-home medication errors. An inverse correlation exists between such errors and good communication. Information-giving by clinicians positively correlates to proper follow-through on prescribed medication administration practices and to higher satisfaction among patients with chronic health conditions; it also correlates with better medical health outcomes

(Drotar 2000; Edwards and Elwyn 2001; Korsch, Gozzi, and Francis 1968; Maly, Bourque, and Engelhardt 1999; Renzi et al. 2002; Riekert and Drotar 2000; L. F. Snow 1993; Tebbi 1993).

The literature also shows that on their own, clinicians are not so good at assessing patient or parent preferences accurately (Robinson and Thomson 2001; Waitzkin 1985). For instance, in a survey study of 425 patient-physician pairs, physicians remained unaware of patient treatment preferences in 45% of cases (Coulter, Peto, and Doll 1994). Much contributes to the problem, including not only provider bias (Butow et al. 1997) but wishful thinking: Enduring personal practitioner-patient relationships in which face-to-face communication provides clinicians with information about patient or parent expectations and desires may be in keeping with U.S. ideals for health care, but high patient volumes and quick staff turnover limit the degree to which such relationships with patients can actually be built (for further background, see Sobo 2004a).

My first thought was that someone somewhere already had created the perfect tool to help providers profile preferences, and that we might use it to tailor information provision and decision-making involvement opportunities to suit each parent's comfort level (although I will use only the term "parent," I also mean guardians as well as adolescent patients; younger patient preferences were off the table for this particular project, largely because of predominating constructions of children's agency and cognitive capacity). Importantly, tailoring does not need to be so individualized that it is inefficient. Individuals can be "segmented" or grouped according to their expressed preferences, and methods of personalization can be systematized; this is termed "mass customization" (Institute of Medicine Committee on Quality of Health Care in America 2001). Population segmentation and mass customization both are recommended by the Institute of Medicine as important care strategies, and by referring to them in my proposal for the project and making evaluative questions responsive to these priorities, I could help ensure the project's appeal to hospital leadership. But, as it turned out, no suitable tool for assessing preferences was available. To help our providers, then, we had to invent out own.

The Solution: Create a New Decision Support Tool

In partnership with the medical and administrative directors of heme-onc, a team that included me as the leader, the medical safety officer (an MD), a health educator (an RN), and three research assistants (RAs) developed the prototype of a simple, easy-to-administer, and effective communication preferences assessment tool: the PIINT©. It is a paper-and-pencil survey that both parents and patients aged twelve years and older can easily self-administer. Completed forms can be kept in the patient chart, where all care team members have access to results.

I review the steps undertaken in the tool's development here because they provide a model for developing and piloting new data collection tools for other projects that readers may be interested in undertaking. They also make clear the immense benefit of working directly with end-users.

Initial Tool Development Steps

Tool development was informed by the PDSA system of RCI, described above. In PDSA, change is evaluated and findings are fed back into a given project, for example as modifications to a form being developed.

And develop a form we did. As a first step in designing our PIINT© survey form, the team created a single-sided one-page document with two "pick one" questions (the final form is seen in Figure 13.1). The first question was adapted from another related tool (Degner, Sloan, and Venkatesh 1997; Pyke-Grimm et al. 1999). The second question presented four information preference statements developed in light of the literature review. Our ideas for how the form might be used were based on our observational knowledge of how heme-onc worked. We definitely wanted it to be fast to fill in.

The team then created a graphic for plotting one's preferences. The goal here was to produce an easily readable visual indicator of the parent's communication preferences—one that a busy clinician might glance at and understand very quickly without having to scrutinize—and to make self-administration more interesting for the parent, thus increasing the return rate.

The PIINT© prototype was reviewed in two focus group meetings (regarding my approach to focus groups, see Chapter 10). First, heme-onc's medical director, a social worker, a parent liaison, and a psychologist participated. The group's main concern was liability; the initial statement, which at first had no contingency clause, was modified to include "when possible" (e.g., "When possible, I want to share in making the decisions"). The information preference statements also were adjusted slightly.

Second, about fifteen members of the hospital's in-house research center, who were intensely familiar with the hospital's culture, reviewed the revised PIINT© prototype. The initial question and its possible responses were seen as too medically oriented; the graphic was seen as too complex. Appropriate revisions were made.

After being revised, the statements were all evaluated for reading ease (word-processing software programs often provide reading grade level

Children's
Hospital
and Health
Center

Your needs matter...

People differ in how much they want to make decisions about their child's health care. People also differ in how much information they want about the care of their child. Your answers to this survey will help Children's staff to understand your needs.

Your needs may change over time. So you can update your answers later if you want to.

1. <u>What is your relation to the patient?</u> (please circle one)

       Mother   Father   Other Female   Other male   I am the patient
                                                    (12 years or over)

2. <u>Which sentence best describes the decision-making role that you *want*?</u>
   "*When possible, _____* " (please circle one number)

   1) I want to leave all decisions about my (my child's) care to the care team. (The care team includes doctors, nurses, and others giving care to the child.)

   2) I want the care team to make the decisions about my (my child's) care. But I want the care team to seriously listen to my views.

   3) I want to share in making the decisions about my (my child's) care with the care team.

   4) I want to make the decisions about my (my child's) care. But I will seriously listen to the care team's advice.

   5) I want to make all decisions about my (my child's) care.

3. <u>Compared to what I want, my decision-making role *right now* is:</u> (circle one)

          Too small   Just right   Too big

4. <u>Which sentence best describes how much information you *want* about your child's care?</u>

   "*When possible, _____* " (please circle one letter)

   a) I want the simplest information you can give me.
   b) I want more than the simplest information. But keep it in everyday terms.
   c) I want more than the simplest information. I also want help to u nderstand
      things in depth.
   d) I want as much in-depth and detailed information as you can give to me.

5. <u>Compared to what I want, the information I get *right now* is:</u> (circle one)

          Too little   Just right   Too much

Continued

STEP TWO:

What <u>number</u> did you circle for question 2 (decision-making)? _____

What <u>letter</u> did you circle for question 4 (information)? _____

1) Find (but do not mark) your <u>number</u> in the top row of the chart below.
2) Then find (but do not mark) your <u>letter</u> in the column on the left side of the chart.
3) Now, <u>mark a big</u> X inside the <u>box</u> where the number and letter row and column <u>intersect.</u>

Your mark will show us your information and decision needs.
We will try our best to meet these needs.

		DECISION ROLE				
		1	2	3	4	5
INFORMATION	A					
	B					
	C					
	D					

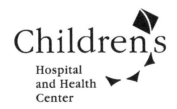

Children's
Hospital
and Health
Center

Figure 13.1 The Patient/Parent Information and Involvement Assessment Tool, or PIINT© (reprinted, with permission, from Sobo 2004a). Question 2 is adapted from Degner, Sloan, and Venkatesh 1997 (cf. Pyke-Grimm et al. 1999).

assessment tools). The statements were simplified to the sixth grade level or lower to ensure that most parents would be able to complete them. Then they were pilot tested.

Prototype Testing with Rapid Cognitive Interviews

The statements on the PIINT© prototype were tested with a convenience sample of twenty-one English-speaking parents (seventeen mothers, two fathers, two female relatives). The sample was recruited from parent lounges, patient rooms, and hospital corridors. Respondents were asked to select one statement from each group, and to talk about their selection process. They were asked to alert us to any problems they had in making their choices, especially problems about wording. These sessions generally lasted about five minutes.

This technique is an adaptation of the **cognitive interview** method (see Chapter 10 regarding its use in participant observation). Cognitive or "think aloud" interviews provide information about how people formulate answers to questionnaires or what they understand particular written materials to mean. Participants are asked to think aloud or narrate their cognitions as they read and react to materials (Aday 1989; Sudman, Bradburn, and Schwartz 1996). This process can take an hour or more, depending on tool length and complexity. Because our form was purposely short, our cognitive interviews were done rapidly. Our method might therefore be termed "rapid cognitive interviewing." A rapid assessment method, it is both appropriate for and well suited to the PDSA process.

More Modifications

Participant comments noted during the interviews were reviewed. We made a few small wording changes in response (e.g., in one statement "final decision"' was changed to "the decisions," for continuity). Not one parent suggested that specific information-type categories would have been helpful; they were satisfied with a global information construct. Finally, just to be thorough, a scatter plot with involvement answers on one axis, and information-related answers on the other, indicated no obvious relationship between involvement and information preference choices. A Spanish-language translation was created using back translation (see Chapter 10).

To broaden the use of the PIINT© to include performance improvement information, after validating the statements, the team added two questions relating to whether decision-making and information preferences are being met. The answers to these questions would allow clinicians to improve the quality of their efforts to fulfill parent preferences (and the hospital also could point to their existence to demonstrate a commitment to this).

A third additional question regarding the respondent's relationship to the patient (which includes the category "self") also was added and the statements modified with parentheses so that an adolescent patient might apply them to him- or herself. The final form is depicted in Figure 13.1.

Administration Ease and Utility Tests

The PIINT© was re-piloted with a larger convenience sample of seventy-nine individuals, this time including Spanish speakers and patients over twelve years of age. This time, the plotting graphic was included on the backside of the single-sheet form. Ease of administration was confirmed for the graphic: The error rate was 5%, which included mostly not filling it in. To fix this problem, "Please turn over" was inserted on the bottom of the front side of the form. A few small wording changes also were made in the graphic's instructions, to improve the clarity of the directions. The initial findings regarding no relationship between statement choices were confirmed.

As a final step in the pilot process, a comparison was made between a convenience sample of English- and Spanish-speaking parents' PIINT© survey answers and the information and involvement answers attributed to them by their (or their child's) assigned nurses. This "agreement study" was undertaken as a type of utility test, so that care team members could see for themselves if the PIINT© was needed. Fifty-one parent-nurse pairs completed the PIINT© process. Results were examined for each parent-nurse pair to ascertain agreement levels, and frequencies for the different types of agreement or disagreement were calculated.

Overall, nurses' assessments matched parents' self-assessments only one-third of the time. Regarding parental involvement preferences, erroneous perceptions on the part of nursing staff were equally likely to be over- or underestimations. However, with regard to information preferences, nurses were more likely to attribute smaller desires to parents than larger desires. (For a full description of findings, see Sobo 2004a.)

Change Instigation

We showed all this and more to the nurses in tables describing frequencies and the results of statistical tests. But the point here is not so much what the data describe quantitatively as their value for instigating a change in the unit's processes. Without them, the staff may not have been convinced of the need for yet another bit of paperwork. But we did have data, and the staff did believe them.

It did not hurt that, based on my observational knowledge of the situation, we highlighted the time pressures nurses are under when presenting the data, which we did in person. Thus, perceptions were mismatched as described above not because the nurses were not good at their jobs but because their jobs were too busy. In this light, our creation of the PIINT© decision aid validated employee claims that they were overworked and under pressure.

At the nurses' and directors' request, the PIINT© tool (see Figure 13.1) was put into use in heme-onc. It was administered by registrars at inpatient admissions and filed in patient charts by heme-onc nurses, where care team members could use it during inpatient care giving.

Epilog

My description has shown how, in a few simple stages or improvement cycles—including a literature review, draft tool generation, two focus groups, statement validation, rapid cognitive interviews, an administration ease test, and confirmation of statement validation, each of which led to improvements in the prototype—a potentially useful tool was created. Contextual knowledge instigated the project, which would never have been conceived without an anthropologically induced awareness of the need for the tool. Contextual knowledge also helped ensure its good reception, not only among the nurses but also among hospital leadership. The story does not, however, have a totally happy ending.

Eventually, financial constraints that led to a series of lay-offs significantly affected follow-through in the long term. Early champions left the organization and with them gone commitment fizzled as knowledge regarding the PIINT© was not maintained. So, in the end, the success of this story was short lived. On the bright side, I have had contact with representatives from a number of other health services organizations that have put the tool into practice.

The lesson regarding staff turnover and recidivism is an important one; I address it briefly below in regard to sustainability (and see Chapter 14). But first, let me provide one last example of focused, rapid, anthropologically informed HSR work.

FREE LISTING FOR RAPID DEMARCATION OF CULTURAL DOMAINS

The next project I describe involved physicians. The main method used was the free list. **Free listing** is an established data collection technique that asks participants to list, freely, terms they associate with a stated topic area or cultural domain (in this case, "competent parents") (de Munck and Sobo 1998; Weller and Romney 1988). Cultural domains are shared, learned understandings of a phenomenon or topic (D'Andrade and Strauss 1992). So, for example, if we wanted to know what illness states people considered common in childhood, we would ask them to freely list all the common childhood illnesses they know. This is much faster than gleaning this information simply by observing who gets sick with what.

However, because free list data consist only of disconnected terms rather than discourse or narrative, unlike focus group or even one-time interview data, without extensive ethnographic background findings they are difficult to make sense of. On its own, then, this method yields little in terms of anthropologically informed insight. One can delimit cultural domain contents, but not their meanings, with free listing alone.

Yet, in certain situations this is all one needs. For instance, clinicians today caution parents against starting infants on solids prior to six months of age. This is all well and good, but some parents may not define solids the same way that providers do. Is infant formula with a little rice cereal mixed in a "solid"? What about soup? According to some parents, no. According to clinicians, yes. With a better understanding of how parents define the solids domain—with emic information—better education messages can be crafted.

Head Bonks Revisited

I mentioned in Chapter 2 the debate at Children's regarding the use of CT or computed tomography scans on children brought in with minor head injuries (MHI) or what our providers called "head bonks." In due time, professional guidelines were issued, complete with an algorithmic pathway describing what doctors should do. These guidelines, published in *Pediatrics* (AAP-AAFP 1999) recommend that children two years or older who present with an MHI with no more than one minute of reported loss of consciousness and who seem "normal" after a clinical examination should be sent home for observation if a "competent" parent (or the equivalent) is available (p. 1409). "Observation" entails "regular monitoring by a competent adult who would be able to recognize abnormalities and to seek appropriate assistance" (p. 1408).

The recommendation assumes consensus among physicians as to what constitutes a competent parent. Or, to put this more anthropologically, it assumes consensus among physicians as to what the "cultural model" or "domain" of parental competence comprises.

Gauging Domain Consensus through the Free-List Technique

I questioned the basis for that assumption, and put together an in-house study protocol to explore this as well as the reasons why physicians may contravene the recommendation for home observation. The study considered cultural domains and social contexts key variables in medical decision-making.

Being relatively new at Children's at the time, I figured that I would interview a few dozen physicians. The proposal was rejected out of hand by my director, who asked me whose budget the money would come from to pay for their time and why I thought they would even make time for the project. Of course they would not; I was new and unknown to them, and the project was far from the clinical trial-type standard. Why not do a survey instead, my boss cheerily suggested. And so I did. In keeping with pragmatic constraints, it was intended to be brief (one page, single sided), anonymous, and self-administered.

I pilot tested my survey with twenty-eight clinicians attending a morbidity and mortality meeting convened by Trauma Services. Feedback on the survey format as well as reliability and validity was provided by the respondents and by physician members of the hospital's Medical Staff Executive Committee. After reviewing this feedback and running preliminary analyses of the data collected, which supported reports of good face validity and reliability, the survey was revised for clarity and completeness. It was then mailed to all physicians affiliated with Children's, although only a subset would eventually qualify for the MHI-specific analysis. My focus here is the survey tool itself and the analysis as these illuminate the free-list method, but I should note that, although a stamped return envelope was included, there was no financial incentive because of our limited budget; regarding ways to maximize mailed physician survey returns (see Dillman 2007; Van Geest, Johnson, and Welch 2007).

The final survey included seven demographic questions, seven Likert-type scaled questions on parental competence decision-making (e.g., "On a scale of one to five ..."), and—to my director's surprise—a free-list section that aimed to elicit ideas regarding parental competence. Although free listing is generally used in person, its productive use in written form with groups for whom systematic interviews are inconvenient or difficult has been established (Fleisher and Harrington 1998). The survey's free-list section consisted simply of a question and an array of blanks to be filled in. The question was:

> Please list, in the order they come to you, *without self-censorship*, as many terms or phrases to describe a "competent" and "responsible" caretaker as you can think of. Be as specific as you can. You will find it helpful to keep in mind a time you had to make this distinction. Your terms will be mostly descriptive. They may have implied opposites (e.g., the opposite of "up" is "down"). They can be negatives (e.g., "not "). Be as specific as you can. Please don't worry how your terms or phrases sound—your answers cannot be traced to you!

Free-list data are words; they are qualitative. The lists elicited are prototypical, reflecting factors that one expects to be present if, in this example, parents are competent. In this, data can be compared to the normative data gleaned from standard focus groups.

However, after terms or "items" are collected, frequencies, ranks, and salience levels are determined using specialized software, for example, ANTHROPAC (Borgatti 1992). An item's rank is its average place in respondent lists. "Salience" refers to the relationship between an item's rank and the varied lengths of the lists in which it was mentioned. An item listed fifth in a ten-item list will have a higher salience than an item listed fifth in a five-item list; the overall salience figure corrects for this.

Free listing identifies the contents of cultural domains and establishes their coherence, confirming similarity, not difference. Therefore, within-group comparisons with statistical tests such as chi-square are not indicated. What is indicated, however, is a qualitative, context-sensitive assessment of the meaning of the rank and salience information and of differences between these for important subsamples.

Analytic Methods

Respondents were divided into subsamples according to gender, training emphasis, specialization, and practice location. The items most commonly listed differed by subgroup in certain respects, and in some cases the proportion of respondents listing an item differed substantially (see Sobo and Kurtin 2003). In keeping with the analytic demands of the method, subsamples with more than fifty members were reduced systematically, with every other or every third respondent included (depending on original subsample size) so that the final subsamples each had less than fifty members. ANTHROPAC software does not allow for more; establishing domain coherence never requires it (Handwerker 1998; Weller and Romney 1988). Still, I scanned the remaining data to assure myself that they were similar to the data that were formally analyzed.

Why, if no more than fifty cases are needed, did all physicians receive surveys? This was in part because some of the other questions would yield useful descriptive data for all physicians surveyed. Had this not been the case, a random sample might have been assembled. Here I should note that the survey sample as a whole was representative of the gender and general training mix of the relevant physician population. Such information increases the face validity of study findings when presented back to physicians and other end-users.

Through a process that might be termed **"data reduction"** and was reminiscent of the process undertaken with the focus group data described in Chapter 10, I condensed the raw item lists. I eliminated spelling or wording distinctions, but not meaning distinctions. So, synonyms such as "caring" and "concerned" were condensed and counted (coded) as one item ("caring & concerned"). But "good with medications" and "keeps appointments" were coded separately because, although both refer to what physicians would term adherence issues, enough respondents listed them with sufficient specificity. Conversely, poor differentiation between "clean," "tidy," "neat," and "appropriately dressed" led to the consolidation of all terms referring to this aspect of appearance.

A total of sixty-four discrete items remained (for a list of these as well as the full list and more details regarding the demographic aspect of the analysis, see Sobo and Kurtin 2003). Later input from two physicians (see below) led to the elimination of two items and the consolidation of two more, for a final total of sixty-one discrete items.

A computer-assisted free-list analysis was then run on the various fifty-case-limited sub-samples' coded data, and item lists generated. Individual lists contained an average of 6.5 items; each subsample group listed an average of fifty-three items (range: forty-seven to fifty-nine). In light of the distinction made between medical and surgical culture in Chapter 5, here I will note that the average length of surgeons' lists was significantly shorter than that of nonsurgeons. Surgeons also were more likely than nonsurgeons to order discretionary CTs.

Once the data were run through the software, I undertook a careful, iterative inspection of coded items to identify possible parental competence subdomains. The entire exercise was informed by the skeletal specifications for parental competence provided in the AAP MHI guidelines. My inspection helped offset the fact that items listed represented various levels of specificity, as will happen when free lists are not collected in person, when researcher guidance or redirection techniques cannot be imposed.

What do I mean by various levels of specificity? For instance, one respondent might list a particular behavior (e.g., drunkenness) and the next might list the class or category that includes that behavior (e.g., substance use). The broader category subsumes the narrower one. Likewise, the broader category is a subdomain of the domain under investigation—parental competence.

The emergent scheme of subdomains and subdomain items was scrutinized during a modified subject review (Patton 1999), in which two physicians individually sorted and grouped the individual items (i.e., they did pile sorts; see Weller and Romney 1988) without seeing my model. They explained to me their views on the items' meanings to physicians and the logic behind their groupings. I adjusted my model slightly in accordance. A third physician (my director and coauthor; see Chapter 14) also participated here, albeit indirectly: His main role in most of our coauthored pieces was troubleshooting from the physician's perspective, identifying statements that the docs would disagree with, whether because they would be incomprehensible (as jargon) or culturally offensive.

I invited only two physicians' help with the formal subject review described above because the domain of parental competence was *not* coherent. Consensus on items making up the domain was not high. Most of the sixty-one factors were listed by fewer than 20% of respondents. And although seven subdomains were identified (see below), not everyone listed an item from each. Thus, parental competence was not, for physicians, a unitary construct.

Had coherence and consensus been high, a full-blown pile-sort exercise would have been undertaken with twenty or so physicians. Proximity data generated would have been subject to multidimensional scaling in which a graphic chart or plot depicting item clusters can be derived from calculations based on how often people lump items together in their piles (Borgatti 1992; Caulkins 1998; Dressler and Bindon 2000; Handwerker 1998; Weller and Romney 1988). A multidimensionally scaled or MDS plot is a type of scatter plot, with x and y coordinates. The MDS plot, with its graphically displayed clusters, can be resubmitted to subjects or, better yet, to another sample from the same population for further interpretation.

To better visualize what multidimensionally scaled pile sort data look like, imagine that we have collected free-list data regarding the domain of "food." After deriving the aggregate list of items, we ask people to lump the items into various piles at their discretion. Once the data that each person's piles contain (i.e., the item names) have been coded and the codes turned into a data set and the data set processed so that proximity data (data regarding how often certain food names turn up in the same pile) have been calculated, we generate an MDS plot displaying the findings (see the references above for detailed information on how to do that).

If college students in the United States, say, were doing the listing and sorting, we might see that various kinds of pizza all show up in one area of the plot, breakfast cereals in another, and so on, with various item clumps representing the basic food groups that U.S. students know to exist. Closer or more tightly clumped items were deemed more similar by participants. Some items might hover in between groups; for instance, flavored yogurt might hover between a dairy product clump and a desserts clump. Such hovering happens when some participants put an item in one pile and others put it in another. Isolated outlier items—items deemed unlike any of the others—also might appear. To interpret the meanings of the clumps and disjunctions, we must take into account what people told us while the items were sorted as well as, when possible, what people say on viewing the MDS plot depiction.

In addition to pile-sort-based multidimensional scaling, other analytic techniques can be applied to free-list data. Further, beside pile sort data, triadic comparisons, in which participants are given data in sets of three items and asked to determine which item is not like the rest, also can be displayed in MDS plots (for more ideas on how to follow up on domain-based investigations, see de Munck and Sobo 1998).

In the project under discussion, data were not coherent and consensus seemed low. Therefore, I did not undertake a full-blown pile sort with physicians. Nor did I undertake to do pile sorts with each separate sub-sample because, following the MHI guidelines, the project's focus was physicians in general. And, as becomes clear below, the lack of consensus was in itself a significant finding.

This lack notwithstanding, there seem to be three broad subdomains that may underwrite physician perceptions of parental competence. In the tabular depiction of these shown in Table 13.1, each broad sub-domain is divided further into the subdomain item clusters it is built from. The distribution of items suggests that specific items may differ with physician characteristics; it also suggests that not all clusters will be relevant to every physician. For illustrative purposes, however, items

Table 13.1 Parental competence free-list subdomains and subdomain item clusters (see Sobo and Kurtin 2003)

I.   Parenting skills
(a)   Parent-child interaction
   Compassionate & empathetic
   Good interaction with child
   Loving & affectionate
(b)   Child health advocacy: Prior
   Good follow up in past
   Good with medications
   Keeps appointments
(c)   Child health advocacy: Present
   Asks (good) questions
   Can repeat instructions
   Caring & concerned
   Compliant & cooperative
   Good historian
   Observant & focused on child's condition
   Pays attention
   Responsive
   Understands instructions

II.   General features
(a)   General disposition
   Adult & mature
   Clean, neat, & appropriately attired
   Detail-oriented & organized
   Skilled communicator

continued

Table 13.1 *(Continued)*

(b) *General cognitive capacity*
Educated & informed
Intelligent

(c) *Environment of care*
Good support system
Married & stable

III. *Essential prerequisites*
Abuse not suspected
No access issues (phone, transport, proximity)
No language barriers
Not impaired (physically or mentally)
Not homeless

---

from the general list of sixty-one (generally those that were higher ranking and had higher salience) were included in the table.

The first broad subdomain, "Parenting skills," was important to the most participants. The three clusters making up this broad area refer to abilities or characteristics that can be appraised directly in relation to a parent's dealings with his or her children. The first cluster ("parent-child interaction") reflects the way a parent deals with a child. The second and third clusters relate to the way the parent performs the child health advocate role in terms of "prior" and "present" thought and action. The former category contains items that are relevant when a physician has a history of service with a given parent or access to a chart with historic information.

The "General features" area comprises three clusters of items that are not specific to the parental role; rather, they are expected of any competent U.S. adult. "General disposition" items define personality traits. *General cognitive capacity* items relate to logical facility. "Environment of care" items have to do with household organization or social arrangements. Such factors may be desired by given physicians, but subject review results suggested that they are not necessary for competent observation.

The final broad area, "Essential prerequisites," comprises factors without which a parent cannot observe to the standard required. One item is "abuse not suspected." If it is, the parent cannot be trusted to carry out the observation task.

What Does Discussion of Free-List Findings Look Like?

My key concern with this study was to gain some understanding of the issues that inform physicians' parental competence decisions. In the specific situation under study, parenting skills items were the most frequently listed and most highly specified. So, in writing up the research I suggested that the attributes of competence highlighted by future guidelines could be based on items in the parenting skills area, such as whether the parent can correctly repeat instructions, or frequency of missed appointments. Without such direction, clinicians are free to define "competence" however they liked.

Findings also suggested that competing models of parental competence exist. Therefore, I suggested that competence attribute items for guidelines might be constructed or selected to speak to the particular type of physician for which the guidelines are intended or the specific setting in which they are to be put into use. For example, pediatric-trained physicians were less interested than adult-trained physicians in whether a parent appeared "caring & concerned" (29% vs. 63%) and more interested in whether a parent "asks (good) questions" (39% vs. 22%). They were more interested in items related to the parent role in consultations, such as "keeps appointments" and "good historian." These items were not among the top items listed by adult-trained physicians. On the other hand, although adult-trained physicians highlighted appearances and passive cognitive features (such as "pays attention"), these did not rank high for pediatric-trained physicians. The same general pattern seems to characterize the contrasts between medical physicians and surgeons, again perhaps because of differing physician-parent contact patterns.

I suggested in my write-up that these things could be borne in mind during a revision of the guidelines. Of course, Children's did not write the guidelines in question. Still, we did have an in-house pathways program for tailoring guidelines to fit our specific circumstances. Information such as this would be taken into account locally to increase the effectiveness of physician practice pathways.

Constructive Criticisms

Project findings pointed to the context-dependent nature of the parental competence construct, which may be deemed present in one context and absent in another. Therefore, although the free-list method is widely accepted as a powerful elicitor of the cognitive cultural domains that help underwrite practice patterns, and the survey approach allowed for the efficient elicitation of data from a hard-to-reach population (busy physicians), it may not have been the best choice in hindsight: It cannot take such contextual shifts into account. Yet, the example demonstrates how, by using a survey format, one can gain entry for a quick qualitative inquiry that questions the definitions taken for granted by medicine. Such research can help ensure that improvement efforts are appropriately targeted.

/ SUSTAINING CHANGE

Applied research seeks to directly effect change for the better. Sometimes, change efforts fail, however. This can be because the categories held to by the target audience are not well understood. Efforts also can fail if a project drops off an organization's leaders' priority list or because champions leave the site. Implementation science, further explored in the next chapter, takes a critical look at what makes for successful—and sustainable—improvement.

To paraphrase Dean Fixsen and colleagues (2005), the goal of sustainability is not only an intervention or change's long-term survival or its embeddedness within a program or organization, but also its continued effectiveness and capacity to adapt within the constantly changing context of health services. Slippage can be limited through performance monitoring, standards enforcement, and creating receptive subcultures (Rosenheck 2001)—all strategies requiring some degree of infrastructure support.

Whether improvements are actively maintained or just passively monitored may make all the difference in long-term success. Sustainability failure is particularly likely if the level of support provided for the intervention during implementation (e.g., enriched clinic staff, research assistants, leadership endorsement) is withdrawn after completion. A successfully implemented intervention designed with follow-up booster activity at certain intervals can better sustain performance improvements; declines are attenuated as a result of a periodic nudge. If we view organizations as complex, adaptive systems—systems that change with their environment and in which patterns (e.g., of outcomes) emerge through the interactions of system agents (e.g., employees) (Plsek 2001, 2003)—cultural factors or processes that promise to be inherently (albeit unintentionally) supportive of the change anticipated can be leveraged with careful planning.

Further, a change in organizational structures (meaning not only the hierarchical relationships between staff but also the built environment in which relationships are enacted and through which they are expressed) can generate and support a change in organizational processes. For example, relocating a worker's office from the end of the hall to a central position often relocates that worker in the social structure of the department. Organizational changes such as this and others must therefore be taken into account when planning for sustainability.

Part V examines organizational factors. It does so not only in the context of research effectiveness but also to help readers understand how anthropologically informed HSR is, itself, organizationally situated.

Power Dynamics:
The Politics of Research

Readers should now have a good grasp on the what, how, and why of anthropologically informed health services research or HSR. This includes some familiarity with not only various anthropologically informed research methods but also the philosophical reasons for using them. Chapters in Part V will support readers in applying these lessons: They address the larger context in which research is designed, executed, and (sometimes) put to use.

Chapter 14 describes, and demonstrates through examples, some of the more political dimensions of the research process, with a special focus on the structuring force of organizational and professional cultures. My own research-based findings are coupled with autoethnographic observations to define and characterize the macro-level factors determining the nature of research as well as the researcher **ethos** or cultural worldview engendered by these. Although much that is described in this chapter might be seen as frustrating, it is essential that researchers enter the field with their eyes wide open.

After examining "how the sausage is made" (as some colleagues in HSR refer to research's backstage doings), Chapter 14 explores the need for protecting the interests of the organizations under study. It also examines how authorship is configured in health services settings as opposed to within academic anthropology and related disciplines. The emphasis throughout the chapter is on how, despite the best of intentions, the choices made and actions taken by researchers, like those of health care providers, are to a certain degree constrained by the options available given the sociocultural environment within which work is undertaken.

Despite the challenges that HSR work entails, it is still a keenly rewarding endeavor. Chapter 15 reminds us of where we started our journey and why, with an exploration of the relationship between storytelling and scholarly work. I present a concrete example of how findings from one project were fed back to project sponsors and unit personnel to foster positive change, after which I review specific suggestions for effective dissemination. The final section of the chapter focuses us back onto the persuasive aspects of dissemination, emphasizing that good storytelling can and should be linked to good scholarship in the interest of measurable improvement or enlightenment—and the fulfillment of a job well done.

CHAPTER 14

Institutional and Other
Sociocultural Challenges to
Doing Good Work

As Clifford Geertz points out, "If you want to understand what a science is, you should look not in the first instance at its theories or findings, and certainly not at what its apologists say about it: you should look at what the practitioners of it do" (1973, p. 5). The rapidly growing science studies literature has, accordingly, dissected and explored the "mangle of practice" (Pickering 1995) through which scientific facts are "fabricated" (e.g., Latour 1999; see also Franklin 1995; regarding culture as practice, see Chapter 6). An important subset of this literature investigates evidence creation and negotiation in health-related laboratory science, clinical trials, and clinical care, relating this to power structures and the social distribution of authority (we examined some of this literature in Chapter 8). But not much has been written about the production of knowledge in health services research (HSR) in general and nothing, bar this book, deals with anthropologically informed HSR specifically.

This chapter examines some key sociocultural features of the contests ongoing in the specific arena of implementation-related HSR. Although scholars in the disciplines of public and community health have for many years studied the implementation of evidence-based behavioral change, the science of doing so in real-world clinical health service settings is so young that agreement on what to call it has not yet coalesced. The terms "translation research" and "quality improvement research" have been suggested. The individuals and organizational units that participated in my investigation of the field use the term "implementation science" (IS), as does the first journal dedicated to the topic (*Implementation Science*, launched in 2006). Accordingly, I use IS-HSR to refer to this area and, to avoid confusion, I refer to researchers in this area as IS-HS researchers.

Elsewhere, I examine the sociocultural context of IS-HSR to help improve how the relationship between structure and agency is theorized as well as to foster the productive application of complexity theory to illuminate organizational issues and the emergence of new disciplinary subfields (Sobo, Bowman, and Gifford 2008). Here, my focus is more pragmatic. I want to help the new researcher find his or her feet on the playing field of HSR. I use this athletic metaphor purposively: More than one participant in my formal research on IS-HSR has informed me that implementation-related HSR is a team sport. Many would add conspiratorially that it is a contact sport to boot.

The defensive attitude that informants expressed with this particular metaphor is not, however, always helpful as it distracts listeners from the first referent, team sports. Indeed, I originally titled this chapter "Playing Well with Others" to convey the importance of teamness. Part of the team process is knowing when and how to capitulate in service of a greater good.

/ RESEARCH ON RESEARCH: WHAT CAN IT TELL US?

I was engaged in contract work for one of the nation's largest integrated health care systems when the opportunity for formal research on research processes arose. The study was undertaken in support of the organization's longstanding commitment to self-improvement through self-scrutiny. One of the organization's IS-HSR service units hosted the research project.

Like the system's other IS-HSR units, the unit I studied has a centrally funded, competitively awarded, potentially renewable four-year program budget to support core administrative functions. All research project costs are paid for with additional competitively derived grants ("soft money," generally budgeted for two to three years). The IS-HSR units in this organization thus serve as central hubs for numerous affiliated researchers—MDs and PhDs from throughout the nation who are recruited by or seek out each unit's directors to collaborate on projects and funding bids. Also like the other IS-HSR centers, this unit is located within one of the system's regional service networks.

One particular interventional pilot project overseen by the unit—the implementation of a computerized disease screening reminder—served as the core case study for the research, and data were drawn from forty-one key informant interviews. My interpretation of the data was informed by my immersion in day-to-day business of the unit. Here I focus on those findings that have pragmatic bearing on the daily conduct of HSR and that show how the broader organizational environment within which IS-HSR takes place inevitably structures IS-HSR processes and, ultimately, its outcomes. Chapter 9 provided foundational knowledge regarding how research teams function; here, I illustrate what it is really like to work in HSR, be it anthropologically informed or otherwise.

There are many HSR sites other than the one I describe and many parts to the HSR system other than the IS branch. But because I believe that similar processes are at play and similar forces are in motion in each of these, the fine-grained, experiential information I provide serves as a useful window into the HSR enterprise. In all parts of this enterprise, at all institutions, workers similarly are driven to maximize their organizationally and professionally determined agendas, given the conditions under which they labor.

Nonetheless, the findings themselves pertain explicitly to IS-HSR. Furthermore, they are site- and study specific. The unit's leaders and I have agreed, therefore, to refer to the host organization and unit generically here and to remove identifiers from participant quotations when they are included below. This pragmatically defensive desire for anonymity reflects some of the very tensions about to be discussed, which are pervasive in HSR. Although the danger of protesting too much was noted by colleagues in the organization who preferred transparency as others hedged and prevaricated about how to position themselves in relation to the findings, the assured commonality of the patterns described cannot be understated. They can be seen throughout the world of HSR—some are seen perhaps even in other fields where the expectation for bringing in grant funding is high or new subdisciplines are emerging.

Portfolio Development Work

Each IS-HSR unit is charged with developing and maintaining a program of research relating to a particular set of diseases or conditions. Each strives to create a well-stocked portfolio of projects, quality improvement processes or products, and publications. Continued funding for the unit depends largely on success in doing so.

Program-building work often begins with a pilot project in a unit's home-base facility. If successful, the pilot is scaled up, pending competitive grant funding, to the regional level and, from there, it can go on to have national impact. Another portfolio-building tactic is to attract others to collaborate or otherwise affiliate their studies with the unit. "Prospecting" was one way in which participants in my research described this process.

In terms of day-to-day work for those in IS-HSR, the need for projects translates to constant activity and a modicum of confusion or indeterminacy. In the first instance, when ideas are just crystallizing and funding is scant or nonexistent, a project may seem very disorganized and undirected. Students or interns who arrange to work on a start-up project in IS-HSR can be quite dismayed when they learn just how disorganized things can be. Those considering a research career can be distressed to find out that investigators actually have to donate their time or work off the clock in some cases to get projects started or completed. This can be stressful for investigators, too.

Indeed, the particular pilot project taken as the core case study for this research—the screening reminder—was at first, in the words of some, a "patchwork": "You know," said one researcher participant, Person X "did it when she could and [person Y] did it when she could … but you know, they also have other competing demands." The respondent went on regarding the difficulties that competing demands entail: "[It] takes your focus away. … 'OK, I'll work on it for an hour' and then, 'Oh, I got called to do this.' And then you have to go back and refresh, and where are you, and start up over again. That's tough."

In part because studies are constantly being initiated, but also because many researchers have multiple affiliations, high workloads are pervasive in IS-HSR. IS-HS researchers report feeling stretched too thin or feeling fragmented. Juggling metaphors ("Too many balls up in the air at once"), spatial metaphors ("She's in multiple places"), and images of excess socializing ("Everybody's really exhausted, you know, or have a really full dance plate") also were offered. People not uncommonly participated in conference calls from cell phones while walking, driving, or otherwise in transit; one call participant dialed in from her seat on an airport shuttle.

Addressing the institutional structuring of such demands was not an option. For one thing, "People are working really long hours. … [B]ecause they feel the projects are important." As well, being busy demonstrates one's commitment to—and capacity for success in—the IS-HSR profession. Time to reflect on the structural causes of overwork is often unavailable anyhow: "I have not met any people who are able to step back long enough to even say, Well, what if we did it this way? They're just—they feel they're under pressure."

IS-HS researchers are acculturated to working hard, even without being paid for it. It helps them amass the research capital (pilot data, publications) necessary to back requests for full-scale research grants and helps enrich their curricula vitae (academic résumés). The financial metaphor here is participant derived: The fruits of their labors were often described in capitalist terms by researchers enrolled as participants in the IS-HSR study. As one explained: "The currency of the land, if you will, is in academic research publication and grants. … [This] satisfies professional needs [And] will inform the field … which itself is currency, if you will, from an academic perspective."

All research conducted through the IS-HSR unit under study, mine included, was funded by the federal government, not by charitable organizations or trusts. In the particular federal arena in question, proposals had to be shaped according to the clinical research model in which more publications lead to more grants. That is, although charitable funding organizations may be satisfied with program improvements, the

National Institutes of Health and its sister institutions generally are not: Dissemination of findings in peer-reviewed media is required. And this fostered and reinforced some of our participants' academic concerns.

The screening project was seen as a promising source for funding and esteem: "Basically it's going to put us on the map as far as, you know, the [funding] committee; they sort of—we live and die by their sword. And hopefully we avoid the sword." Note the knightly imagery, connoting the program's honor and chivalry as well as the sovereign power of the funder; the mapping metaphor references (in the broader discourse not reproduced here) the age of exploration, when new worlds were still being discovered.

One reason for all of the age-of-discovery-imagery that I encountered was the nature of IS-HSR. It is a fledgling field, emerging somewhere in the interstices between quality improvement (QI) and research proper (see Chapter 8). As one participant said, explaining IS-HS researchers' position as what he termed "bridge professionals":

> You live in two worlds and you're not necessarily well accepted by either of them. So you're treated with some degree of suspicion by your research buddies [laughs]. In fact I had somebody just say, "That's not research the way I define research. Why are you doing that?" And I have to do my little stump speech to make them understand that, you know, we're not the dumbed-down health services researchers. We are venturing into new territory where, frankly, we're making new discoveries and new insights.

Another metaphor sometimes offered was that of a new product or corporation; my field notes contain many references to "spreading the brand name." For instance, to this end, the unit's personnel orchestrated the use of its logo on poster presentations and project materials. Unit-logo coffee mugs also were distributed. Attempts to foster brand-name recognition is not uncommon in scholarly circles today: At one point during the drafting of this text, the board of the Society for Medical Anthropology was considering creating a logo and identity-confirming promotional items to sell. Such merchandising can be considered a fourth step in the professionalization process, although it traditionally is taught to have three (inception of a membership organization, a journal or media outlet for dissemination, and conferences or meetings for networking and sharing findings; see Chapter 8).

Grantland

"Grantland" represents a necessary landscape of reified wishes in which investigators carefully craft messages to foster an award or continued beneficence. The link between grant timelines and requirements (e.g., for pilot data) and the shape of the pilot intervention project was clearly articulated by participants. For example, one IS-HS researcher explained that projects in general "take place on the time cycle of grant renewals." Another mused, "I think that it drives it. ... The—I mean it starts with some of the timing about it. ... There are some tactical effects."

Grant applications must be carefully timed, so that a research group does not, in effect, compete with itself. A strategic, long-term plan for stepped and sequenced applications existed in the unit. Delaying a grant application for a full-scale screening intervention would sabotage this, setting back not only the screening project but others queued to apply for funding.

So, despite the confusing first few months and requests from collaborators and junior research team members to delay, the pilot project barreled ahead according to a schedule devised by counting back from the full grant's due date. To amass enough pilot data to submit a large grant application by the next due date, this was seen as the only option ("There's no chance it's going to get funded unless we have three months' data"). The findings here come from notes taken in regular, everyday, business-related group meetings between consented participants; they directly reflect actual interactive behavior.

Grantsmanship is about more than just timelines. It is also about skillful framing: Said an interviewee, "When we're going for funding it's portrayed as an implementation research project, loudly and boldly, because that's the audience that we're speaking to. ... Once you obtain the funding you can tailor the message of how the project is portrayed mostly at the site to ... retain buy in." Framing (or reframing) is sometimes deployed in program grant-writing and yearly reports. For example, one IS-HS researcher said in a meeting that a certain component of a planning document existed, "in grantland. It's constituted in our various strategic plans."

Navigating grantland requires skills not learned in school, according to wisdom shared, with laughter, during a meeting regarding a regional project. One IS-HS researcher joked in another such meeting about using the "underside" of his mind in strategizing. Creativity is required, and respected: "We know that this is a game and that, [if] we play well, we get the grant." Another, noting how high the stakes were, said on a conference call, "This is no game playing; this is reality."

Recruiting Collaboration: Beyond the Good Team Player Approach

Despite the need for projects and the possibility of justifying them in reference to theoretical debates within IS-HSR, "doing the right thing" was a common catch-phrase for all participants. Enacting a cross-culturally common rhetorical pattern that F. G. (Freddy) Bailey has meticulously described (1983) and that we reviewed in Chapter 2, most referred their actions to the overall mission or core values of the organization, appealing to culturally self-evident, incontestable imperatives. For instance, IS-HS researchers could justify the screening program as "a way to reach and test people that should be getting tested but aren't" or even as just being "good for patients."

In aligning themselves with QI and patient care goals, the IS-HS researchers distanced themselves from what clinical and operational collaborators saw as the disinterested nature of research (and see Chapter 9). But although they and collaborators thereby shared core values, each had differing means of promoting and measuring improvement. To collaborators, research work usually took too much time, yielding too little too late, primarily benefiting the research community at best, or individual researcher's careers at worst.

The IS-HS researchers were well aware of this perception and the subcultural differences indexed: "If you're seen as research, you're seen as somebody who comes in and imposes yourself, tries something out, picks up your marbles and leaves. And so you're very unpopular." Therefore, in addition to adopting the good team player persona suggested in Chapter 9, something more subversive—but equally well intentioned—is called for:

> We go into some sites and it's like, don't call this a research project, because no one's going to pay attention to you. ... So we've had these euphemism phrases that we've come up with so, for our [x] project we don't say "This is research." ... We go there and say, "Well this project focuses on improving the health and well being of [patients]." It's kind of the marketer coming out in me and in us. ... It's just word games with people, but you find a message that they will respond to—that resonates with them—and then we stick with it.

In the struggle to distinguish the project in question from clinical-trial-type research, this IS-HS researcher avoided the term "research" with clinical stakeholders, favoring alternate labels—labels that some argue better describe the quality-related aspects of what IS-HSR seeks to accomplish. This type of well-intentioned reframing helps IS-HS researchers make progress with their projects.

Well-meant reframing can backfire when an IS-HSR team's motives are overtly read as game playing or if intentions are unclear. For example, territoriality may be provoked among clinical collaborators if the IS-HS researchers' words or actions are interpreted as ploys to achieve traditional research (as opposed to QI) ends. When this happens, collaborators may use language strategically also, seeking to subvert IS-HSR work by attacking it either within the clinical care paradigm as not putting patients first, or within the clinical research paradigm as poorly designed, not evidence-based, unscientific, or not up to institutional review board (IRB) standards.

For instance, one collaborator, who was not a researcher, used such rhetoric when explaining his group's opposition to the pilot intervention team's push for a change in the screening reminder. It was her personal perception that this subverted the actual project leader's authority. This collaborator told the interviewer:

> [This screening reminder is] completely evidence-based. We looked at a whole [region's] data on what factors really would provide meaningful additional need for screening. Not something that was somebody's opinion. ... [The IS-HSR unit just had] a strong opinion about something that needed to be added for which they had no information or data. ... [Our] approach was to take it carefully and evaluate it and their approach was to add it now and be done with it.

Team Turnover

HSR units' personnel lists are, in my experience, often in flux and that of the unit under study was no exception. Two in five (44%, $n = 14$) participants were considering a job change when interviewed (only thirty-two of the forty-one participants were asked; I added the question after initial interviews and observations suggested it needed asking). Importantly, researchers were overrepresented here: Although accounting for only three in ten (31%) of those asked, they accounted for half (50%, $n = 7$) of the "yes" answers. Indeed, seven of the ten researchers asked said "yes."

These numbers are small and using percentages can therefore be seen as misleading; the proportion is not predictive. However, researchers do change jobs quite a lot. One reason for their overrepresentation among interviewees thinking about a job change was the mismatch between the organization's and academia's agendas. One organizational leader who was deeply supportive of IS-HSR asked: "How do you engage researchers and academically oriented people to do system-oriented work when you have two different sets of rules and really two cultures?"

Turnover also resulted from strategic processes entailed in building research careers, including the prospecting process (see above). Most health services researchers are not permanent organizational employees. Like academic institutions, the organization in question has "unfunded lines" for research professionals, who build their own salaries through grant procurement. This does ensure "some degree of competition [in funding] merit review. We need to be rigorous; we need to apply essentially the [logic of the] marketplace," as one participant put it. But market logic cuts two ways: Researchers are somewhat itinerant; they may switch primary affiliations when offered something better.

In managing their evolving research portfolios, IS-HS researchers sometimes put career needs before team or organizational needs. They may withhold information regarding long-term plans so that it cannot be used against them. Often such information omission leads to blind-siding; however, certain signs may be indicative of potential switch-ups. For instance, a fellow researcher's lack of follow-through can signal that an affiliation change or percent-time reduction on a given project is soon to come, as can more-frequent-than-usual travel. Such signs were observed several times over the course of this research; progress on various projects was hampered while career moves were negotiated.

Similarly, because grant competitions are stiff and grants come and go, IS-HS researchers may have extra grants in review at any given moment. Chapter 9 noted that researchers have to be "nimble" (a common term in HSR; used also by participants in the present project). Researchers must be able to quickly revise percent times itemized on particular projects in addition to bringing in research assistance as needed. But replacement personnel may lack the original investigators' skills and knowledge; highly rated proposals may not be as well executed as originally planned. Further, institutional knowledge maintenance can suffer. At the time I first drafted this paragraph, seven of ten IS-HSR units were undergoing core personnel transitions.

Common Themes and Institutional Responses

Although not all of the following themes were explored fully above (see also Sobo, Bowman, and Gifford 2008), my IS-HSR research showed overall that institutional factors—particularly funding mechanisms and their entailments—structure and ensure high workloads (e.g., administrative burdens, grant timelines, and the related pressure for projects). Attentions are divided—and morale and functionality compromised—not only by the high number of disparate projects undertaken but also by other affiliations and duties that membership in the IS-HS researcher's career world demands.

IS-HSR programs are challenged, then, not only by local contingencies but also by inbuilt or structurally driven system processes, such as those related to researchers' maintenance of academic status or program review and funding. Top-notch IS-HSR demands high productivity as part of the market mechanism used to distribute grant monies; this creates a cycle in which overstretched researchers can short-change funded projects (e.g., through reactive work strategies or percent-time reallocations) to foster new ones. Products are sometimes created to satisfy funders, reviewers, or gatekeepers rather than because of intrinsic scientific merit or ultimate applied use. In addition, as forecasted in Chapters 1 and 8, the marginal position of IS-HSR in relation to the broader health research industry creates and maintains conflicts for the IS-HSR researchers, and a good deal of time is spent negotiating these.

In my analysis, I purposefully involved several of the participants who were observed and interviewed. Specifically, I presented findings to five key stakeholders and incorporated their feedback (sometimes as authors) in the articles and presentations resulting from the work. In addition, these stakeholders responded dynamically to what was essentially an ongoing discussion, making changes in the program's internal, organizational practices and in some of the ways that program personnel interacted with external stakeholders.

For example, a more precise task and time accounting scheme was instituted to reduce difficulties in prioritization. To improve the project team's ability to follow through on research findings, direct contacts with operational leadership both at the national and regional level were greatly deepened.

I was very glad for the collaboration this work represented. Social links led to the direct application of a number of the findings that might otherwise have simply languished in shelved reports or been read and regarded by audiences that, no matter how important to me, are not in the position to apply them (i.e., if only published in anthropological journals).

Having said that, my colleagues' responses to the data and their reactions in terms of action were influenced greatly by their own structural positions within the host organization and their professional needs. Not all of my conclusions saw the light of day, and the vetting process often resulted in dismay as well as delay.

/ INSTITUTIONAL LOYALTIES

One of the challenges of IS-HSR is that, to do it, researchers must have some allegiance to the organization to be served. Interests can be vested because one's paycheck comes through the organization or because of the organization's gatekeeping function in regard to the research in question. Without an organization's blessing, we will not have safe passage within it to conduct our studies. This makes it good to play nice.

Of course, playing nice is not hard. We work in HSR to make positive things happen. We believe in the product we sell. We believe in showing the truth of a situation that needs improvement so that change for the better can be made to happen. The problem, then, is not one of sociality or maintaining optimism but rather one of social expectations. The problem stems from concerns over how far the limits of truth-telling can stretch.

Organizational Face-Saving

Data collection for the research described above mostly took place in summer 2005. On my computer desktop now sits what I hope is the final prepublication version of an article regarding the project that I began writing in spring 2006. The article has several coauthors, which, as readers will know by now, is quite typical in this kind of work. None are anthropologists, but that is for the best: Being pushed by colleagues to clarify myself for the HSR audience rather than relying on obfuscating jargon no doubt helped strengthen this article immensely, as it has others.

Requests for translation were especially prominent in comments on my initial efforts to cross disciplinary publication divides. However, with this particular manuscript, their frequency and vigor seemed strangely renewed. Further, challenges emanated even for fairly straightforward terms, such as "reframing," used impartially in the social sciences to describe the omnipresent practice of strategically representing an idea or event to others. This and related terms were misread by some coauthors and other insiders who previewed the article as denoting improper conduct among study participants. That was an unwarranted conclusion. Nonetheless, I altered my phrasing accordingly.

Being misread by colleagues and organizational members is bad enough, but the consequences of being so badly misconstrued by outsiders once findings were published could have been dire. Reputations—both individual and organizational—might have been damaged and legal action—however unsustainable—could have been threatened. Concern over such consequences explains why, despite careful caveats made in every publication dealing with this project explaining that the processes and patterns reported pervade the industry, any section of the article that had the slightest chance of being misinterpreted by a reader had to be redrawn (yes, reframed)—or cut out of the story completely. Doing so took over a year because of the time coauthors needed to frame their responses. Although the type of time scarcity described above did play into this, so too may have certain coauthors' hesitance to confront the issues that the article raised.

In summer 2007, after intense discussions, one coauthor suggested we consult (and thereby add as coauthor) another colleague. I complied. The article was submitted in early fall, revised in keeping with reviewer requests, resubmitted in late winter, and recommended for publication in late spring 2008—bringing the timeline to about two and one-half years post-data collection. The bulk of time elapsed while waiting for responses from the various coauthors (not reviewers for the journal, as sometimes is the case).

Much to my chagrin, as soon as publication was recommended, the article was brought back to the starting line by a coauthor who not only wished to wordsmith it all over again but also saw the need for others higher up in the organization to read and comment. This individual's stand at the eleventh hour was annoying at best. It can only be understood in light of the context of this coauthor's professional life. In the time since the article was drafted, vetted, submitted, revised, resubmitted, and recommended, there had been several authorial affiliation changes as well as numerous changes in the host organization, including personnel turnover in important offices and shifts in the political landscape. And this was what drove my coauthor's apparent madness—which was quite logical after all, when understood in context.

I cannot deny that it is, frankly, inefficient and frustrating to keep adding authors, soliciting new readers, and receiving revisions. Having to reframe statements that readers familiar with sociology and anthropology would not deem problematic does try my inner social scientist's patience. But in the end, because my preference is to see the implicated findings disseminated and acted on rather than hidden under wraps, my willingness to engage in such extended vetting and reframing is expedient. That is what counts.

Without such attention to detail, the findings described might be taken out of context to draw inaccurate conclusions regarding the host organization. The problem of representation has received a great deal of attention in anthropology. In addition to epistemological concerns (see Chapters 6 and 8), scholars have debated the ethical aspects of disseminating findings. The American Anthropological Association's Committee on Ethics has prepared a brief regarding the need to consider the potentially negative impact of the publication of factual data on the study population (Watkins 2008). Our ethical obligations to those studied—even when those studied are part of a large integrated health care organization—cannot be taken lightly.

But there is more at stake here than the ethical concern to do the right thing. Helping the organization save face through careful word selection helps me maintain good relations with collaborators within the organization and, by extension, with the organization itself. It would be unethical for me to omit mention of my vested interest in maintaining these ties. In light of the findings presented in the foregoing section and my pledge to illuminate the tensions inherent in attempting to make a living doing anthropologically informed HSR, I must not downplay the link between the article in question's evolution and my own organizationally and professionally structured desire for career advancement. As more than one participant in my IS-HSR research noted, the coin of the realm—and this is so in my profession as in theirs—is measured out in terms of research publications. Investing several years in a potential publication only to see it disowned because of one wrong word choice was not, therefore, a strategically sensible option for me.

My colleagues, too, have vested interests that go beyond simple organizational face-saving. They do not want the article to go to press without having had key stakeholders in the screening program process read it. This is not only because these individuals might have helpful edits but also because they may feel left out or disrespected if not included. This could affect program roll-out or progress for my colleagues. Moreover, the key stakeholders may be called to task by the media, their constituents, or even governmental agencies for challenges we report. This could cause them problems if they do not have ready answers based on prior knowledge of the article and its contents.

For all of the reasons above, to make absolutely certain that readers get the story right, I continued to work with my colleagues on the article's language. Lest one point has been lost let me reiterate: This does not mean hiding dirty laundry. My colleagues on the project at hand are keen to learn from past experiences. The aim of their program is service improvement. The host organization, like many health service organizations both major and minor, is keen on transparency. But through a publication, the public may learn of some of this particular organization's challenges. Because the public may not have the contextual background to properly interpret the challenges reported, message control is paramount. The amount of time added in this case is on the high side. But some delay should always be expected so that any potential sensitivities may be identified and diffused. Simply put, except in the direst circumstances (i.e., when essential ethical standards actually are being flouted and no other recourse is at hand), it is neither smart nor effective to make key stakeholders feel bad.

In addition to paying careful attention to every word the article contains, action taken in response to findings is now described in the body of the article (which did achieve publication by the time the present book was copyedited; see Sobo, Bowman, and Gifford 2008). By making this addition, the screening program's directors could show the powers that be how proactive the program is. They could demonstrate that the program has evolved. They also could make moral claims regarding their belief in transparency and commitment to health care improvement.

Whims of Leadership

In addition to the kind of internal politics described in regard to grant-getting, research, and publication, researchers need to be aware of organizational leadership's priorities in general. These do sometimes change quickly, for example, in response to accreditation reports, congressional decisions, new industry requirements, or what might be termed "industry trends." Also, critical incidents can be major forces in fostering intense shifts of interest to particular safety issues. In my experience, I have seen such disparate things as oral health, care pathways or guidelines, wait times, employee-driven improvement studies, wrong-site surgery, medical record documentation practices, patient identification, pain management, and patient satisfaction variously prioritized by those in top command. It is good to be flexible and to have the nimbleness necessary to respond as needed.

Safety was a big issue when the Institutes of Medicine released their report *To Err Is Human*, documenting the human and financial costs of safety problems such as harmful medical errors and providing a state-of-the-art review of how to prevent them (Kohn, Corrigan, and Donaldson 2000). Interest has remained relatively high, but distraction is inevitable. Having said that, a big attentional booster shot was delivered in summer 2007 when it was announced that Medicare would no longer reimburse for the treatment of preventable hospital-acquired illness, injury, or infection. That is, the costs of treating problems like bedsores, injuries caused when patients fall out of bed, complications from inpatient medication dosage errors or from administering the wrong medicines, and surgical sponges forgotten in the body will now have to be absorbed by hospitals themselves for patients that would otherwise have been covered by Medicare. Private insurers may soon follow suit. Safety is now back on the radar in a big way. Although this will generate some wonderful new studies and fuel much positive action, any such change in priorities will ripple down through an organization, affecting even the types of topics that are seen to merit a research focus. In-house researchers may find themselves pulled now—or pushed—to do more safety research—and less research of another kind.

Some shifts in priority are slow or incremental; others can be fast and seem almost whimsical. In-house researchers have joked in my presence about being windblown.

Recall how busy many IS-HS researchers are. In the words of one researcher who participated in the study described above, perceived whims of leadership complicated the task of juggling "the 40 balls that I keep in the air." There was a common perception that leadership did "change the rules on us a lot; which they've been changing the rules every year since I've been here." Because of changes, "You go from being the top dog, the honor student, to being nearly expelled; and then back up to being honor student." Performance anxiety was palpable, but the researchers I talked with seemed willing to move with the organization, even if sometimes a bit resentfully, in the interest of doing good work.

Authorship

The IS-HSR units described above each have at least one core IS-HSR specialist working to coordinate the IS-HSR efforts of the unit and its affiliates. The specialists, and other officially junior researchers as well as some staff members, spend a great deal of time drafting grant proposals and preparing posters, presentation papers, and articles for senior collaborators to finalize. This is not uncommon in health services and medical research (see Flanagin et al. 1998). But it seemed strange to me when I joined in full in 1999. Indeed, on entry, I experienced a kind of culture shock adjusting to the standards for authorship.

I am not sure how I cottoned onto it, but sometime before my first article bearing the Children's affiliation was published, it occurred to me that I needed to list my boss as coauthor. My reaction, as I digested this realization, was somewhat akin to moral horror. I genuinely like this boss, who continues to mentor and collaborate with me. He is wise and well respected. He took good care of his employees and had high ethical standards for himself as well as those around him. However, he had not actually done anything authorial on the project in question—at least as my home discipline of anthropology would have seen it.

As I took in the fact that my boss was everyone's coauthor, I also began to notice how many projects listed his name as principal investigator, even though others seemed to be doing the work and had written the proposals. I built up a head of resentment. Surely, this was not right.

I managed to repress some of my anger: I did not want to jeopardize my job. And for at least that first publication I could rationalize including his name because, after all, I had joined that project late and did not know what my boss had actually set in motion before I took the reins. This was despite some doubts: The publication in question was completely my doing, anthropological in scope, and not a listed deliverable but instead penned by me as an add-on.

For the next publication, however, I saw no route to easy acquiescence. It was true that my boss was the one who requested that I investigate something to do with minor head injury (costs for treatment of which seemed to outweigh any health outcomes benefits, as previously noted). He did make a few suggestions regarding how I might best glean information from relevant physicians (using a self-administered survey rather than attempting face-to-face interviews; see Chapter 13). He did request permission from the relevant clinical and administrative leaders for me to attend a meeting where I could pilot my survey. These were all crucial actions. However, they were not the actions of an author—at least not anthropologically speaking.

In anthropology, single authorship is the norm. Times are changing slowly as more and more of us venture into collaborative work, but the norm still holds, as demonstrated in the questions my own collaborations have generated in recent reviews of my performance at the university where I now work. This norm is partly the legacy of the lone fieldworker tradition and the independent nature of most ethnographic undertakings. At least until recently, analysis was done in the head of the fieldworker and in his or her head alone. In this, anthropology is more like philosophy or mathematics than patient care or other endeavors where no one person can do it all.

Someone who helps an anthropologist gain access to a community, or provides information on approaches that a community may be most receptive to, or pays for the work, or even helps generate ideas on topics to work on is not, in anthropology, thereby an author. There are ways to acknowledge technical and other forms of assistance—but they do not include space in the by-line. Spurring ideas, administering surveys, copyediting penultimate drafts—these things garner hourly pay or a drink at the pub rather than authorship. Even someone who helps the anthropologist improve his or her ideas by making a cutting or insightful comment during a conversation concerning the work or after reading a draft of an article gets no more than an acknowledgment in the published version. Space on the by-line would be out of the question except for someone who participated fully in conceiving and writing the article. This does mean that getting an acknowledgment in an anthropological publication is itself something of an accomplishment.

It is not that authorship is highly guarded by anthropologists in any active sense. It's more that it is very rarely requested without good reason and, as such, it is not a topic given much overt consideration.

Moreover, unlike in medical journals, because coauthorship generally ends at two or three when it does occur in anthropology, there has been no need as yet for journal editors to take a stand or set any limits. Biomedical journals now often ask for signed author statements, many with space to detail the actual contribution that was made and affirm that authorship is warranted. Some actually limit the number of authors who can be listed. For instance, a journal I recently submitted to had only six author slots. This might seem ample to anthropologists, but the number of collaborators in medical research can run to double digits.

Anthropology is lacking in any agreed-on code for authorship standards, in part because authorship has rarely been an area of disputation and thus has not been an area in which standards have needed delineation. Collaboration in anthropology that might lead to concerns over authorship has generally been limited to teacher-student collaboration, not collaboration among putative equals who might dispute rights. Perhaps because of the increase in perceived needs to publish and an increase in student status as compared to their instructors, some are beginning to call for codified ethical standards (see, for example, Seidmann 2006).

However, anthropology's common-law standards are similar to those of other social sciences. For example, according to the British Sociological Association or BSA, which codified authorship expectations in 2001:

> Authorship should be reserved for those, and only those, who have made significant intellectual contribution to the research. Participation solely in the acquisition of funding or general supervision of the research group is not sufficient for authorship. Honorary authorship is not acceptable.
>
> 1. Everyone who is listed as an author should have made a substantial direct academic contribution (i.e. intellectual responsibility and substantive work) to at least **two** of the four main components of a typical scientific project or article:
>   a) Conception or design
>   b) Data collection and processing
>   c) Analysis and interpretation of the data
>   d) Writing substantial sections of the article (e.g., synthesising findings in the literature review or the findings/results section)
> 2. Everyone who is listed as an author should have critically reviewed successive drafts of the article and should approve the final version.
> 3. Everyone who is listed as author should be able to defend the article as a whole (although not necessarily all the technical details). (2001; emphasis in the original)

An editorial written by Sally Macintyre when she was Editor-in-Chief of *Social Science & Medicine* also noted confusion on the part of submitters regarding what constituted authorship (and on "the requirement for originality"; 1997, p. 1).

Such problems have only recently come to plague the social sciences, in part because of the recent increase in collaborative and interdisciplinary work. But in medicine, Uniform Requirements for authorship were put in place in 1978 by the International Committee of Medical Journal Editors (ICMJE). Even when not interdisciplinary, medical research is generally a team undertaking involving many individuals and, as such, it makes sense that authorship would become an issue there first.

What did the ICMJE recommend? Something much like the BSA standards, which, to be fair, were influenced by those of the ICMJE (listed in the BSA guideline document's references section; the Committee of Publication Ethics, another medical journal editors' group, also is suggested as a resource).

Although the Uniform Requirements have by now been around for a long time, the context in which publishing happens has changed. In the late 20th century, increasing pressure among academics to publish to advance in their careers spurred an onslaught of dodgy submissions meant only to please tenure and promotion committees and ensure the renewal of contracts. Alternately, as revealed to me through my participant observation regarding the amalgamation between Children's and the region's School of Medicine, clinicians seeking to advance their credibility in the university world also may claim undue authorial credits. Concurrently, they may be offered them, for political reasons, by the real authors or their agents (e.g., authors' bosses).

This kind of bequeathed authorship is politely called "honorary" or "courtesy" authorship (or, less politely, "cosmetic"). It can be opposed to the kind generally undertaken by my masters-prepared colleagues at Children's, which is politely termed (when termed at all) "ghost." These individuals remained unacknowledged in the by-lines because, after all, their careers did not depend on it, they were paid for it, and they were uninterested, or so it was said. An additional factor here is that, as contract staffers, they often had moved on to implement other projects by the time a given article was published.

A review of peer-reviewed articles in medical journals showed that one in five articles included honorary authors. Ghost authors contributed to or wrote one in ten articles (Flanagin et al. 1998). In another research study, common reasons given for including honorary authors had to do with repaying favors, encouraging collaboration (including not wanting to offend bosses), maintaining good working relationships, and increasing the potential for a manuscript's acceptance by including famous names (Bhopal et al. 1997).

My understanding of these issues was enhanced by my IS-HSR research. Recall my mention above of the way that the IS-HSR specialists spent so much time writing grant proposals and preparing posters, presentation papers, and articles for senior collaborators to finalize. They even drafted text for some letters of commitment, to be signed by collaborators or officials.

Information on text production and authorship that I collected during that project corroborated what the emerging literature on scholarly writing tells us happens. But I also learned concretely through my experience over time in HSR to view authorship through a functionalist lens.

That is, authorship may also be a key mechanism for holding research projects together because of the gatekeeping function that courtesy authors hold. For example, in one organization, when an essential collaborator who had been asked to review two conference abstracts (proposals) failed to respond, project leaders decided to add her name anyhow. Her authorship implied her endorsement of the work, and although someone would eventually have to call her to get her permission to use her name, so long as she approved the work it could and would be used despite the fact that approval would have been her only tangible authorial contribution.

In sum, authorship decisions have a lot to do with power dynamics and dependencies. As a senior leader at Children's advised me when I mentioned to him that the senior-most leader wanted to "collaborate" with me on an article, "You don't say no to the CEO." By that time, I had become accustomed to the cultural norms promoting honorary and ghost authorship. I saw our exchange as conspiratorial, and I think he did too. Yet our insider cultural critique was not really subversive; it did not change the course of my actions.

Although I did, eventually, acculturate to this type of norm, the depth of my anguish in the first year of my work at Children's is etched on an old backup CD that includes a special folder called "authorship." In the folder are several documents regarding authorship criteria, including some of the articles just cited and published criteria that were, in practice, being flouted.

Gaps between written policy and actual process are not unusual. Even when accurately documented in policy form, common practice can evolve. Or, as in this situation, laws, policies, standards, and such are generated under what might be termed "border" or "frontier" conditions, in which one group's standard is contradicted by another's, or where a shift in norms is happening quickly but not smoothly or uniformly. Policy here (e.g., the Uniform Requirements) is meant to help.

As part of my own attempt to foster adherence to written standards, in an act of great cultural incompetence, I created an authorship handout for distribution at a staff meeting. I still feel palpable relief, when I think about this plan, that I never actually followed through. Eventually, I realized that a far better thing to do was to adapt to established local norms—at least in the near term—and experience the lessons that first-hand participant observation can teach.

I have so far shared a good number of the key lessons that my participant observation within HSR has taught me. We have peeked behind the curtain of the research endeavor to examine some of its sociocultural structuring. The next and final task before us is to explore how, in the present cultural context of health services, anthropologically informed HSR findings are best disseminated. For it is in doing so—and thereby touching the lives of others—that even the hard parts of working in HSR can come to have their deepest meaning.

CHAPTER 15

/ Framing Our Message: Telling Stories, Making Action

When I worked in clinical trials, a PhD nutritionist on another project asked for some resources regarding breastfeeding. I found some classic anthropological works for her. A week or so later, in passing, I asked her what she thought of them. My question was met with her own, which went something like this: "Why do you anthropologists write such darn long papers?"

The nutritionist's point was that the essays I gave her may have contained interesting, even helpful, information, but she had not figured out how to parse that out. She was not versed in the anthropological genre of descriptive writing, which can go on for pages and pages before any generalization gets made. And sometimes, no generalization is actually forthcoming. Local practices are described as just that, with no take-home lessons or messages appended.

How does the health services research or HSR administrator or program head or policymaker—or researcher—deal with that? What can he or she do with a publication whose author never stops talking and yet refuses to take an actionable stand? In this chapter, I explore the options and make some suggestions of my own for broadcasting anthropologically informed messages so that they not only can be heard but can also end in action.

/ KNOWING AND REACHING YOUR AUDIENCE

Recall the hematology and oncology (heme-onc) work reviewed in Part IV regarding parent concerns and preferences. I drew out the links between the findings and the methods used to derive them; I demonstrated the anthropologically informed nature of study results.

But how did I treat the findings when reporting to heme-onc directors? How did I frame them for hospital leadership? Not the same way I framed them for this book's readers—and not the same way I framed them for publication as research articles. What is the key inference to make here? Know your audience.

Importantly, my internal report on the initial heme-onc project (which will be our example here) began with an executive summary that was two pages long. While it was, in that, a bit longer than most, it had many bulleted points, which is common for the genre. They focused on action recommendations that were easy to see and understand.

It is up to us to provide actionable, data-driven ideas; readers or employers have neither the time nor the desire to dig for needles in haystacks, let alone pearls of wisdom. We must overtly declare our value to them by providing specifics on what can or should be done. Moreover, it is good for these ideas to come from us not only so that key puzzle pieces are not overlooked by audience members too busy or whatnot to read our full write-ups but also so that any action taken will be anthropologically informed. Who knows better what knock-on ramifications a given change may make than the investigator who has either participated in a population's life world extensively or had enough extra-project experience to infer with enough precision what that life may be like?

Thus, although the body of the report (which was actually several dozen pages) presented parents' key concerns as parents expressed them, the executive summary did not. For that (see Table 15.1), I grouped parents' concerns in terms of the 2001 Institute of Medicine (IOM) report's then-very-popular quality domains: safety, effectiveness, efficiency, timeliness, patient centeredness, and equity (Institute of Medicine Committee on Quality of Health Care in America 2001). Importantly, the terms used in the recommendations were active, specific, and directive. I underlined and bolded key instructions. There was no need for anyone to second-guess.

Although some would see the representation of the data in IOM terms as having done violence to the emic point of view, I saw it more as building a crosswalk between the parent's perspective and bureaucratic imperatives. In making the translation, I was able to help leadership as well as my quality management colleagues more efficiently incorporate parents' voices into the aims and objectives of future quality improvement work. New projects would be easier to justify in relation to one or more of the domains, especially when resources were requested.

More immediately, in talking about the project with heme-onc leaders and core staff, some red flags were noted. For instance, when we told them a few of the stories that parents had told us, consciousness was raised in the unit about the need for standardization—even for techniques that do not necessarily need to be standardized from the medical perspective. Efforts by supervisors to impose standardization can seem totalitarian, but in this case the nurses learned, through direct feedback of project findings, that families could be confused and frightened by the lack of uniformity. Therefore, the nurses took it on themselves to

Table 15.1 Parent concerns by quality domain (see Sobo et al. 2002)*

1. Safety
   - Improve the coordination, consistency, and reliability of medication administration across shifts, at care transitions, and at discharge.
   - Insure that a specific and scripted medication review consistently occurs at the time of discharge from the hospital or clinic.
   - Provide more detailed and specific information/resource materials regarding medication, (e.g., re: side effects, adverse drug reactions, complementary and alternative medicine, what to do if when a child vomits after having taken their medication).
   - Provide, or assist parents in the development of, tools to facilitate accurate medication administration and compliance (e.g., lists with pronunciations; date and time calendars).
2. Effectiveness
   - Improve communication between clinicians (e.g., nurses and nurses; nurses and physicians).
   - Provide additional medication administration training for after discharge.
   - Provide, or assist parents in the development of, tools to facilitate accurate medication administration and compliance (e.g., lists with pronunciations; date and time calendars).
3. Efficiency
   - Reduce long wait times (Infusion Center specifically cited).
   - Provide pagers to families while they are waiting for services, or results to become available.
   - Review patient flow to optimize a patient's access to care.
   - Improve availability of and accessibility to test results.
4. Timeliness
   - Provide pain relief in a more timely fashion.
   - Review patient flow to optimize a patient's access to care.
5. Patient Centeredness
   - Standardize all nursing procedures and techniques so that patients and families experience consistency, predictability, and equality in the care that is being provided.
   - Improve communication between clinicians and families (e.g., more direct time and contact with physicians; require staff to introduce themselves when entering the room and explain what they are going to do and why; provide parents with a greater understanding of what to expect, and when to expect it).
   - Develop a tool to segment our families by information needs or preferences in conjunction with the degree of responsibility they would like to take for any decisions related to their child's medical care.
   - Improve availability of and accessibility to test results.
   - Provide Internet access for families to access on-line resources (e.g. PubMed, web pages).
6. Equity
   - Enhance existing translation services so that we can increase our ability to provide a consistent high level of care to all of the patients and families that we serve.
   - Standardize all nursing procedures and techniques so that patients and families experience consistency, predictability, and equality in the care that is being provided.

*Where relevant, recommendations are included in two categories.

promote standardization when possible (e.g., in regard to how the skin is prepared for an injection). This effort was extended to include physician practices, when possible (e.g., in regard to face masks, necessary for some patients but which doctors would continue to wear with subsequent patients, frightening them and their families needlessly).

This demonstrates how measures to promote improvement can be facilitated by the type of data collected. Qualitative data that takes narrative form can be helpful in encouraging care team and other organization members to empathize with the families served. That is, relevant and representative stories can be deployed strategically in the context of well-framed overall dissemination of findings so that members of an organization or target audience more fully absorb the main points made by participants. This, in turn, helps mobilize action.

PACKAGING STORIES IN AN ACTIONABLE FORMAT

Chapter 2 reviewed the power of stories, establishing a precedent for systematically collecting and analyzing them if we are to truly understand today's health services delivery challenges. Toward this chapter's end, I will talk about stories' content. Before doing so, however, it is crucial to discuss how to package the master stories in which individual tales are embedded—how to frame one's total research narrative. Why? Because if we are to tell good stories—stories that will catch the ear of the health services world—we have to be willing to package them in an actionable format. Telling it like it is is useless unless we also tell something of what it all means: Recommendations must be made and they must be made in a way that makes them useful.

Recall the short length of the executive summary in the heme-onc case. Aim for brevity always, because the health care workday demands it. Nobody has the leisure to read a forty-page anthropology article, let alone an ethnographic monograph. Although the length issue in publications is to some degree decided for us by length limits in health care–relevant journals (3,000 words or twelve pages is not unusual), one answer to the accusation that we write too much is to confine long-winded descriptive sections to a data appendix, if that is allowable. In the case described above for heme-onc, the report's body was essentially that. It also formed the basis for the subsequent publication, because of the degree of detail it contained, and was made available to the interested organizational reader.

Another tactic that can make even a semi-long article seem short is avoiding jargon. There is no use for words that confuse or stymie readers (let alone coauthors; see Chapter 14). Although some might say that the use of technical terms promotes more specific and focused thinking, this is important within and not between fields when discussions are not theoretical or methodological. That is, save the technical erudition for peers. For the commissioning audience, communicate in as straightforward a way as possible. Some mechanics have started using illustrations when explaining to consumers which valves were checked or belts were changed. Some pharmacies have streamlined prescription vial labeling. We must do the same, simplifying when possible in an effort to democratize the knowledge that we have to share—and in an effort to make sure that it is remembered and perceived of as useful.

A key aspect of the ethnographic tradition entails sharing with readers the richness of what we find. But nothing dulls a point like repetition. Although it is difficult to eject quotations lovingly elicited from our participants, it gets easier to do if one thinks of such quotes as photographs in an overly chatty office-mate's chunky vacation photo album or part of a too-friendly neighbor's substantial family reunion slide show. Keep only those quotations that are necessary to make your point. And, whenever possible, use a case study or story that sums up the meanings you wish to convey in a narrative format. Stories stir up emotions in a way that hanging quotations or dry facts—even ethnographic facts—generally cannot do. Even when merely suggestive or indicative rather than statistically significant and predictive, findings linked together in a storyline that stimulates emotions can motivate audience members to act on a researcher's data-based suggestions. Emotion compels us to get things done.

Reports are not the only way to get one's story heard; in fact, presentations will have more power in the immediate organization you seek to affect. A good story can be told in person. Others can repeat it with ease. Avoiding jargon certainly helps here, but so does crafting memorable and appropriately evocative sound bites and creating eye-catching visual illustrations that others will want to share. In HSR, it is neither unusual nor unethical for one's boss or director to borrow one's presentation to use for presenting the same material to his or her own boss, or peers. Indeed, such reuse often signifies a job well done.

To ensure that a presentation is useful (or reused), create it in a common medium, such as PowerPoint. Make it short. Make it visually appealing. Use the relevant organization's logo and a plain professional rather than faddish distracting template.

Some common rules of thumb for content are to use no more than five lines of text per slide and to use short phrases rather than sentences. Do not include quotes to be read; rather, put up pictures to express meanings symbolically and read your quotations (which may be reproduced on a handout that has other study information or transcribed into the speaker's notes plane of the presentation program, if there is one). Be sure to end the presentation with a short list of action recommendations, or proof of improved outcomes if you have it.

If you have an employer or client who will want to give the presentation him- or herself (and sometimes this is the best way to ensure recommendations are acted on), provide notes so that he or she will not be caught short in trying to reproduce the presentation. It is also good to provide notes so that anyone who views the presentation on-line or without your narration will be able to follow the presentation's argument. This dissemination model is different from the one prominent in academia, but intellectual property is much less of an issue in the health services arena, where the focus is not on who did a thing but what it can do.

Finally, whether disseminating findings on paper or in a presentation, an appeal to finances never hurts. For instance, the screening program that I described in the last chapter was promoted first and foremost as a cost-efficient strategy: Treating patients early is less expensive than treating patients who discover their disease or gain access to care late in the game. Importantly, the screening program would not result in cost savings, such as might have been the case for, for example, decreasing computed tomography or CT scanning for minor head injury (see Chapter 13). On the contrary, getting more people into treatment now meant budgets would be affected now. It was important to anticipate and troubleshoot financial objections so that answers might be stockpiled for use in presentations promoting the screening program. For instance, some skeptics worried about whose budget the screening test kits or extra screening-related counseling hours would come from, but being prepared with answers helped offset such nay-saying.

/ STORYTELLING AND SCHOLARLY WORK

I mentioned that a few relevant and representative stories might be told in the context of a well-framed report or presentation to aid the target audience in making meaning from the findings. Psychologist Stephen Denning explains, "Storytelling is natural and easy and entertaining and energizing. Stories help us understand complexity. Stories can enhance or change perceptions. Stories are easy to remember. Stories are inherently non-adversarial and non-hierarchical. They bypass normal defense mechanisms and engage our feelings" (2001, p. xv). All well and good, but how do these ideas fit with the ideals of or figure into high-quality scholarly research, even under our revised definition of "science"?

Sitting around telling stories is not the sign of good scholarship, and I hope that the preceding chapters made a clear demonstration of and a compelling argument for the necessity of giving the most considered attention to our methods as we attentively and systematically operationalize our variables and collect and analyze our data. The evidence base for anthropologically informed research is not anecdotal.

Having established the importance of a methodical and methodologically motivated approach, I hope also to have convinced the reader that research does not take place in a vacuum. Moreover, we cannot responsibly ignore the contexts in which research results are released. Research that nobody pays attention to cannot make an impact. Concurrently, for better or for worse, researchers who cannot tell good stories are less likely to be read or heard than those who can, whatever the quality of the research product. And stories are the stock and trade of anthropologically informed research: Enacted or told by our research participants, stories are part of the outwardly "great blooming, buzzing confusion" (James 1918 [1890], p. 488)—the cultural world—from which we extract data. We have them, so we should use them. In this, we can take a leaf from the ethnographic tradition.

Ethnography (the Noun)

Clifford Geertz's popularization of "thick description" (see Chapter 2) was, in the eyes of at least one of my medical colleagues, synonymous with anthropology. For Geertz, ethnography was anthropology's key branch; it seeks to "uncover the conceptual structures that inform our subjects' acts" (1973, p. 27).

As Geertz has written, after Weber, because "man is an animal suspended in webs of significance he himself has spun ... the analysis of [culture is] therefore not an experimental science in search of law but an interpretive one in search of meaning. It is explication" (1973, p. 5). Ethnographies are written to provide readers "access to the conceptual world in which our subjects live so that we can, in some extended sense of the term, converse with them" (p. 24). Put slightly differently, ethnographic writing exists "to make available to us answers that others ... have given, and thus to include them in the consultable record of what man [*sic*] has said" (p. 30).

Through ethnography, anthropologists—ethnographers—proffer for the rest of us (or anyhow intend to or try to proffer or present) a given group's conceptual world, seen and experienced from the inside. As journalist Anne Fadiman said when describing, to an interviewer, her experience examining a case of clinical misunderstanding in which culture played a role, "I pulled on the thread and the thread became a string and the string became a rope, and then I tugged really hard on the rope and I discovered that it was attached to the entire universe" (Anderson [2001], as cited in Taylor 2003).

Ethnographers do, of course, have other aims than exposing cultural universes. However, ethnographic storytelling is a powerful way to help evoke in the reader a holistic understanding of what it might be like to be a member of a given cultural group at a given time in history—of what it means to be, for example, a parent of a child with cancer or Down syndrome, a person asked to sign a consent form for surgery, a provider asked to incorporate yet another screening test reminder (and a time-intensive one at that) into an already packed clinic visit, or a nurse attempting to infer how involved a particular patient might like to be in his or her own care. In this, its evocative dimension, much of good ethnography entails good writing—or telling a good, research-based story.

It was not always thus. Evocation was not always an ethnographic goal. Early ethnography generally consisted mainly of lists of "culture traits" or blow-by-blow recounts of ritual sequences, some of which lasted for days. In part, this reflected early anthropology's keen desire to establish the scientific or at least systematic nature of the discipline. As such, early anthropologists often followed what they viewed as a scientific style of data presentation. Further, there was little appreciation for cultural dynamism or change (except for the hope that non-Europeans would evolve to be more "civilized"). Practices or viewpoints that seemed modern or looked borrowed were often simply ignored as inauthentic in the ethnographer's quest to document "traditional" lifestyles.

All told, early ethnography was often dry and nearly always nonreflexive. Today, however, anthropologists recognize the authorial power of the ethnographer as well as the benefit of a story well told.

Much of the impetus that came for reconsidering the act of "writing culture" and acknowledging the power and representational issues entailed in ethnographic writing came from outside anthropology at first. For instance, in the art-and-literature world, postmodernism had taken hold; this entailed disillusion with positivist science for not living up to its promises as well as some suspicion (which would increase in the late 20th century; see Chapter 8) regarding the notion of one scientifically discoverable and verifiable truth or reality. Postmodernism openly discussed the role of the author in delimiting and defining the boundaries and terms of a given debate through choices regarding word use, which topics to cover, and which to ignore; as well, it promoted more subjective approaches. Inspired, a number of cultural anthropologists published what were to become a highly influential set of essays regarding the power dynamics at play in the ethnographic endeavor (Clifford and Marcus 1986). The creative aspect of writing in anthropology was highlighted.

Some of today's impetus toward more humanistic writing also stemmed from the huge market success of books like Anne Fadiman's aforementioned best seller, *The Spirit Catches You and You Fall*

Down (1997), a heartbreaking, award-winning story about an adverse series of encounters between a Hmong family and the biomedical and social services systems in the United States. Anthropologists are sometimes embarrassed by the fact that this best-selling book, which deals directly with key anthropological issues, was written by a journalist. They also have expressed concern with the problematic way in which certain anthropological concepts, such as the culture concept itself, are represented. But *The Spirit Catches You* is, nonetheless, an excellent read.

In her astute critique of the book, Janelle Taylor queries its author Anne Fadiman's success in reaching both the biomedical community and the public at large with an anthropologically influenced message, and doing so in a way that was far more effective than any anthropologist to date (barring perhaps Margaret Mead). Taylor notes that one reason for this—and a key reason indeed—has to do with the compelling narrative drive that Fadiman's authorial choices such as regarding genre, plot, and motive give to the story (Taylor 2003).

As Taylor shows, *"The Spirit Catches You* is so influential as ethnography because it is so moving as a story; it is so moving as a story because it works so well as a tragedy" (2003, p. 159). That is, it sets up an essential tension between two goods, implying an inevitable (tragic) outcome. Through this narrative device, tragedies arouse emotions (e.g., pity, fear) and allow us to engage in catharsis, by which we purge such emotions. This is one of the "narrative pleasures" of the tragedy genre. It is a pleasure that even academics can succumb to although, as Taylor notes in regard to her own experience, and by extension that of many academics who read Fadiman's book, "indulging in narrative pleasures [is] quite at odds with the theoretical principles that I admire." Earlier, she had defined these, and so "good" anthropology, as able to articulate an understanding of culture as complex, processual, and performative (p. 160; and see Chapter 6).

This antagonism notwithstanding, Fadiman's book sold. It touched hearts—probably millions. Perhaps, muses Taylor, its narrative and others like it work "through a special form of shamanic activity. Storytellers, like shamans, specialize in producing those trancelike states in which invisible and mute souls show themselves, and speak" (2003, p. 173). Taylor likens being engrossed in a book or a story with being caught by "the spirit." The experience of reading a really good book is thereby "powerfully real" (p. 174).

To get our own work to speak to readers in so powerful a fashion would be wonderful indeed. But who among us is not also concerned, as Taylor is, with theoretical principles, including those related to what can rightly constitute data or findings. One may be left wondering, "Is it not disingenuous to tell a story rather than to present hard facts?" But remember, we tore down the myth of hard facts in Chapter 8. More to the point here is the question: "Can a story represent a finding?" My answer is: Yes, it can, if it is indeed representative of a project's overall conclusions and if it has been carefully captured, preserved, and retold—that is, if anthropologically informed methods are carefully and thoughtfully employed for collecting it.

Stories for Change

Taylor advises that we offer up our research participants' stories "not as solid lumps of congealed truth, but as goads to curiosity, invitations to make meaning" (2003, p. 179). This parallels the advice that business consultant and psychologist Stephen Denning gives to those in the corporate world who need to foster organizational change (2001).

Denning describes the "springboard story": a specific type of story that facilitates change by providing listeners with a new way to see their worlds, allowing them to imagine how the story might play out for them. That they do so actively is part of the power of this technique. Importantly, rather than placing the audience as spectators, which is what Denning suggests that typical, quantitative presentations do, storytelling makes audience members participants in the action. They get "inside the story, projecting themselves into the situation, living the predicament of the protagonist, feeling what he or she was feeling, experiencing the same hopes and fears" (2001, p. 69). The listener then assumes a vested interest in seeing that things work out for the best.

Springboard stories can be complete, with a beginning and an end, in which case the audience will re-create them, mentally, as they think about how the stories might play out in their own circumstances (e.g., "here in the surgical unit" or "here in heme-onc"). Stories that do not have an actual ending can be useful, too, if the storyteller suggests a good ending and then tells the audience that this can happen only if certain, specified conditions are put into place (Denning 2001, p. 33).

This facilitation of foresight or future-mindedness underlies the utility of telling a story at the start of a presentation rather than after presenting disjointed data. It in part explains how springboard stories can shift the discussion from whether to believe in particular findings or recommendations to how to react to or implement them. Such shifts, and the way that they cause listeners to view all subsequent information delivered through what Denning calls "the prism of the living story" (2001, p. 150), can be crucial to a presentation's success. My initial quote of Denning referred to the nonadversarial climate set up by stories, which "bypass normal defense mechanisms" (p. xv). Rather than feeling under attack, which is often the first response audience members have when their normal modes of operation are questioned, listeners will prioritize the values activated by the story and use those to organize their reactions or discussion.

This is not necessarily a good thing in itself. What if the data are bad or bogus and the conclusions spurious? What if the recommendations are flawed? History is strewn with the wreckage that comes when the wrong story gets followed. We want research to be strenuously evaluated. However, let us suspend disbelief for a moment, assuming that our research is robust and our recommendations make sense: Let us assume that lessons like those in this book have been followed and the scholarship is sound. All things being equal, is it not better to have one's message heard?

Again, all things being equal—with incontrovertible research findings and recommendations—the anthropologically informed researcher is well-prepared to get through to listeners. Doing research the anthropological way inherently creates intimate relationships and enables the researcher to gain experiential knowledge. This fosters real commitment to one's findings. I have never met an anthropologist who does not believe in the stories he or she gets the honor of telling. Doubts do arise, but that is part of the analytic process; the overarching story that emerges in the final analysis, and the stories that can be recounted from the field, are always sincerely imparted. Denning has noted the importance of conviction for making storytelling effective: "The deep feelings of the storyteller will seep into the story, and from there into the minds of the listeners, and so help take the audience to the level where deep meaning resides" (2001, p. 147).

As Taylor notes in concluding her exposition of the Fadiman book, "The meanings that we make set the course for the actions that we take; they matter enormously" (2003, p. 179). This is perhaps nowhere so true as it is in regard to health services process design, program creation, and policy-making. Stories are powerful and, when illuminated or supported by other forms of data, they are an excellent part of the health services researchers' armamentarium. Those who excel in anthropologically informed data collection and analysis are in the best position to provide them.

Afterword

In this book, Elisa Sobo shows that modern medical institutions—urgently dynamic, combined or separate modern hospitals, medical schools, and research establishments—are composed of specialists with different vocations fortified by sometimes apparently diverse theoretical, vocational, and personal beliefs as well as perhaps contradictory goals and primary values. These individuals struggle both to advance their own goals and to adapt to each others' agendas and professional cultures. Each seeks to ensure his or her own success. Cooperative research in such institutions requires, above all, a flexible and nimble mindset. If circumstances prevent you from conforming, you have no option other than to be clever (or correct?).

It is always a pleasure to finish reading an important book that transforms one's own subject. But exactly what kind of pleasure does this book offer? It is not a sense of final achievement, an experience of self-conscious complacent relief (Been there! Done that!). It is not a text one can put on the shelf and contemplate with the satisfaction of having completed or achieved an intellectual duty. It is not a text one can notice occasionally with its companions, part of an army of past achievements (and sometimes temporary failures to understand).

This book is different. It is a book that is never closed in the sense of finally being absorbed and finished. It is a desktop-and-satchel book, not a left-on-the-shelf book. It is a book that tells a set of complex stories about past events that are relevant to the *present* but that nevertheless, like all good science, social or natural, tells its real story by posing questions to and about the future. Even within curative medicine, diagnosis shares with ethnography important implications for the future as well as a statement about the past. Each carries within it prognosis as a main output. Sobo's book is an object lesson in the virtues of her key (and highly sophisticated) use of the anthropological method of qualitative participant observation and her simultaneous control (in the medical arena) of more conventional natural science methods of precise mathematical and objective isolation. She at once lives, describes, and analyzes her own experience and puts it in the context of the "other," whether patient or colleague. One might use the metaphors of thorough, broad, contextual analysis, on the one hand, and deep, invasive surgery, on the other.

The book engaged me, and will engage others also, in Sobo's consciousness in and of at least two overlapping sets of experiences. Sobo shows how to understand health service practice and research by consciously engaging with them; at the same time, she reflexively observes herself and fellow qualitative social scientists alongside and always in close cooperation with clinically oriented practitioners. She recognizes and creatively combines the merits and overcomes the inevitable blind spots of everyone from detached natural scientists to empathetic curers, healers, and carers. She draws on experience in teaching, practice, and research that, as her accomplishments in the field and in print, in both pragmatic and research appointments indicate, is almost certainly unique in both depth and diversity.

The important (if perhaps somewhat arrogantly expressed) question posed by Nobel Prize–winner Crick, with which Sobo starts her account, shows his own inevitably limited awareness and a certain unwillingness to recognize his and his fellow prize winners' indebtedness to their colleague Rosalind Franklin who demonstrated, with her remarkable photographic skill, the spiral of DNA before they themselves discovered it and proved its importance. Clearly, scientific discovery is dependent on more than the activities of scientists sticking closely (one might even say religiously?) to protocol. Medical science requires the kind of understanding and empathy that Sobo displays, alongside insight and expert, but not dogmatic, control of both technical methods and the context in which research is conceived and practiced. Sobo's methods, her intelligent application of them, and her reporting of the findings arising from them transform blueprints into kaleidoscopic images, and kaleidoscopic images into fully layered *contour maps* of method and practice available for practitioners, observing participants, and potential patients.

Ronnie Frankenberg
Emeritus Professor and Honorary Life Fellow,
Hon D.Sc. Keele University, UK
October 2008

References

Abu-Lughod, L. (2005). Should Anthropologists Abandon the Concept of Culture? Yes: Writing against Culture. *Taking Sides: Clashing Views in Cultural Anthropology.* R. L. Welsch and K. M. Endicott, eds. Dubuque, IA, McGraw Hill: 49–57.

Aday, L. A. (1989). *Designing and Conducting Health Surveys: A Comprehensive Guide.* San Francisco, Jossey-Bass.

AAP-AAFP (American Academy of Pediatrics Committee on Quality Improvement and American Academy of Family Physicians Commission on Clinical Policies and Research) (1999). The Management of Minor Closed Head Injury in Children. *Pediatrics* 104(6): 1407–1415.

AOA (American Osteopathic Assocation) (n.d.). What Is the American Osteopathic Association (AOA)? Washington, DC, American Osteopathic Association, Department of Government Relations. Available online at http://www.osteopathic.org/pdf/about_the_aoa.pdf (accessed August 28, 2008).

Baer, H. A. (1989). The American Dominative Medical System as a Reflection of Social Relations in the Larger Society. *Social Science & Medicine* 28(11): 1103–1112.

Baer, H. A., M. Singer, and J. H. Johnson (1986). Toward a Critical Medical Anthropology. *Social Science & Medicine* 23(2): 95–98.

Baer, H. A., M. Singer, and I. Susser, I. (1997). *Medical Anthropology and the World System: A Critical Perspective.* Westport, CT, Bergin & Garvey.

Bailey, F. G. (1983). *The Tactical Uses of Passion: An Essay on Power, Reason, and Rationality.* Ithaca, NY, Cornell University Press.

———. (2001). *Treasons, Strategems, and Spoils: How Leaders Make Practical Use of Beliefs and Values.* Boulder, CO, Westview Press.

Basch, C. (1987). Focus Group Interview: An Underutilized Research Technique for Improving Theory and Practice in Health Education. *Health Education Quarterly* 14(4): 411–448.

Becker, H. S. (1996). The Epistemology of Qualitative Research. *Essays on Ethnography and Human Development.* R. Jessor, A. Colby, and R. Schweder, eds. Chicago, University of Chicago Press: 53–72.

Behar, R. (1996). *The Vulnerable Observer: Anthropology that Breaks Your Heart.* Boston, Beacon.

Bellin, E. and N. Neveloff Dubler (2001). The Quality Improvement-Research Divide and the Need for External Oversight. *American Journal of Public Health* 91(9): 1512–1517.

Bentley, M. E., R. Y. Stallings, and J. Gittelsohn (1994). The Structured Observation Technique for the Study of Health Behaviour. *Studying Hygiene Behaviour: Methods, Issues, and Experiences.* S. Cairncross and V. Kochar, eds. New Delhi, India, Sage: 102–120.

Berliner, H. (1975). A Larger Perspective on the Flexner Report. *International Journal of Health Services* 5(4): 573–592.

Bernard, H. R. (1995a). Qualitative Data, Quantitative Analysis. *Cultural Anthropology Methods* 8(1): 9–11.

———. (1995b). *Research Methods in Anthropology: Qualitative and Quantitative Approaches*. Walnut Creek, CA, AltaMira.

Bernard, H. R., Ed. (1998). *Handbook of Methods in Cultural Anthropology*. Walnut Creek, CA, AltaMira.

Bernard, H. R. and G. W. Ryan (1998). Text Analysis: Qualitative and Quantitative Methods. *Handbook of Methods in Cultural Anthropology*. H. R. Bernard, ed. Walnut Creek, CA, AltaMira: 595–646.

Bernstein, J. (1973). II. The Secret of the Old One. *New Yorker*, March 17, p. 44.

Berwick, D. M. (1996). A Primer on Leading the Improvement of Systems. *British Medical Journal* 312: 619–622.

———. (2005). Broadening the View of Evidence-Based Medicine. *Quality and Safety in Health Care* 14: 315–316.

Betancourt, J. R., J. E. Carrillo, and A. R. Green (1999). Hypertension in Multicultural and Minority Populations: Linking Communication to Compliance. *Current Hypertension Reports* 1(6): 482–488.

Bethell, C., L. Simpson, D. Read, E. J. Sobo, J. Vitucci, B. Latzke, S. Hedges, and P. S. Kurtin (2006). Quality and Safety of Hospital Care for Children from Spanish-Speaking Families with Limited English Proficiency. *Journal for Healthcare Quality* (Web Exclusive) 28(3): W3.2–W3.16. Cited material used with permission.

Bhopal, R., J. Rankin, E. McColl, L. Thomas, E. Kaner, R. Stacy, P. Pearson, B. Vernon, and H. Rodgers (1997). The Vexed Question of Authorship: Views of Researchers in a British Medical Faculty. *British Medical Journal* 314(7086): 1009–1012.

Bogdan, R. C. and S. K. Biklen (1992). *Qualitative Research for Education: An Introduction to Theory and Methods*. Boston, Allyn and Bacon.

Borgatti, S. B. (1992). ANTHROPAC 4.0. Columbia, SC, Analytic Technologies.

Boster, J. S. (1985). Requiem for the Omniscient Informant: There's Life in the Old Girl Yet. *Directions in Cognitive Anthropology*. J. W. D. Dougherty, ed. Urbana, University of Illinois Press: 177–198.

Bourgois, P. and N. Scheper-Hughes (2004). Comments on "An Anthropology of Structural Violence." *Current Anthropology* 45(3): 317–318.

Brach, C. and I. Fraser (2000). Can Cultural Competency Reduce Racial and Ethnic Disparities? A Review and Conceptual Model. *Medical Care Research and Review* 57(Suppl. 1): 181–217.

Brink, P. J. and N. Edgecombe (2003). What Is Becoming of Ethnography? *Qualitative Health Research* 13(7): 1028–1030.

British Sociological Association (2001). Authorship Guidelines for Academic Papers. Available online at http://www.britsoc.co.uk/Library/authorship_01.doc (accessed December 29, 2006).

Brown, E. (1979). *Rockefeller Medicine Men*. Berkeley, University of California Press.

Brown, P. (1995). Naming and Framing: The Social Construction of Diagnosis and Illness. *Journal of Health and Social Behavior* (extra issue): 34–42.

Browner, C. H. (1999). On the Medicalization of Medical Anthropology. *Medical Anthropology Quarterly* 13(2): 135–140.

Brumann, C. (2005). Should Anthropologists Abandon the Concept of Culture? No—Writing for Culture: Why a Successful Concept Should Not Be Discarded. *Taking Sides: Clashing Views in Cultural Anthropology*. R. L. Welsch and K. M. Endicott, eds. Dubuque, IA, McGraw Hill: 58–66.

Butow, P., M. Maclean, S. M. Dunn, M. H. N. Tattersall, and M. J. Boyer (1997). The Dynamics of Change: Cancer Patients' Preferences for Information, Involvement, and Support. *Annals of Oncology* 8: 857–863.

Campbell, M. and F. Gregor (2004). *Mapping Social Relations: A Primer in Doing Institutional Ethnography*. Walnut Creek, CA, AltaMira.

Carthey, J. (2003). The Role of Structured Observational Research in Health Care. *Quality and Safety in Health Care* 12(Supp. II): ii13–ii16.

Cassell, J. (1991). *Expected Miracles: Surgeons at Work*. Philadelphia, Temple University Press.

Castaneda, C. (2002). *Figurations: Child, Bodies, Worlds*. Durham, NC, Duke University Press.

Catlin, A., C. Cowan, S. M. Dunn, M. Hartman, S. Heffler, and National Health Expenditure Accounts Team (2008). National Health Spending in 2006: A Year of Change for Prescription Drugs. *Health Affairs* 27(1): 14–29.

Caulkins, D. (1998). Consensus Analysis: Do Scottish Business Advisers Agree on Models of Success? *Using Methods in the Field: A Practical Introduction and Casebook*. V. C. de Munck and E. J. Sobo, eds. Walnut Creek, CA, AltaMira: 179–195.

Chrisman, N. J. (1977). The Health Seeking Process: An Approach to the Natural History of Illness. *Culture, Medicine and Psychiatry* 1(4): 351–377.

Christakis, D. and F. Rivara (1998). Pediatricians' Awareness of and Attitudes about Four Clinical Practice Guidelines. *Pediatrics* 101(5): 825–830.

Clark, J., D. Potter, and J. McKinlay (1991). Bringing Social Structure Back into Clinical Decision Making. *Social Science & Medicine* 32(8): 853–866.

Clark, L. and L. Hofsess (1998). Acculturation. *Handbook of Immigrant Health*. S. Loue, ed. New York, Plenum: 37–59.

Clark, L., R. C. de Baca, K. Reidy, and M. Turner (2002). Is Cultural Competence All about Language? Data from Two Medicaid Managed Care Systems Serving Latinos. Paper presented at the 101st Annual Meeting of the American Anthropological Association, New Orleans, LA, November 20–24.

Clements, F. E. (1932). Primitive Concepts of Disease. *University of California Publications in American Archaeology and Ethnology* 32(2): 185–252.

Clifford, J. and G. E. Marcus, Eds. (1986). *Writing Culture: The Poetics and Politics of Ethnography*. Los Angeles: University of California Press.

Coulter, A., V. Peto, and H. Doll (1994). Patients' Preferences and General Practitioners' Decisions in the Treatment of Menstrual Disorders. *Family Practice* 11(1): 67–74.

Crispell, D. (1994). Pet Projections. *American Demographics* 16(9): 59.

D'Andrade, R. (1995). *The Development of Cognitive Anthropology*. Cambridge, Cambridge University Press.

D'Andrade, R. and C. Strauss, Eds. (1992). *Human Motives and Cultural Models*. Cambridge, Cambridge University Press.

Davidson, S. J. (1993). Closing the Loop: Discard Bad Apples or Continuously Improve EMS? *Quality Management in Prehospital Care*. R. Swor, ed. St. Louis, MO, Mosby Lifeline: 55–69.

De, D. and J. Richardson (2008). Cultural Safety: An Introduction. *Paediatric Nursing* 20(2): 39–43.

Degner, L. F., J. A. Sloan, and P. Venkatesh (1997). The Control Preferences Scale. *Canadian Journal of Nursing Research* 29(3): 21–43.

Demers, R., R. Altamore, H. Mustin, A. Kleinman, and D. Leonardi (1980). An Exploration of the Dimensions of Illness Behavior. *Journal of Family Practice* 11: 1085–1092.

de Munck, V. C. (1998). Participant Observation: A Thick Explanation of Conflict in a Sri Lankan Village. *Using Methods in the Field: A Practical Introduction and Casebook*. V. C. de Munck and E. J. Sobo, eds. Walnut Creek, CA, AltaMira: 39–54.

de Munck, V. C. and E. J. Sobo (1998). *Using Methods in the Field: A Practical Introduction and Casebook*. Walnut Creek, CA, AltaMira.

Denning, S. (2001). *The Springboard: How Storytelling Ignites Action in Knowledge-Era Organizations*. Woburn, MA, Butterworth-Heinemann.

Dennis, K. (2004). Helping Families with Children with Down Syndrome Navigate The Health Care System. (Findings from an Exploratory Study.) San Diego: Center for Child Health Outcomes; Children's Hospital and Healthcare Center.

Dillman, D. A. (2007). *Mail and Internet Surveys: The Tailored Design Method 2007 Update with New Internet, Visual, and Mixed-Mode Guide.* New York, Wiley.

Dingwall, R. (2008). The Ethical Case against Ethical Regulation in Humanitities and Social Science Research. *21st Century Society* 3(1): 1–12.

Donabedian, A. (1966). Evaluating the Quality of Medical Care. *Milbank Memorial Fund Quarterly* 44(3), Suppl.:166–206.

———. (1988). The Quality of Health Care: How Can It Be Assessed? *Journal of the American Medical Association* 260: 1743–1748.

Dressler, W. W. and J. R. Bindon (2000). The Health Consequences of Cultural Consonance: Cultural Dimensions of Lifestyle, Social Support, and Arterial Blood Pressure in an African American Community. *American Anthropologist* 102(2): 244–260.

Dreyfus, H. L. (1987). From Socrates to Expert Systems: The Limits of Calculative Rationality. *Bulletin of the American Academy of Arts and Sciences* 40(4): 15–31.

Drotar, D., Ed. (2000). *Promoting Adherence to Medical Treatment in Chronic Childhood Illness: Concepts, Methods, and Interventions.* Mahwah, NJ, Lawrence Erlbaum Associates.

Dunbar, R. (1996). *Grooming, Gossip, and the Evolution of Language.* Cambridge, MA, Harvard University Press.

Durkheim, É. (1915). *The elementary forms of the religious life : A study in religious sociology* (translated from the French by J. W. Swain). London, G. Allen & Unwin.

Edwards, A. and G. Elwyn (2001). Developing Professional Ability to Involve Patients in Their Care: Pull or Push? *Quality in Health Care* 10: 129–130.

Ehrlich, P. R. (2006). *Human Natures.* New York, Penguin Books.

Fadiman, A. (1997). *The Spirit Catches You and You Fall Down: A Hmong Child, Her American Doctors, and the Collision of Two Cultures.* New York, Noonday Press.

Fairhurst, K. and G. Huby (1998). From Trial Data to Practical Knowledge: Qualitative Study of How General Practitioners Have Accessed and Used Evidence about Statin Drugs in Their Management of Hypercholesterolaemia. *British Medical Journal* 317: 1130–1134.

Farmer, P. (2004). An Anthropology of Structural Violence. *Current Anthropology* 45(3): 305–325.

———. (2005). *Pathologies of Power: Health, Human Rights, and the New War on the Poor.* Los Angeles, University of California Press.

Fixsen, D., S. Naoom, K. A. Blase, R. M. Friedman, and F. Wallace (2005). *Implementation Research: A Synthesis of the Literature.* Tampa, University of South Florida, Louis de la Parte Florida Mental Health Institute, The National Implementation Research Network.

Flanagin, A., L. Carey, P. B. Fontanarosa, S. G. Phillips, B. P. Pace, G. D. Lundberg, and D. Rennie (1998). Prevalence of Articles with Honorary Authors and Ghost Authors in Peer-Reviewed Medical Journals. *Journal of the American Medical Association* 280(3): 222–224.

Fleisher, M. S. and J. A. Harrington (1998). Freelisting: Management at a Women's Federal Prison Camp. *Using Methods in the Field: A Practical Introduction and Case Book.* V. C. de Munck and E. J. Sobo, eds. Walnut Creek, CA, AltaMira: 69–84.

Flores, G., D. Gee, and B. Kastner (2000). The Teaching of Cultural Issues in U.S. and Canadian Medical Schools. *Academic Medicine* 75: 451–455.

Fluehr-Lobban, C. (2006). *Race and Racism: An Introduction.* Lanham, MD, AltaMira.

Foster, G. M. (1976). Disease Etiologies in Non-Western Medical Systems. *American Anthropologist* 78(4): 773–782.

Foster, G. M. and B. G. Anderson (1978). *Medical Anthropology.* New York, Alfred A. Knopf.

Frankenberg, R. and J. Leeson (1976). Disease, Illness and Sickness: Social Aspects of the Choice of Healer in a Lusaka Suburb. *Social Anthropology and Medicine.* J. B. Loudon, ed. New York, Academic Press, vol. 13: 223–258.

Frankenberg, R., I. Robinson, and A. Delahooke (2000). Countering Essentialism in Behavioural Social Science: The Example of "The Vulnerable Child" Ethnographically Examined. *Sociological Review* 48(4): 586–611.

Franklin, S. (1995). Science as Culture, Cultures of Science. *Annual Review of Anthropology* 24: 163–184.

Fuller, K. (2002). Eradicating Essentialism from Cultural Competency Education. *Academic Medicine* 77(3): 198–201.

Galanti, G. A. (1997). *Caring for Patients from Different Cultures: Case Studies from American Hospitals*. Philadelphia, University of Pennsylvania Press.

Gallese, V., L. Fadiga, L. Fogassi, and G. Rizzolatti (1996). Action Recognition in the Premotor Cortex. *Brain* 119(2): 593–609.

Galtung, J. (1969). Violence, Peace, and Peace Research. *Journal of Peace Research* 6(3): 167–191.

Gawande, A. (2007). A Lifesaving Checklist. *New York Times*, December 30, Opinion section.

Geertz, C. (1973). *The Interpretation of Cultures*. New York, Basic Books.

———. (1983). *Local Knowledge: Further Essays in Interpretive Anthropology*. New York, Basic Books.

Glaser, B. and A. Strauss (1965). *Awareness of Dying*. Chicago, Aldine.

———. (1967). *The Discovery of Grounded Theory: Strategies for Qualitative Research*. New York, Aldine de Gruyter.

Golden, P. M. (1976). *The Research Experience*. Itasca, IL, F. E. Peacock Publishers.

Goldschmidt, W. (2006). *The Bridge to Humanity: How Affect Hunger Trumps the Selfish Gene*. New York, Oxford University Press.

Good, B. J. (1994). *Medicine, Rationality, and Experience: An Anthropological Perspective*. Cambridge, Cambridge University Press.

Good, B. J. and M. J. D. Good (1993). Learning Medicine: The Constructing of Medical Knowledge at Harvard Medical School. *Knowledge, Power, and Practice*. S. Lindenbaum and M. Lock, eds. Los Angeles, University of California Press: 81–107.

Good, M. J. D. (1998). *American Medicine: The Quest for Competence* (with a new preface). Los Angeles, University of California Press.

Gottschalk, L. and G. Gleser (1969). *The Measurement of Psychological States through Analysis of Verbal Behavior*. Berkeley, University of California Press.

Grady, K. A. and B. S. Wallston (1988). *Research in Health Care Settings*. Newbury Park, CA, Sage.

Green, E. C. (2001). Can Qualitative Research Produce Reliable Quantitative Findings. *Field Methods* 13(1): 3–19.

Green, G. and E. J. Sobo (2000). *The Endangered Self: Managing the Social Risk of HIV*. London, Routledge.

Green, L. (2004). Comments on "An Anthropology of Structural Violence." *Current Anthropology* 45(3): 319–320.

Hahn, R. A. (1984). Rethinking "Disease" and "Illness." *Contributions to Asian Studies: Special Volume on Southasian Systems of Healing* 18: 1–23.

Hahn, R. A. (1995). *Sickness and Healing: An Anthropological Perspective*. New Haven, CT, Yale University Press.

Handwerker, W. P. (1998). Consensus Analysis: Sampling Frames for Valid, Generalizable Research Findings. *Using Methods in the Field: A Practical Introduction and Casebook*. V. C. de Munck and E. J. Sobo, eds. Walnut Creek, CA, AltaMira: 165–178.

Hart, E. (2001). System Induced Setbacks in Stroke Recovery. *Sociology of Health and Illness* 23(1): 101–123.

Health Resources and Services Administration (2001). Cultural Competence Works: Using Cultural Competence to Improve the Quality of Health Care for Diverse Populations and Add Value to Managed Care Arrangements. Washington, DC, U.S. Department of

Health and Human Services. Available online at ftp://ftp.hrsa.gov/financeMC/cultural-competence.pdf (accessed November 1, 2008).

Heggenhougen, H. K. (2004). Comments on "An Anthropology of Structural Violence." *Current Anthropology* 45(3): 320–321.

Hill, J. (2005). Finding Culture in Narrative. *Finding Culture in Talk: A Collection of Methods*. N. Quinn, ed. New York, Palgrave Macmillan: 157–202.

Hodgson, I. (2000). Ethnography and Health Care: Focus on Nursing. *Forum Qualitative Sozialforschung/Forum: Qualitative Social Research* [on-line journal available at: http://qualitative-research.net/fqs] 1(1): twenty-five paragraphs.

Holmes, O. W. (1888 [1861]). Currents and Counter-Currents in Medical Science. *Medical Essays, 1842–1882*. Boston, Houghton, Mifflin.

Huby, G. (1999). Contesting Needs: Entitlement to Welfare Benefits for People with HIV/AIDS in Lothian, Scotland. *Anthropology and Medicine* 6(1): 143–152.

Huby, G., E. Hart, C. McKevitt, and E. J. Sobo (2007). Addressing the Complexity of Health Care: The Practical Potential of Ethnography. *Journal of Health Services Research and Policy* 12(4): 193–194.

Inhorn, M. (2006). Defining Women's Health. *Medical Anthropology Quarterly* 20(3): 345–378.

Institute of Medicine Committee on Quality of Health Care in America (2001). *Crossing the Quality Chasm: A New Health System for the 21st Century*. Washington, DC, National Academies Press.

James, W. (1890 [1918]). *The Principles of Psychology*. New York, Henry Holt and Company.

Janzen, J. M. (1978). *The Quest for Therapy in Lower Zaire*. Berkeley, University of California Press.

Katz, D. A. (1999). Barriers between Guidelines and Improved Patient Care: An Analysis of ACCPR's Unstable Angina Clinical Practice Guideline. *Health Services Research* 3–4: 377–389.

Katz, P. (1999). *The Scalpel's Edge: The Culture of Surgeons*. Needham Heights, MA, Allyn & Bacon.

Kaufman, S. (2005). *… And a Time to Die: How American Hospitals Shape the End of Life*. New York, Scribner.

Kirk, J. and M. L. Miller (1987). *Reliability and Validity in Qualitative Research*. Newbury Park, CA, Sage.

Kirmayer, L. (2004). Comments on "An Anthropology of Structural Violence." *Current Anthropology* 45(3): 321–322.

Kleinman, A. (1978). Concepts and a Model for the Comparison of Medical Systems as Cultural Systems. *Social Science & Medicine* 12: 85–93.

———. (1981). *Patients and Healers in the Context of Culture: An Exploration of the Borderland between Anthropology, Medicine, and Psychiatry*. Los Angeles, University of California Press.

Kohn, L. T., J. M. Corrigan, and M. S. Donaldson, Eds. (2000). *To Err Is Human: Building a Safer Health System*. Washington, DC, National Academies Press.

Korsch, B. M., E. K. Gozzi, and V. Francis (1968). Gaps in Doctor-Patient Communication: 1. Doctor-Patient Interaction and Patient Satisfaction. *Pediatrics* 42(5): 855–871.

Kristal, A. R., R. E. Patterson, M. L. Neuhouser, M. D. Thornquist, D. Newmark-Sztainer, C. L. Rock, M. C. Berlin, L. J. Cheskin, and P. J. Schreiner (1998). Olestra Postmarketing Surveillance Study: Design and Baseline Results from the Sentinel Site. *Journal of the American Dietetic Association* 98(11): 1290–1296.

Kroeber, A. L., C. Kluckhohn, A. G. Meyer, and W. Untereiner (1952). *Culture: A Critical Review of Concepts and Definitions*. Cambridge, MA, Peabody Museum.

Kroeber, A. L., and T. Parsons (1958). The Concept of Culture and of Social System. *American Sociological Review* 23: 582–583.

Kronenfeld, D. B. (1996). *Plastic Glasses and Church Fathers*. New York, Oxford University Press.

Kuhn, T. S. (1996 [1962]). *The Structure of Scientific Revolutions*. Chicago, University of Chicago Press.

Kuzel, A. J. (1992). Sampling in Qualitative Inquiry. *Doing Qualitative Research*. B. F. Crabtree and W. L. Miller, eds. Newbury Park, CA, Sage: 31–44.

Lambert, H. (2006). Accounting for EBM: Notions of Evidence in Medicine. *Social Science & Medicine* 62(11): 2633–2645.

Lambert, H. and C. McKevitt (2002). Anthropology in Health Research: From Qualitative Methods to Multidisciplinarity. *British Medical Journal* 325: 210–213.

Langley, G. J., K. M. Nolan, and T. W. Nolan (1992). *The Foundations of Improvement*. Silver Spring, MD, API Publishing.

Langness, L. L. (2005). *The Study of Culture*. Novato, CA, Chandler and Sharp.

Latour, B. (1999). *Pandora's Hope: Essays on the Reality of Science Studies*. Cambridge, MA, Harvard University Press.

Lawlor, M. C., and C. F. Mattingly (2001). Beyond the Unobtrusive Observer: Reflections on Researcher-Informant Relationships in Urban Ethnography. *American Journal of Occupational Therapy* 55(2): 147–154.

Leape, L. L. and D. M. Berwick (2005). Five Years after "To Err Is Human": What Have We Learned? *Journal of the American Medical Association* 293: 2384–2390.

Leichter, H. M. (2003). "Evil Habits" and "Personal Choices": Assigning Responsibility for Health in the 20th Century. *Milbank Memorial Fund Quarterly* 81(4): 603–626.

Leininger, M. (2002). Culture Care Theory: A Major Contribution to Advance Transcultural Nursing Knowledge and Practices. *Journal of Transcultural Nursing* 13(3): 189–192.

Lipman, T. (2000). Power and Influence in Clinical Effectiveness and Evidence-Based Medicine. *Family Practice* 17(6): 557–563.

Lock, M. (2002). *Twice Dead: Organ Transplants and the Reinvention of Death*. Los Angeles, University of California Press.

Loustaunau, M. O. and E. J. Sobo (1997). *The Cultural Context of Health, Illness and Medicine*. Westport, CT, Bergin & Garvey. Copyright 1997 by Martha O. Loustaunau and Elisa J. Sobo. Cited material reproduced with permission of Greenwood Publishing Group, Inc., Westport, CT.

Lupton, D. (1994). *Medicine as Culture: Illness, Disease and the Body in Western Societies*.

Macdonald, M. E., F. A. Carnevale, S. Liben, and S. R. Cohen (2005). Critically Caring: Displacing and Re-Placing Parenthood in a Pediatric Intensive Care Unit. Paper read at the 104th Annual Meeting of the American Anthropological Association. Washington, DC, November 30–December 4.

Macdonald, M. E., S. Liben, F. A. Carnevale, J. E. Rennick, and S. R. Cohen (2007). Office or Bedroom? A Disconnect between Family Culture and Professional Culture in the PICU. Paper read at the 5th World Congress on Pediatric Critical Care. Geneva, June 24–28.

MacIntyre, A. (1985). *After Virtue: A Study in Moral Theory*. London, Duckworth.

Macintyre, S. (1997). Conventions, Ethics and Laws in Journal Publishing. *Social Science & Medicine* 45(1): 1–2.

Mainland, D. (1966). *Health Services Research I & II*. New York, Milbank Memorial Fund.

Malinowski, B. (1989 [1967]). *A Diary in the Strict Sense of the Term* (reissued with a new introduction by Raymond Firth). Stanford, CA, Stanford University Press.

Maly, R. C., L. B. Bourque, and R. F. Engelhardt (1999). A Randomized Controlled Trial of Facilitating Information Giving to Patients with Chronic Medical Conditions: Effects on Outcomes of Care. *Journal of Family Practice* 48(5): 356–363.

Manderson, L. and C. Smith-Morris, Eds. (Forthcoming). *Chronic Conditions, Fluid States: Globalization and the Anthropology of Illness*. Piscataway, NJ, Rutgers University Press.

Martin, E. (1987). *The Woman in the Body: A Cultural Analysis of Reproduction*. Boston, Beacon Press.

Martin, E. (1994). *Flexible Bodies: Tracking Immunity in American Culture from the Days of Polio to the Age of AIDS*. Boston, Beacon Press.

Martin, J. (1982). A Garbage Can Model of the Research Process. *Judgment Calls in Research*. J. E. McGrath, J. Martin and R. A. Kulka, eds. Beverly Hills, CA, Sage: 17–39.

Mattingly, C. (1998). *Healing Dramas and Clinical Plots: The Narrative Structure of Experience*. Cambridge, Cambridge University Press.

Maxwell, J. A. (1992). Understanding and Validity in Qualitative Research. *Harvard Educational Review* 62(3): 279–300.

———. (1996). *Qualitative Research Design: An Interactive Approach*. Thousand Oaks, CA, Sage.

Mays, N. and C. Pope (2000). Qualitative Research in Healthcare: Assessing Quality in Qualitative Research. *British Medical Journal* 320: 50–52.

McCarthy, T. and K. L. White (2000). Origins of Health Services Research. *Health Services Research* 35(2): 375–387.

McLean, A. (2007). *The Person in Dementia: A Study of Nursing Home Care in the US*. Toronto, Broadview Press.

Mead, M. (1932). An Investigation of the Thought of Primitive Children, with Special Reference to Animism. *Journal of the Royal Anthropological Institute of Great Britain and Ireland* 62: 173–190.

Mechanic, D. (1962). The Concept of Illness Behavior. *Journal of Chronic Diseases* 15: 189–194.

Miles, M. B. and A. M. Huberman (1984). *Qualitative Data Analysis: A Sourcebook of New Methods*. Newbury Park, CA, Sage.

Milstein, A., and M. Smith (2006). America's New Refugees: Seeking Affordable Surgery Offshore. *New England Journal of Medicine* 355(16): 1637–1640.

Moerman, D. (2002). *Meaning, Medicine, and the "Placebo Effect."* Cambridge, University of Cambridge Press.

Mol, A. (2002). *The Body Multiple: Ontology in Medical Practice*. Durham, NC, Duke University Press.

———. (2006). Proving or Improving: On Health Care Research as a Form of Self-Reflection. *Qualitative Health Research* 16(3): 405–414.

Morgan, D. L. (1997). *Focus Groups as Qualitative Research*. Thousand Oaks, CA, Sage.

Moynihan, R. (2006). Scientists Find New Disease: Motivational Deficiency Disorder. *British Medical Journal* 332: 745.

Murphy, R. (2001). *The Body Silent: The Different World of the Disabled*. New York, W.W. Norton & Company.

Mykhalovskiy, E. and L. Weir (2004). The Problem of Evidence-Based Medicine: Directions for Social Science. *Social Science & Medicine* 59: 1059–1069.

Nichter, M. (2000). *Fat Talk: What Girls and Their Parents Say about Dieting*. Cambridge, MA, Harvard University Press.

Nichter, M. and M. Nichter (1996). *Anthropology and International Health: Asian Case Studies*. Amsterdam, Gordon and Breach.

O'Connor, B. B. (1995). *Healing Traditions: Alternative Medicine and the Health Professions*. Philadelphia, University of Pennsylvania Press.

Office of Behavioral and Social Sciences Research, National Institutes of Health. (December 2001). Qualitative Methods in Health Research: Opportunities and Considerations in Application and Review. Washington, DC, National Institutes of Health. Available online at http://obssr.od.nih.gov/Documents/Publications/Qualitative.PDF (accessed November 1, 2008).

Oldani, M. (2004). Thick Prescriptions: Toward an Interpretation of Pharmaceutical Sales Practices. *Medical Anthropology Quarterly* 18(3): 325–356.

Parker, M. and I. Harper (2005). The Anthropology of Public Health. *Journal of Biosocial Science* 38: 1–5.

Parker, R., D. Baker, M. Williams, and J. Nurss (1995). The Test of Functional Health Literacy in Adults: A New Instrument for Measuring Patients' Literacy Skills. *Journal of General Internal Medicine* 10(10): 537–541.

Patton, M. Q. (1990). *Qualitative Evaluation and Research Methods*. Newbury Park, CA, Sage.

———. (1999). Enhancing the Quality and Credibility of Qualitative Analysis. *Health Services Research* 34: 1189–1208.

Payer, L. (1988). *Medicine and Culture: Varieties of Treatments in the United States, England, West Germany and France*. New York, Henry Holt and Company.

Pelto, P. J. and G. H. Pelto (1996). Research Designs in Medical Anthropology. *Medical Anthropology: Contemporary Theory and Method*. C. Sargent and T. Johnson, eds. Westport, CT, Praeger: 293–324.

Pelto, P. J. and G. H. Pelto (1997). Studying Knowledge, Culture, and Behavior in Applied Medical Anthropology. *Medical Anthropology Quarterly* 11(2): 147–163.

Phillips, D. C. (1990). Subjectivity and Objectivity: An Objective Inquiry. *Qualitative Inquiry in Education: The Continuing Debate*. W. Eisner and A. Peshkin, eds. New York, The Teachers College Press: 19–37.

Pickering, A. (1995). *The Mangle of Practice: Time, Agency, and Science*. Chicago, University of Chicago Press.

Plsek, P. (2001). Appendix B: Redesigning Health Care with Insights from the Science of Complex Adaptive Systems. *Crossing the Quality Chasm: A New Health System for the 21st Century*. Institute of Medicine Committee on Quality of Health Care in America. Washington, DC, National Academies Press: 309–322.

———. (2003). Complexity and the Adoption of Innovation in Health Care. Paper presented at Accelerating Quality Improvement in Health Care: Strategies to Speed the Diffusion of Evidence-Based Innovations, convened by the National Institute for Health Care Management Foundation and the National Committee for Quality Health Care, Washington DC, January 27–28.

Pool, R. and W. Geissler (2005). *Medical Anthropology*. New York, Open University Press.

Potter, V. (1971). *Bioethics: Bridge to the Future*. Englewood Cliffs, NJ, Prentice-Hall.

Prussing, E., E. J. Sobo, E. Walker, K. Dennis, and P. S. Kurtin (2004). Communicating about Complementary/Alternative Medicine: Perspectives from Parents of Children with Down Syndrome. Ambulatory Pediatrics. *Ambulatory Pediatrics* 4(6): 488–494.

Prussing, E., E. J. Sobo, E. Walker, and P. S. Kurtin (2005). Between "desperation" and Disability Rights: A Narrative Analysis of Complementary/Alternative Medicine Use by Parents for Children with Down Syndrome. *Social Science & Medicine*. 60(3):587–598.

Pyke-Grimm, K., L. Degner, A. Small, and B. Mueller (1999). Preferences for Participation in Treatment Decision Making and Information Needs of Parents of Children with Cancer: A Pilot Study. *Journal of Pediatric Oncology Nursing* 16(1): 13–24.

Quinn, N. (2005). How to Reconstruct Schemas People Share, from What They Say. *Finding Culture in Talk: A Collection of Methods*. N. Quinn, ed. New York, Palgrave Macmillan: 35–81.

Renzi, C., A. Picardi, D. Abeni, E. Agostini, G. Baliva, P. Pasquini, P. Puddu, and M. Braga (2002). Association of Dissatisfaction with Care and Psychiatric Morbidity with Poor Treatment Compliance. *Archives of Dermatology* 138(3): 337–342.

Richardson, P., E. J. Sobo, and E. Stuckey (2003). Standardized Approaches to Clinical Care: Pathways and Disease Management. *Child Health Services Research: Applications, Innovations, and Insights*. E. J. Sobo and P. S. Kurtin, eds. San Francisco, Jossey-Bass: 275–309.

Ridley, M. (2003). *The Agile Gene*. New York, Perennial.

Riekert, K. A. and D. Drotar (2000). Adherence to Medical Treatment in Pediatric Chronic Illness: Critical Issues and Unanswered Questions. *Promoting Adherence to Medical*

Treatment in Chronic Childhood Illness: Concepts, Methods, and Interventions. D. Drotar, ed. Mahwah, NJ, Lawrence Erlbaum Associates: 3–32.

Rizzolatti, G., L. Fadiga, V. Galesse, and L. Fogassi (1996). Premotor Cortex and the Recognition of Motor Actions. *Cognitive Brain Research* 3(2): 131–141.

Robinson, A. and R. Thomson (2001). Variability in Patient Preferences for Participating in Medical Decision Making: Implication for the Use of Decision Support Tools. *Quality in Health Care* 10(Suppl. 1): i34–i38.

Romanucci-Ross, L. (1977 [1969]). The Hierarchy of Resort in Curative Practices: The Admiralty Islands, Melanesia. *Culture, Disease and Healing: Studies in Medical Anthropology*. D. Landy, ed. New York, Macmillan Publishing: 481–487.

Romney, A. K. and S. C. Weller (1988). Predicting Informant Accuracy from Patterns of Recall among Individuals. *Social Networks* 4: 59–77.

Rosenheck, R. (2001). Stages in the Implementation of Innovative Clinical Programs in Complex Organizations. *Journal of Nervous and Mental Disease* 189: 812–821.

Rous, T. and A. Hunt (2003). Governing Peanuts: The Regulation of the Social Bodies of Children and the Risks of Food Allergies. *Social Science & Medicine* 58(2004): 825–836.

Ryan, G. W. and H. R. Bernard (2003). Techniques to Identify Themes. *Field Methods* 15(1): 85–109.

Sackett, D. L., W. M. C. Rosenberg, J. A. M. Gray, R. B. Haynes, and W. S. Richardson (1996). Evidence Based Medicine: What It Is and What It Isn't. *British Medical Journal* 312: 71–72.

Sargent, C. and T. Johnson, Eds. (1996). *Medical Anthropology: Contemporary Theory and Method* (revised edition). Westport, CT, Greenwood Publishing Group.

Sargent, C. and N. Stark (1989). Childbirth Education and Childbirth Models: Parental Perspectives on Control, Anesthesia, and Technological Intervention in the Birth Process. *Medical Anthropology Quarterly* 3(1): 36–51.

Savage, J. (2000). Ethnography and Health Care. *British Medical Journal* 321: 1400–1402.

Segal, D. A. and S. J. Yanagisako (2005). *Unwrapping the Sacred Bundle: Reflections on the Disciplining of Anthropology*. Durham, NC, Duke University Press.

Seid, M., E. J. Sobo, L. Reyes, and J. W. Varni (2004). Barriers to Care for Children with Special Health Care Needs: Development and Validation of the Barriers to Care Questionnaire. *Ambulatory Pediatrics* 4(4): 323–331.

Seid, M., J. W. Varni, P. Gidwani, L. Reyes Gelhard, and D. Slymen (n.d.) Problem Solving Skills Training Plus Asthma Home Visits Improved Child Health-Related Quality of Life in Vulnerable Families of Children with Asthma: Report of a Randomized Trial. Unpublished manuscript.

Seidel, J. V. (1998). Qualitative Data Analysis, www.qualisresearch.com (originally published as Qualitative Data Analysis, in *The Ethnograph v5.0: A Users Guide*, Appendix E, Colorado Springs, CO: Qualis Research).

Seidmann, R. M. (2006). Authorship Credit and Ethics in Anthropology. *Anthropology News* 47(1): 29, 31.

Sharp, L. (2006). *Strange Harvest: Organ Transplants, Denatured Bodies, and the Transformed Self*. Los Angeles, University of California Press.

Shekelle, P. G., R. L. Kravitz, J. Beart, M. Marger, M. Wang, and M. Lee (2000). Are Nonspecific Practice Guidelines Potentially Harmful? A Randomized Comparison of the Effect of Nonsepecific Versus Specific Guidelines on Physician Decision Making. *Health Services Research* 34(7): 1429–1448.

Sinclair, S. (2000). Disease Narratives: Constituting Doctors. *Anthropology & Medicine* 7(1): 115–134.

Singer, M. (1986). Developing a Critical Perspective in Medical Anthropology. *Medical Anthropology* 17(5): 128–129.

————. (1992). Theory in Medical Anthropology. *Medical Anthropology* (Special Issue: *The Application of Theory in Medical Anthropology*, M. Singer, ed.) 14(1): 1–8.

Singer, M., Ed. (1998). *The Political Economy of AIDS*. Amityville, NY, Baywood Publishing Company, Inc.

Singer, M. and H. Baer (2007). *Introducing Medical Anthropology: A Discipline in Action*. New York, AltaMira.

Smedley, B. D., A. Y. Stith, A. R. Nelson, and Committee on Understanding and Eliminating Racial and Ethnic Disparities in Health Care, Board on Health Sciences Policy, Institute of Medicine, Eds. (2003). *Unequal Treatment: Confronting Racial and Ethnic Disparities in Health Care*. Washington, DC, National Academies Press.

Smith-Morris, C. (2006). "Community Participation" in Tribal Diabetes Programs. *American Indian Culture and Research Journal* 30(2): 85–110.

Snow, C. P. (1993 [1959]). *The Two Cultures*. Cambridge, Cambridge University Press.

Snow, L. F. (1993). *Walkin' over Medicine*. Boulder, CO, Westview Press.

Sobo, E. J. (1993a). Bodies, Kin, and Flow: Family Planning in Rural Jamaica. *Medical Anthropology Quarterly* 7(1): 50–73.

————. (1993b). Inner-City Women and AIDS: The Psycho-Social Benefits of Unsafe Sex. *Culture, Medicine and Psychiatry* 17(4): 455–485.

————. (1994). Attitudes toward HIV Testing among Urban Impoverished African-American Women. *Medical Anthropology* 16(2): 17–38.

————. (1995). *Choosing Unsafe Sex: AIDS-risk Denial among Disadvantaged Women*. Philadelphia, University of Pennsylvania Press.

————. (1996a). Abortion Traditions in Rural Jamaica. *Social Science & Medicine* 42(4): 495–508.

————. (1996b). Pregnancy Loss in Rural Jamaican Tradition. *Pregnancy Loss Cross-culturally*. R. Cecil, ed. Oxford, Berg Publishers: 39–58.

————. (1997). Self-Disclosure and Self-Construction among HIV-Positive People: The Rhetorical Uses of Stereotypes and Sex. *Anthropology & Medicine* 4(1): 67–87.

————. (2001). Rationalization of Medical Risk through Talk of Trust: An Exploration of Elective Eye Surgery Narratives. *Anthropology & Medicine* 8(2/3): 265–278.

————. (2004a). Nurses' Knowledge of Parent or Patient Communication Needs in a Pediatric Cancer Unit: Room for Improvement. *Journal of Nursing Care Quality* 19(3): 253–262.

————. (2004b). Theoretical and Applied Issues in Cross-Cultural Health Research. *Encyclopedia of Medical Anthropology: Health and Illness in the World's Cultures* (Vol. 1). C. Ember and M. Ember, eds. New York, Kluwer Academic Publishers: 3–11.

————. (2005). Parents' Perceptions of Pediatric Day Surgery Risks: Unforeseeable Complications, or Avoidable Mistakes? *Social Science & Medicine* 60(10): 2341–2350.

————. (2007). Mastering the Health Care System for Children with Special Health Care Needs. *Optimizing Care for Young Children with Special Health Care Needs: Knowledge and Strategies for Navigating the System*. E. J. Sobo and P. S. Kurtin, eds. Baltimore, Paul H. Brookes Publishing Co., Inc. 209–234. Cited material reprinted/adapted with permission.

————. (n.d.). Caring for Children with Special Healthcare Needs: "Once We Got There, It Was Fine." *Chronic Conditions, Fluid States: Globalization and the Anthropology of Illness*. L. Manderson and C. Smith-Morris, eds. Piscataway, NJ, Rutgers University Press.

Sobo, E., G. Billman, L. Lim, W. Murdock, E. Romero, D. Donaghue, W. Roberts, and P. S. Kurtin (2002). A Rapid Interview Protocol supporting Patient-centered Quality Improvement: Hearing the Voice of the Parent in a Pediatric Cancer Unit. *The Joint Commission Journal on Quality Improvement* 28(9): 498–509.

Sobo, E. J., C. Bowman, and A. Gifford (2008). Behind the Scenes in Healthcare Improvement: The Complex Structures and Emergent Strategies of Implementation Science. *Social Science & Medicine* 67(10): 1530–1540.

Sobo, E. J., C. Bowman, J. Halloran, G. Aarons, S. Asch, and A. Gifford (2008a). Enhancing Organizational Change and Improvement Prospects: Lessons from an HIV Testing Intervention for Veterans. *Human Organization* 67(4): 443–453.

Sobo, E. J., C. Bowman, J. Halloran, S. Asch, M. Goetz, and A. Gifford (2008b). "A Routine Thing": Clinician Strategies for Implementing HIV Testing for At-Risk Patients in a Busy Healthcare Organization (and Implications for Implementation of other New Practice Recommendations). *Anthropology & Medicine* 15(3): 213–225.

Sobo, E. J. and P. S. Kurtin (2003). Variation in Physicians' Definitions of the Competent Parent and Other Barriers to Guideline Adherence: The Case of Pediatric Minor Head Injury Management. *Social Science & Medicine* 56(12): 2479–2491.

Sobo, E. J. and M. Loustaunau (Forthcoming). *The Cultural Context of Health, Illness and Medicine* (2nd Ed.). Westport, CT, Bergin & Garvey.

Sobo, E. J. and C. L. Rock (2001). "You Ate All That!?": Caretaker-Child Interaction during Children's Assisted Dietary Recall Interviews. *Medical Anthropology Quarterly* 15(2): 222–244.

Sobo, E. J., C. L. Rock, M. L. Neuhouser, T. L. Maciel, and D. Neumark-Sztainer (2000). Caretaker-Child Interaction during Children's 24-Hour Dietary Recalls: Who Contributes What to the Recall Record? *Journal of the American Dietetic Association* 100(4): 428–433.

Sobo, E. J. and B. L. Sadler (2002). Improving Organizational Communication and Cohesion in a Health Care Setting through Employee-Leadership Exchange. *Human Organization* 61(3): 277–287.

Sobo, E. J. and M. Seid (2003). Cultural Issues in Health Services Delivery: What Kind of "Competence" Is Needed, and from Whom? *Annals of Behavioral Science & Medical Education* 9(2): 97–100.

Sobo, E. J., M. Seid, and L. R. Gelherd (2006). Parent-Identified Barriers to Pediatric Health Care: A Process-Oriented Model and Method. *Health Services Research* 41(1): 148–172.

Sobo, E., D. Simmes, J. Landsverk, and P. Kurtin (2003). Rapid Assessment with Qualitative Telephone Interviews: Lessons from an Evaluation of California's Healthy Families Program & Medi-Cal for Children. *American Journal of Evaluation* 24(3): 399–408.

Sofaer, S. (1999). Qualitative Methods: What Are They and Why Use Them? *Health Services Research* 34(5/II): 1101–1118.

Spradley, J. (1979). *The Ethnographic Interview*. New York, Holt, Rinehart and Winston.

Starr, P. (1982). *The Social Transformation of American Medicine*. New York, Basic Books.

Strauss, A. and J. Corbin (1998). *Basics of Qualitative Research: Techniques and Procedures for Developing Grounded Theory*. Thousand Oaks, CA, Sage.

Sudman, S., N. M. Bradburn, and N. Schwarz (1996). *Thinking about Answers: The Application of Cognitive Processes to Survey Methodology*. San Francisco, Jossey-Bass.

Sullivan, M. (2003). The New Subjective Medicine: Taking the Patient's Point of View on Health Care and Health. *Social Science & Medicine* 56: 1595–1604.

Taylor, C. (1992). The Harp that Plays by Itself. *Anthropological Approaches to the Study of Ethnomedicine*. M. Nichter, ed. New York, Gordon and Breach: 127–148.

Taylor, J. S. (2003). The Story Catches You and You Fall Down: Tragedy, Ethnography, and "Cultural Competence." *Medical Anthropology Quarterly* 17(2): 159–181.

Tebbi, C. (1993). Treatment Compliance in Childhood and Adolescence. *Cancer* 71(Suppl. 10): 3441–3449.

Todd, H. F. and J. L. Ruffini (1979). *Teaching Medical Anthropology: Model Courses for Graduate and Undergraduate Instruction* (Society for Medical Anthropology Special Publication No. 1). Washington, DC, Society for Medical Anthropology.

Traweek, S. (1988). *Beamtimes and Lifetimes: The World of High Energy Physicists.* Cambridge, MA, Harvard University Press.

Tylor, E. B. (1871). *Primitive Culture.* London, John Murray.

Ulrich, R. S. (1984). View through a Window May Influence Recovery from Surgery. *Science* 224(4647): 420–421.

———. (2006). Evidence-Based Healthcare Architecture. *Lancet* 368(Suppl. 1): S38–S39.

van der Geest, S. and K. Finkler (2004). Hospital Ethnography: Introduction. *Social Science & Medicine* 59(10): 1995–2001.

Van Dongen, E. (2007). Farewell to Fieldwork? Constraints in Anthropological Research in Violent Situations. *On Knowing and Not Knowing in the Anthropology of Medicine.* R. Littlewood, ed. Walnut Creek, CA, Left Coast Press: 160–171.

Van Geest, J. B., T. P. Johnson, and V. L. Welch (2007). Methodologies for Improving Response Rates in Surveys of Physicians: A Systematic Review. *Evaluation & the Health Professions* 30(4): 303–321.

Virchow, R. L. K. (1985 [1848]). The Charity Physician. *Collected Essays on Public Health and Epidemiology.* L. J. Rather, ed. Canton, MA, Science History Publications, vol. 1: 33–36.

Vivier, P. M., J. A. Bernier, and B. Starfield (1994). Current Approaches to Measuring Health Outcomes in Pediatric Research. *Current Opinion in Pediatrics* 6: 530–537.

Vuckovic, N. (1999). Fast Relief: Buying Time with Medications. *Medical Anthropology Quarterly* 13(1): 51–68.

Waber, R., B. Shiv, Z. Carmon, and D. Ariely (2008). Commercial Features of Placebo and Therapeutic Efficacy. *Journal of the American Medical Association* 299(9): 1016–1017.

Wacquant, L. (2004). Comments on "An Anthropology of Structural Violence." *Current Anthropology* 45(3): 322.

Waitzkin, H. (1985). Information Giving in Medical Care. *Journal of Health and Social Behavior* 26(June): 81–101.

———. (2000). *The Second Sickness: Contradictions of Capitalist Health Care* (revised and updated edition). New York, Rowman & Littlefield.

Watkins, J., for the AAA Committee on Ethics (2008 [January 18]). Briefing Paper on Consideration of the Potentially Negative Impact of the Publication of Factual Data about a Study Population on Such Population (Draft for comment). Available online at http://www.aaanet.org/committees/ethics/bp4.htm (accessed May 14, 2007).

Weakland, J. H. (1951). Method in Cultural Anthropology. *Philosophy of Science* 18(1): 55–69.

Weller, S. C. and A. K. Romney (1988). *Systematic Data Collection.* Newbury Park, CA, Sage.

Werner, O. and H. R. Bernard (1994). Ethnographic Sampling. *Cultural Anthropology Methods* 6(2): 7–9.

Werner, O. and G. M. Schoepfle (1997). *Systematic Fieldwork* (Vol. 1). Newbury Park, CA, Sage.

Whelan, C. and H. H. Woo (2004). Mister or Doctor? What's in a Name? *Medical Journal of Australia* 181(1): 20.

Williams, M., R. Parker, D. W. Baker, N. S. Parikh, K. Pitkin, W. C. Coates, and J. R. Nurss (1995). Inadequate Functional Health Literacy among Patients at Two Public Hospitals. *Journal of the American Medical Association* 274(21): 1677–1682.

Wolf, E. (1982). *Europe and the People without History.* Los Angeles, University of California Press.

Worhol, R. R. (1992). As You Stand, So You Feel and Are: The Crying Body and the Nineteenth-Century Text. *Tattoo, Torture, Mutilation, and Adornment: The*

Denaturalization of the Body in Cultural Context. F. E. Mascia-Lees and P. Sharpe, eds. Albany, State University of New York Press: 100–125.

Young, A. (1983). The Relevance of Traditional Medical Cultures to Modern Primary Health Care. *Social Science & Medicine* 17(16): 1205–1211.

———. (1986 [1976]). Internalising and Externalising Medical Belief Systems: An Ethiopian Example. *Concepts of Health, Illness, and Disease: A Comparative Perspective.* C. Currer and M. Stacey, eds. Oxford, U.K., Berg: 137–160.

Index

Note: Italicized page numbers indicate figures and tables.

About the Author

Elisa ("EJ") Sobo, professor of anthropology at San Diego State University, is a sociocultural anthropologist specializing in health, illness, and medicine. Her current research focus is on the United States, but she has also worked in Jamaica and the United Kingdom. Beyond methods, her work has concerned reproductive and other health traditions, HIV/AIDS, pediatric health, health-care consumerism, organizational culture and organizational change and improvement, and food, weight, and nutrition.

A recognized expert in her field, Dr. Sobo has worked both in academia and in health care. She is on various journal editorial boards, including for *Anthropology & Medicine* and *Medical Anthropology* and she is the Book Reviews Editor for *Medical Anthropology Quarterly*. She has served as an elected member of the board for the Society for Medical Anthropology in addition to having served on the Royal Anthropological Institute's Medical Committee in the United Kingdom.

Among Dr. Sobo's numerous publications are *Choosing Unsafe Sex: AIDS Risk Denial among Disadvantaged Women* (University of Pennsylvania Press, 1995) and the coauthored book, *The Endangered Self: Managing the Social Risks of HIV* (Routledge, 2000). She has also coedited *Optimizing Care for Young Children with Special Health Care Needs: Knowledge and Strategies for Navigating the System* (Brookes Publishing, 2007), *Child Health Services Research: Applications, Innovations, and Insights* (Jossey-Bass, 2003), and *Using Methods in the Field: A Practical Introduction and Casebook* (AltaMira, 1998). Dr. Sobo is currently working on a second edition of her coauthored textbook, *The Cultural Context of Health, Illness and Medicine* (Bergin & Garvey, first edition 1997) as well as beginning new research on medical tourism.